# New Medicine *for a* New Millennium

A Memoir Looking
Front to Back in Time
at a Black Woman's Life
in Medicine

SYLVIA MUSTONEN, DO

*New Medicine for a New Millennium: A Memoir Looking Front to Back in Time at a Black Woman's Life in Medicine*



For information about this title or to order other books and/or electronic media, contact the publisher:
Atkins & Greenspan Publishing
TwoSistersWriting.com
18530 Mack Avenue, Suite 166
Grosse Pointe Farms, MI 48236

ISBN 978-1-956879-25-4 (Hardcover)
ISBN 978-1-956879-26-1 (Paperback)
ISBN 978-1-956879-27-8 (eBook)
Printed in the United States of America

All the stories in this work are true.

Cover Art: Illumination Graphics
Cover and Graphic Design: Illumination Graphics

All photographs are part of the Mustonen family's private collection.

# *Dedication & Acknowledgments*

The dedication is two-tiered. The first tier is to my dear grandchildren, Ezekiel and Magdalana.

I will speak to them as they read my life.

Dear Ezekiel and Magdalana,

Here is all the stuff that you did not know about me. These are the factoids and bits of information about my life as a person and as a doctor that we never got to really discuss. I want you to know these things and learn from them and hopefully avoid the mistakes I made. I want you to be passionate about your family, focused on your future, and proud to be an American who is an African American.

Most grandchildren learn about their grandparents in bits and pieces, and it may be hard for you to see me as an adolescent at age 16, a television news reporter at age 24, a married woman at age 26, a medical student at age 30, a mother to your mother and Aunty Ophelia, or a working physician at age 45. You don't know me until I am well past all those mile markers of life and I only show up to do grandmotherly things.

So, here is a more holistic and inclusive picture of me, my thoughts, and my life, wherein I share the path of your life for a while. I give this to you with all my love, and I hope it will help, guide, and entertain you.

Be proud of who you are and who your ancestors and relatives are—good, bad, or ugly, they all contributed something of value to you and to the making of you.

Perhaps this will be inspirational or not. I know that it became clear to me that my purpose, as it is written in the traditions of

Kwanzaa, was to leave a written record. As it is said, those who do not know their history, are doomed to repeat past mistakes in their future.

And, by the way, my dear grandchildren, other people are going to read this, too, so you need a leg up on them if they come asking you about your "cra' cra' Gramma."

The second tier of this dedication is to all those who have inspired me, mentored me, stirred me up, booted me along, criticized me, praised me, cuddled me at every step in my life.

I must give specific thanks to: my writing mentor Nanette DePriest; my publisher Elizabeth Ann Atkins; long-time friends Sharon and Erik Smith; Gerard and Mary Jean Teachman; Dawn and Rick Strasser; my physics instructor at Central Michigan University; my chemistry instructor at Montcalm Community College; my therapist Michele Turner; Claudette Harris, who provided the direction to Nanette and Elizabeth; my youngest daughter Veronica, who always gave me just what I needed when I needed it the most; my oldest daughter Ophelia, who showed me her world and made me "woke;" and Dr. Mary Segars D. Theol., for giving me Power; Linda Huckleberry; Hazel Turmo; Daisy, the MA at Northwest General Hospital; and my cat Lady Jane for giving me constant companionship.

# CONTENTS

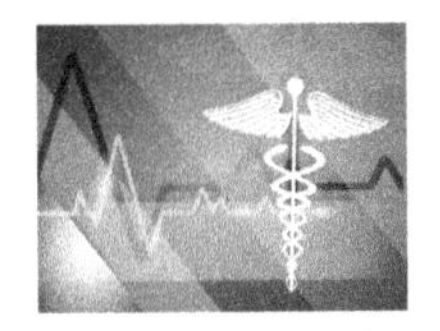

# INTRODUCTION

Here is the story of my life as a young woman in Detroit, navigating the tribulations of Black life in that city.

Here is the roundabout, sometimes deflected, meandering path to medical school. Here is my story about encountering racism and sexism in training and in practice—and rising above it.

Here is the story of my interracial marriage that struggled and foundered on the rocks of every kind of problem except racism.

Here, I share my experiences as a patient, sitting on the other end of a stethoscope, facing my own medical frailties.

Here are my ideas for the necessary revolution in health care, the future of medicine and the improvement of medical education, and my ideas on reparations, and other problems in white and Black American culture today

Here is what pressured me to record my life before I die. The ferocity of the COVID-19 pandemic drove home the reality of all our mortality as I watched friends, neighbors, strangers, famous and infamous people sicken and die.

If COVID-19 was the engine that drove my work, then the direction of the journey is to convince every doctor—whether newly graduated or gradually slumping toward retirement—as well as everyone who has ever been a patient, to join in the disruption of the American health care patriarchy and bring an end to the harm it has caused in the name of wealth over health.

I persisted in the face of it all, as my therapist once said.

Hear me here.

**Sylvia Mustonen, DO**

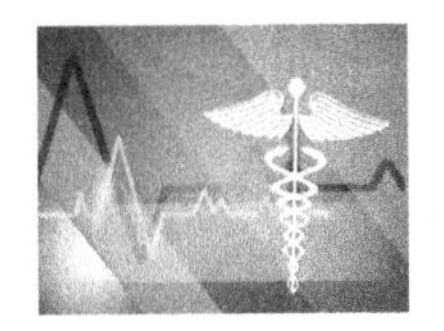

# PREFACE

It makes no sense to take a person through four years of undergraduate school, four years of medical school, two to six years of residency and fellowship, just to have him or her sit behind a desk and pass people through the grinder of primary health care. That grinder gobbles up 25 to 30 people a day for no benefit to any of those patients, but rather for the benefit of the "owners" of health care, which are our government, the insurance companies, and pharmaceutical companies, in the name of profit.

That is what happens in health care, especially in family medicine in America. Once upon a time, I was one of those people running the grinder for the benefit of the "owners" and to the detriment of the patients.

Now I am a retired curmudgeon, and I will say what I wish about the profession I love, and I will tell the story of ME. I also write about my ideal medical clinic and the fictional nation of the New Republic of Covert, where everybody is happy. They are that way because they live the way I tell them to.

My ideas are my visionary take on what we might do differently in medical care and education. Remember that I said different, which is not always better.

I will throw in some thoughts on the practice of medicine, ideas about the future of medicine, and take time to touch on racism and sexism as I have seen and experienced it.

It is my hope to join my voice to the rising tide of righteous indignation at the hijacking of American health care by the patriarchy of health care, which pursues wealth over the goal of health. I hope all who read this will awaken to their own power and ask the questions and take the steps to stop the nonsense that: gives us health disparities, overspending, fraud, racism, and sexism; deprives men and women in health care of work-life balance; fosters inadequate payment models; and allows government micromanipulation of care and caregivers in the pursuit of "quality metrics" instead of quality of life.

I was sober when I wrote all of this. If it sounds like I was high or crazy, just remember that I may have been angry at our political situation, disappointed in how Black Americans are treated, saddened in my personal life, having happy dreams, or ecstatic over some marvelous discovery in science and medicine. In other words, I am just a Black woman living her life and absorbing it all.

As they say in some places I have been, take what you like and leave the rest behind.

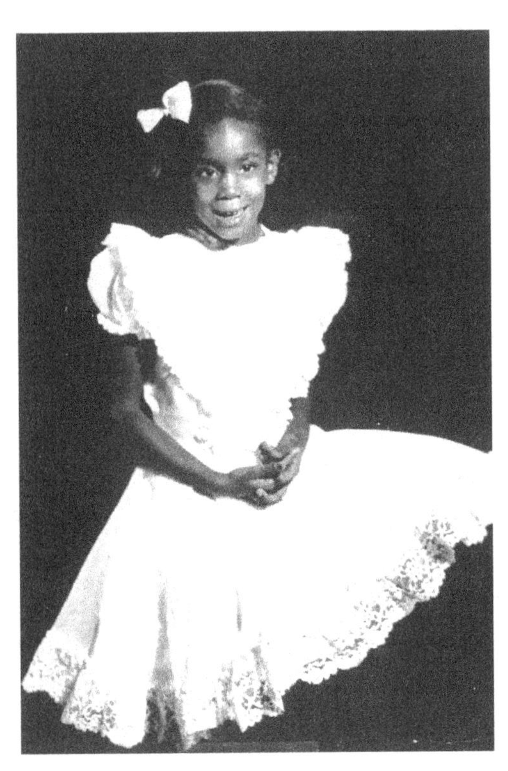

# SECTION ONE
# BEFORE I BECAME A PHYSICIAN

**Following the Steps of a Dead White Man**

I am a DO—Doctor of Osteopathic Medicine—which has a distinct philosophy. Here are the principles from our founder, A.T. Still, MD.

**Some Principles From Our Founder**

- The body is a unit.
- Structure and function are interrelated.
- The body is self-regulating and self-healing.
- Rational application of these principles is the foundation of the profession.

Andrew Taylor Still, MD, DO, was the first Osteopathic physician. I really did not know anything about the profession of Osteopathy, but I knew I wanted to be a physician.

When I was about 15, the flu hit Detroit and everyone got sick in our house. I lived on Trowbridge with my grandparents and my mother. Mom called our family doctor, Garnet T. Ice, MD, and he made a HOUSECALL!

**Inspired by a Living Black Man**

I saw this impressive, elegant, professional, stately Black man walking down our staircase after having taken care of me, Mom, and both grandparents, and I was in awe of his intelligence, carriage, grace, and bearing. At that point, I knew I wanted to be a physician. He was my first family doctor and he took care of me in the kindest, most professional and fatherly way.

Perhaps because my own father was absent at key points in my life, it was easy for me to see myself as his child. He was well known and respected in the city of Detroit, and I can only imagine how hard it must have been for him to be as successful as he was, given the difficulties of racism in medicine at the time. Many years later, I had a chance to actually meet his daughter, who was also a physician. I shared this story with her when we were at a medical conference, to let her know how her father inspired me. Truly, we are all interconnected, and life has a plan for each of us. I feel that some power has brought me full circle!

**Crushed by a Black Man in High School**

No one encouraged me to become a physician. In fact, my high school counselor, who was also a Black man, told me that my science grades were not great, so I should learn to type, get a job, and meet someone and get married.

He was wrong, but he was right. I flunked Algebra 1 and 2, and Geometry 1, and had to retake all of them. But my grades in all other areas were outstanding. He said I was not smart enough to be a doctor because I was weak in math. Numbers truly frightened me, but I could handle all the other subjects. He must have felt that was not enough. Writing now what he told me then makes me wonder how many other people have had a dream crushed in the middle of adolescent vulnerability?

I was crushed and I believed him, but I never let the flame of desire for a career in medicine ever go out.

I drew inspiration from A.T. Still. He was the son of a Methodist preacher, and also was a physician in the Union Army during the Civil War. He had much loss in his life; his first wife and two children, then three more children with his second wife—all died. He was drummed out of his church because they felt laying on of hands to cure a person was tantamount to declaring oneself equal to Jesus Christ. He opened clinics and later founded the first college of Osteopathic medicine, only to have one of his students steal his teachings and set up an alternative school in Iowa. He was never wealthy, but he was visionary and focused. None of these setbacks deterred him. My setbacks seemed minor compared to his.

He was a very observant man and studied anatomy in nature's lab, by cutting open and dissecting the animals he hunted for food as a child, and by watching how people were treated in those days of medical care. The medications were mostly alcohol, opium, and mixtures of both. Amputation was the method by which most trauma was treated. People were being hacked and poisoned in the name of medicine.

He became convinced that there was a better way, and that way did not involve crude removal of body parts or potions of poisonous materials such as alcohol and mercury, or ingestion of addictive materials such as opium and codeine, the two most popular drugs of the day.

He discovered that he could use his hands to "adjust" people's anatomy and thereby improve blood flow to their damaged body parts and they would get well. No one believed him at first. His only adherents were mostly just the people whom he treated. Word of mouth spread about his abilities. He attracted not only patients, but also followers who wished to learn what he did. Eventually, he moved to Kirksville, Missouri and opened a clinic, and then he opened a school. In the late 1890s, he was teaching not only men, but also women how to do what he had developed, and it was called Osteopathy. He was wild, wonderful, weird, and a most remarkable role model for me.

He was blunt and outspoken, so he was someone whose personality resonated with my own personality. Being fed a stream of negative information will either crush a person, or turn a person into a determined SOB. That description was him then, and it is me now.

This led me to explore the art of caring, the science of medicine, and the power of touch.

## MICHIGAN STATE UNIVERSITY, COLLEGE OF OSTEOPATHIC MEDICINE

### A Black Girl Meets Two Osteopaths

The first time I met an Osteopathic physician was when my husband and I moved out of Detroit and into a small town called Sheridan, Michigan in 1970. Actually, we lived in a smaller town called Crystal, but my husband's office was in Stanton, which was the county seat, and Sheridan was a mere three miles or so down the road, highway M66. That town was home to Dr. Henry Beckmeyer and Dr. Robert Ricketts, two Osteopathic physicians who practiced medicine and surgery, respectively.

Beckmeyer became my family doctor and Rickett became my surgeon. Beckmeyer delivered my first child, and Ricketts delivered, by C-section, my second child. Beckmeyer took out my tonsils, Ricketts took out my gallbladder and tied my tubes. Both of them treated me with the best of care, and with respect.

They were totally old school physicians—patronizing, patriarchs of wealth, filled up with and enjoying their status in the community to the hilt. But they followed the beliefs of the profession and they treated me as a human being, looking past my gender and color in the days when most folks would consider gender or color to be social handicaps.

We all lived in the world of the 1950-60s white version of America, except that some of us were in the background. That background was composed of women, all Black people, Indigenous people, any foreign person, any gay or trans persons, any poor person, anybody who was physically not perfect, all non-Christians, and especially, every Jew.

I was a special Black woman because my husband was a white man. That forced the local society of Montcalm County to make a decision about either letting me in or keeping me out. Most of them decided to let me in because I was with Arney. I understood that and took it and ran with it.

When I told Beckmeyer and Ricketts that I wanted to go to medical school, they both volunteered to write letters of recommendation for me, and were even more excited to know that I planned to attend Michigan State University's College of Osteopathic Medicine, which was brand new, having just opened in 1969.

The Michigan State University College of Osteopathic Medicine (MSUCOM) graduated small classes of students—men and women, Black and white, older and younger—and all were committed to staying in Michigan to practice.

These two white, male privileged members of the establishment and patriarchy saw in me the light and spirit of the profession, saw that I possessed a desire to help people, and saw that I had a wealth of intelligence and energy. They encouraged and supported my intention, and without them, my life would have taken a drastically different direction.

> Honesty, open and full on the part of the patient,
> Intention that is pure on the part of the physician,
> Develops trust in the doctor-patient relationship,
> That trust allows for real communication, which is the basis for all healing.
> —Sylvia Mustonen, 2020

My husband and I had just fled from riot-torn Detroit, a couple of interracial city slickers, and those two men showed me that the Osteopathic profession transcended the false construct of race. I think A.T. Still would have been proud of them.

If I were going to be a doctor, I was going to be a DO.

**My Family History, As Best As I Know**

I am a Black person, and we Black people came from Africa, brought here as slaves on ships as part of the Triangle Trade, which operated between Europe, Africa, and the Americas. Our family records are sparse and much depends on word of mouth. By the way, I say "Black" to contrast with "white" in my writing, and I understand the words as a cultural/ethnic designation, not racial. Some Black people were very light in skin color, and the color of your skin is not the prime decider of your Blackness, in my opinion.

This rendition of my ancestry is from Gwyn Kirksey, my dear cousin in Houston, Texas.

My mother left me the Malone Family history records, all that she had. It starts Generation One, circa 1819, Generation Two, 1850, Generation Three, 1850-1900, Generation Four, 1920-1960.

I will share it with you:

According to the records from 1819, the earliest known ancestor of the Malone family was an Indian named Buck. The family site was Dresden, Tennessee. Buck had one child by a Black woman, whose name was unknown. Circa 1850, two white families bought children from this union—one white family was the Malones who bought Talt Malone. He was the first named Talt. The other white family—the Bayliss family—bought Talt's brother, Atlas Bayliss. According to the records, the Malones did not know until about 1980 that the families had been separated in slavery. June Brown Garner learned of this when one of the Bayliss family saw her column in *The Detroit News* and called her. I called her my Aunt June, but she was actually my grandmother's second cousin.

Talt Malone married Jane Edwards. He also married another woman whose name is unknown. Their children were Simpson Malone, Queenie Malone, Walter Malone, Donnie Malone, and Woodridge Malone.

*Generation Three, 1850-1900*

Simpson Malone married Vela Wilkerson and had six children: William; Wilma (Wiggins Wright); Albert and his twin Donnie, who died as an infant; Talt; and June (Brown Hutchinson Garner).

Vela Wilkerson, my maternal grandmother, has a family line traced back to Hayes Guerin, in 1820 on Ancestry.com.

Queenie married Hugh Hayes in 1905 and had seven children: Jennie Lee, Helen (Gwen Pritchett's maternal grandmother), Dorothy, Effie (Helen named my mother after Effie—Effie died when she was still attending college), Virginia (died as an infant), Hugh Jr., and Charles.

*Generation Four, 1920-1960 – Simpson Malone's Children*

Wilma Malone, first born, married Jimmy Wiggins and had a son named Jimmy Jr. She then married William Wright.

William Malone, second born, married twice—Connie Colman and Laverne Nelson. He had three children, two with Connie—William II and Linda—and one with Laverne—Denise Ruth Malone (who married Willie Wheaton).

Donnie Malone, third born, twin of Albert, died early.

Albert Malone, third born, married Della, and they adopted a daughter named Reeva.

Talt Malone, fifth child, married Flora Lancaster and had two children, Talt II and Sheila Malone.

June Malone, sixth child, married Max Brown and had one child, Sylvia Brown Hutchinson (Mustonen). Sylvia and I were raised together. I lost contact with Sylvia when I moved to Texas in 1979. I have been trying to contact her. She did show up on my ancestry chart as a second cousin.

It gets a little confusing because Talt appears so many times, but that is the way it shows on the records. June's parents were Simpson and Vela Malone. I remember them well from when I lived with Aunt June. They were so loving; he always called her "Sugar," and she called him "Honey." The Queenie Malone Hayes line leads to my mother, and her mother, Helen. Queenie was my great-grandmother. I hope this info helps you fill in some gaps in the generations.

*Generation Five, 1960-2000*

Talt Malone II married a Native American-Indian woman from Uruguay and had a son, Talt III (we called him Tico).

Sheila Malone married Sanders Earl McLaughlin and had a son and daughter—Scott McLaughlin, born October 22nd, 1975, and Sasha Alayna McLaughlin, born December 22nd, 1978.

This family has members who work at the University of Michigan's IT department, for Zipcar as a fleet manager and as a salesperson. Their matriarch and my cousin, Sheila, was a graduate of the University of Michigan, worked as a consultant for the Spaulding for Children adoption agency, and with her degree in psychology, worked as a consultant with administrative-level social workers in every state in the Union.

Sylvia Brown, adopted by George Hutchinson, married to Arney Mustonen, had two daughters, Ophelia and Veronica.

Linda Malone married Charles Hale and had two children.

William Malone II married twice and had Marcus and Monica with his first wife, then married Denise Carr and had a daughter, Mikayla Joelle.

Denise Ruth Malone Hawkins Wheaton married twice. Her first husband, Jesse Hawkins, was a skilled tradesman who worked at the Dodge Main auto plant in Detroit. She had a son with him, Jesse Hawkins, Jr. She married a second time to Willie Cornelius Wheaton, an educator who recruited, taught, and counseled more than 65 thousand high school dropout students to return for diploma completion. Their son is Jonathon Malachai Wheaton.

*Generation Six, 2000-Present*

Talt Malone III married and had two children, April Malone and DeAngelo Malone.

Scott McLaughlin married three times: first, Lane Smith, with whom he had one child, Sean Smith-McLaughlin, born September 12th, 1997; second to RayShaun McLaughlin, with whom he had DeShaun McLaughlin, born June 13th, 1998; and lastly, to Charne Gillam, having one child, Zay'den McLaughlin, born October 18th, 2013.

Sasha married Rico Womble, having three children: Jordan Womble, born August 15th, 2003, Brandon Womble, born January 7th, 2005, and Aaron Womble, born May 7th, 2008.

Jessie Hawkins married Alexzandria Jones, and they have two children, Jessie Hawkins Jr., and daughter, Leslie.

Jonathon Malachai Wheaton married Alberta Katrice Morgan and had one son, Malachai William Wheaton, Jr. Jonathon was active in real estate, and Alberta Katrice was a school principal and IT director for ATS Educational Services.

Veronica married and with her husband had a son, Ezekiel, and a daughter, Magdalana.

Queenie Malone, child of Talt Malone and Jane Edwards, married Lester Hayes and had a child, Helen Hayes.

Helen Hayes married Barrett and had a child, Effie Barrett.

Effie Barrett married twice, first to Pritchett, and then to Kirksey. She had a daughter, Gwyn Pritchett, and a son, Wade Kirksey.

Gwyn Pritchett, who lives in Houston, Texas, married three times: first to Byrd, and had three sons, Juan, Tony, and Lamarr. Then she married Franklin and had two sons, Ahmad and Brandon. Her third marriage was to Muhammad.

Wade Kirksey never married, and lives in Idaho.

I am so thankful to Gwyn for sharing what she has about my maternal side of the family. Gwyn and I were together, off and on, while her mother was getting divorced from Pritchett, and before her brother, Wade, was born. She frequently stayed with me and my mother—who at that time was married to George Hutchinson—at our home on Fischer in Detroit, between 1947 and 1958.

**Dora Wilkerson and Vela Malone**

Vela Wilkerson Malone, my maternal grandmother, was born as a free person, but her mother, Dora, was born a slave. I recall visiting my great-grandmother when I was 10 or 11 years old. For some reason, Vela wanted to return to see her mother. Perhaps Dora was ill; I cannot recall the reason, only that Vela and I took a train out of Flint, Michigan down to Erin, Tennessee.

Erin is in the northwest section of the state and remains a quaint, small southern town today. We managed to get to Dora's house, and it was the most underwhelming, unprepossessing structure I had ever seen. But what I was seeing was a modified slave shack. I could only compare it to the grand home my grandmother lived in and so it fell way below my standards as I compared it to Grandmother Vela's "palace." Her home was three stories, with five bedrooms, four bathrooms, a large front and back yard, and room graciously appointed with a fireplace and bookcases filled with books and curios.

A slave shack was one room with an out-house a few steps away and a fireplace for all heating, cooking, and nighttime illumination. The more fortunate had a lamp.

It was maybe 20 feet by 15 feet, one story, with an open,

wood-burning fireplace in the center across from the entry (there was only one entry), and to the left side was a sleeping pallet; to the right side was the dining table and a chair. It had no closets, no counters, no running water, no indoor plumbing, no electric lights, and no interior heating system other than the fireplace. The floors and walls were bare and there was one window. The outhouse was down the hill. The well was up the hill. The chamber pot was by the bed. Great-grandmother Dora had one kerosene lamp on the table, but she did not illuminate it until it was truly dark outside.

Vela introduced me to Dora. I only remember she was small and had shiny eyes. Much later I realized those eyes were cloudy with cataracts, so God Only Really Knows (GORK) what she saw when she looked at me. We ate and then they sent me to the outhouse to take care of my night business and put me to bed on the pallet. I fell asleep watching those two grand dames of our family talk, illuminated in the flickering smoky light of the fireplace. I could not hear the words, but I could feel their conversation was reaching some kind of resolution and closure. They carried on far into the night, long after I fell asleep.

The next day, we wandered around her place, and walked up the hill and looked around. We trudged through town to pick up a few items, but I truly think the walk was to show off her prosperous daughter and great-granddaughter to the Blacks and whites in Erin. I played; they talked. That evening, Vela and I went back to the train station and back home to Michigan.

Dora died. Vela died. I never knew what they had to resolve, but my recall of that night remains vivid today. It was thrust back on me when I had occasion to visit the Smithsonian in Washington, D.C. There was a mock-up recreated slave cabin, and when I saw it, all the visuals of that one night in Dora's house flooded back to me, bringing tears and deep feelings for which I have no name. I stood there and cried till my eyes ran from wet to dry, but weeping silently while other visitors walked around me, clearing away from me, knowing I was enveloped in deep, emotional, vivid memories.

Sometimes I wonder if I am as strong as either of those women, both who survived unimaginable outrages and obstacles. I think I am not as strong as they were, but that is OK because I know I am strong in other ways, more suitable for the times in which I live. I do not know what dreams or aspirations they may have had. No one bothered to spend time talking to little children; children were seen, not heard, and were taught not to participate in family discourse. Their hopes, dreams, and ambitions are lost to me and that is one reason I write this overly long journal, so that you, my dear grandchildren, will know my thoughts, dreams, and ambitions, and form ambitions of your own.

Later after my grandmother Vela died, I found in her home a white, milk glass lamp base for a kerosene lantern. It was the one used by my great-grandmother Dora to illuminate her home. I kept that piece of family history because it is so symbolic and so connective for me and all my children and grandchildren.

Slaves owned nothing, not even their own bodies, so being able to have an item that was in our family—even though it is just a simple milk glass base used for a kerosene lamp—is a big deal. Other families may have portraits, jewels, and rare antiques, while we only have this one item. But it is part of who I am, and who you are, and it symbolizes our family's travels and travails in this country.

I realized that I came from honest country folks who never had much of anything, and were on their own for so much you may take for granted today, like access to health care, a good education, safe living quarters, possessions, and a free future.

Seeing that place in Tennessee and knowing how my progenitors lived and lacked and suffered may have given me some of my ambitions. At first, I wanted to be an oceanographer because I saw Jacques Cousteau's wonderful series of sea exploration on television, but I could not swim and had no vision of being like him. Then I saw Dr. Ice make that house call and I knew I could be as he was.

I wanted to be a physician when I was 15 (in 1959). No one thought I could or should, and I was rerouted, redirected along other pathways for many years. My life as a physician was in my future, but it was a tortuous path. Like the future of medicine, the changes that are coming will take us all along that twisty path.

Join me.

## DIGRESSION #1: TRENDS IN THE FUTURE OF MEDICINE

Anyone who is a futurist predicting what will happen in medicine, might be half blind if he or she is not also a physician.

All the futurists I have read and who have not been doctors have predictions based on great science, but they overlook one important fact. That fact is that future trends in American health care will be driven by money—making it, getting it, keeping it, and avoiding spending it on patient care.

I made this list in 2015:

1. MD and DO schools and professions will merge.
2. DO and DC professions merge.
3. Physicians will become augmented cyborgs.
4. Medical school enrollment will be open to all who can afford it.
5. Hospitals will deploy robots instead of nurses for the majority of care.
6. Nursing homes will also become automated.
7. Government will drop Medicaid and move to Medicare for all.
8. The EVE—Extra-Uterine Viability Environment—device will be invented.
9. More physicians will move to total concierge medicine.
10. Physicians will form independent corporations.
11. NPs will become totally independent health providers.
12. Physician Assistants will become health providers in underserved areas.
13. Patients will be able to order their own labs and X-rays without an order from a physician.
14. Substance abuse treatment centers will be funded by the federal government as a result of dropping Medicaid funding.

15. The medical record will be a video document.
16. The biophysical basis for OMT will be discovered.
17. Biophysical markers for mental health disorders will be discovered.
18. A device that obtains objective measurement of somatic and visceral pain will be developed.
19. A cure for HIV will be developed.
20. A cure for diabetes will be developed.
21. The etiology of autism, irritable bowel disorders, attention deficit/ hyperactivity disorder, celiac disease, Alzheimer's, and other neurodegenerative disorders will be proven to be an environmental/toxic etiology.
22. The male contraceptive will be developed.
23. There will be vaccines for cancer of the lung, bowel, bladder, breast, prostate, and bone.
24. Tort reform will encompass a national no-fault initiative.
25. Mega retailers will install self-care automated medical diagnosis and treatment centers based on super Artificial Intelligence (AI) computer interfaces.
26. Free standing cash/credit, imaging/radiology centers will become common in all states.
27. The Family Independence Agency, a racist failure, will cease to exist.
28. Behavioral health treatment, which is just a system of catch-and-release for the poor, will be dismantled and enfolded into general medical care.

As this narrative goes along, I will revisit many of these predictions along the way, wherever appropriate.

The outgrowth of those future predictions was another list I made on February 1st, 2016, where I tried to identify what was wrong with the American health care system.

I had been retired for two years at the time I created this list that follows, and had time to reflect on all the faults that I encountered as both a patient as well as a physician.

1. It is expensive to operate and run.
2. It is costly to use.
3. There are poor outcomes for most health measures.
4. The system measures the wrong outcomes.
5. Access is limited for many.
6. There are huge financial interventions by national and state governments, but poor results for the expenditure of money.
7. Medical diagnostic errors occur frequently.
8. Medication errors abound.
9. Pharmaceuticals are too expensive.
10. There is inadequate oversight for the purchase of durable medical goods and devices.
11. Contentious tort and litigation contribute to the rise of defensive medicine practices.
12. An uneducated and medically naïve population is easily swayed by false medical claims and clever advertising.
13. Medical scientific research is compromised by funding sources that have slanted agendas and for-profit motivation.
14. Digital record keeping is a mess because patients do not own their records, and the EMR is primarily a tool for billing, not population health data gathering.
15. Patients lack responsibility for their care.
16. There is no national incentive to strive for true health and wellness.
17. Providers fight for "territory" within medical license boards and treatment guidelines.
18. Medical science and technology outstrip medical license boards and treatment guidelines.
19. The driving motive is profit.
20. Minorities have limited access to medical schools due to faulty recruitment strategies and high tuition.
21. Expensive medical schools limit the supply of trained professionals.

22. Professionals graduating from medical school lack adequate cultural competency.
23. Legislation about medicine is rarely proactive, usually reactive, and mainly punitive.
24. National licensure is virtually non-existent but highly necessary.
25. Outdated models of how care is to be provided still predominate.
26. The FDA is slow and toothless.
27. Our politicians are in the pockets of those who want to continue with our current methodologies.
28. There are multiple competing systems of health insurance.

There is no emphasis on health; the emphasis is on profit.

There is no concern for care; there is only concern for meeting false and artificial goals.

There is no system; there is just a patchwork of competing companies and institutions.

It is a profit-driven patchwork.

WE'RE BACK . . .

**June and Her Parents, Vela and Simpson Malone, and My Dad, Max Brown**

My mother, June Bell Malone Brown Hutchinson Garner, was a wonderful woman. It took me more than 60 years to come to this conclusion, because I spent a lot of time being angry with her. She married abusive men who disappointed her, abandoned me, and hurt both of us. I spent a lot of time seeking her love, which she had, but could not freely give.

She married her first husband, Max Brown, in 1944, and she said she did it to get out of the house. She was living with her parents, Vela and Simpson Malone on 239 Trowbridge Street in Detroit.

She was a party animal, and Max was party central. They hooked up, got married, then she got pregnant, and he left her when I was three months old. In 1946, she found herself back in her parents' home, and this time with a baby. She officially divorced Max on April 15th, 1946. She had repeatedly asked him for support, but all he provided was 30 dollars—once. He provided no contact, no money, no interest in her or me.

I lost all contact with him until I was in my fifties. June's life must have been bitter raising me; I can only guess. She was stuck with me, back with her prideful, secret-alcoholic mother and hard-of-hearing father, both of whom were expecting her to care for them because she was the youngest child. They must have been disappointed in her because her efforts now had to be directed to caring for a child instead of caring for them.

So, June lived with her parents—my grandparents, who were hard working people. Simpson Malone had just retired from the Ford Factory. I am not sure if he worked in the River Rouge or at the factory in Highland Park on Woodward, but he would come home so dirty from working—his job was a hammer man—that Grandmother Vela would send him straight to the bathroom to wash up before letting him go through the rest of the house.

A hammer man was the person who broke the cast off the engine block when it came off the formation press. Imagine swinging a 20-pound hammer for eight hours a day, six days a week. That was my grandfather's job. When he moved his family from Tennessee to Michigan, he also built his own home; the first one on Stanford Street, then he bought the property on Trowbridge. He was trained as a finish-carpenter when he lived in Erin, Tennessee, and waited until he was in his thirties before he married Vela, who was 18.

Vela was a drinking woman in her later years, but did so in secret because church women are not supposed to be alcoholics. I remember watching her in the kitchen, cooking really delicious meals, but always sipping from the glass of clear liquid on the top of the stove control panel. Later I discovered that glass of "water" she had was actually gin and rock candy in the glass, and she sipped from it regularly. The rock candy concealed the alcohol smell on her breath. You see how clever your relatives were?

The Malone house on Trowbridge was huge back in the day. The basement had a small apartment that Vela rented out, while she and Simpson lived on the main level. June and I lived on the second floor, and the attic had another small bedroom, plus an open area that was used to store clothes my grandmother was storing to send to Africa as part of the church's missionary work.

Her church, Ebenezer AME, participated in clothing drives for the people in Africa, and she was in charge of those efforts. She was also famous in her church for her social activities, always throwing garden parties and soirées of one kind or another. She hosted our yearly Thanksgiving dinners for the longest time and insisted that all her children and grandchildren show up. She also had a large living room with a baby grand piano and a small electric organ. She had collected all the great works of literature, because society women were supposed to display their education. That is amazing to write because she had only an eighth grade education. But she valued knowledge and, later in life, she took her high school studies and passed her GED exam to earn her degree. What an inspiration she was to us all.

The book collection surrounded the wood burning fireplace. They were all hard cover, some leather bound, and all were beautiful in my eyes because they were my tickets to paradise: worlds of adventure, channels of learning, and places of escape.

I doubt that she read any of them, but I sure did. As an only child, those books were my escape from the drudgery of life and school. Defoe, Bulfinch, Hobbes, Shakespeare, those great authors of the western world were available in hardcover in that living room. She also had a collection of knick-knacks and warned me not to touch them because they were not toys, but collectibles. I touched them one day and she saw me and said, "Go get a switch from the lilac bush; don't bring a small one."

I got the switch and she beat me with it for touching her stuff.

Never touched her stuff again. I also picked up her phrase, "It's not a toy," and recall using those words repeatedly with you, Ezekiel and Magdalana, when I was your babysitter from 2014 to 2019. The words were from my grandmother and I was just passing the pain along down the line. Please forgive me for that.

As bad as that was, I loved my grandmother because she paid attention to me. Grandfather sat in his rocker recliner, hard of hearing from years of being in a factory, and quietly enjoyed his home, children, and grandchildren. I recall he smiled a lot. He and Vela would share breakfast with me on Saturdays with stacks of pancakes covered in Alaga syrup and lots of butter. Alaga is still in business as an online product. It was popular in the Black community starting in 1906, and displayed "The Sweetness of the South" as its motto.

I think it was nothing more than colored cane syrup, but it was cheap and showed two hands shaking each other.

Vela and Simp (his nickname) sat on either end of the table and I was in the middle sharing the fluffy, hot pancakes with the *way* too sweet syrup, and the butter just dribbling and pooling off the stack of pancakes. There was also thick-cut bacon on the plate, or sausage links, but always a piece of breakfast pork to start the day. I do not know where my mom was, but I was at the table with my grandparents getting a dose of the sweetness of the South and totally enjoying it.

In the summer, they had a garden. It was more like a small, compact farm. The backyard was very large, and one section was devoted entirely to Vela's rose garden. She prided herself on having one of every kind of popular rose bush—must have been more than 20. In addition, she had Grandfather build her a rock garden snuggled up to the side of the garage. She planted hanging plants and tall cultivars with brilliant flowers of all kinds in it. The lilac bush was tucked next to the steps at the back of the kitchen entry. It was the most wonderful-smelling shrub, with profuse blooms all spring. Even though it was the source of switches that Grandmother used to punish me, I still loved the bush and its perfume.

The front porch was large with a swing set, a couple of chairs, and two large concrete planters on the front steps. They always held geraniums in profusion. The front beds of the house held tulips and flowering shrubs. She loved those plants, so did I, and so did my mother. I am sure that my love of vegetable and flower gardening came from my grandparents, and for that I am so grateful.

Grandfather had the vegetable garden that produced foods he would have loved in Tennessee. He had one patch on the south side of the garage, in the back along the fence by the alley, and it ran all the way over to the neighbor's fence.

In case you don't know, an alley is a street that ran between the backs of houses on contiguous city blocks. The purpose was to provide a place for trash and garbage pick-up, but it was also the other "playground" in many neighborhoods for poor Black children. Most communities no longer build these. They were a secret world for me to harness my imagination, where I got to play on my own or connect with other kids out of sight of our parents.

Simpson's garden was probably 30 feet by 30 feet, and that was mainly the corn patch. Anything tall was grown there. In addition to corn, he grew pole beans, okra, tomatoes, green peas, and cucumbers. He always told me to plant white corn because yellow corn was for hogs, and white corn was for people. His pride and joy was the watermelon. The fence on the right side of the house, between us and the neighbors, was devoted to The Melon.

He and Vela were both from Erin, Tennessee. It was west of Nashville and tucked close to the northern border of the state. It was small when they married, and it is small now. The population in 2010 was 1,324 souls. They have an Irish Day parade on the third Saturday in March; the place was named in honor of the Irish homeland, also known as Erin. They married when he was 30 and she was 18.

In those days, it was not unusual for men to be older when they married, and to marry a much younger woman. The reasoning was that a man who wanted to be successful, needed to have the wherewithal to support a family, and that took time to get education or training. After accomplishing some kind of skill, a man then tried to marry a younger woman which meant that she would probably be able to have lots of children. The role of children was to support their parents in their old age. Recall that, in those days, there was no social security and this was also life in the South for Black people. The social safety net talked about today was non-existent then.

He had trained as a carpenter and had built a fine home down South, but racism and economics caused them to move to Detroit after five of their children were born in the South. My mother was their only child born in the North in 1923. Grandfather went to work at Mr. Henry Ford's factory for five dollars a day, a lot of money in the mid-twenties. Ford's policy helped the company get record profits. That pay was twice what any other company was paying and he was paying to all men who were willing to work—Black, as well as white.

Vela's and Simpson's gardening habit in the North was a fortunate holdover from their life in the South, as it allowed them to grow food for their family during the Great Depression. They never forgot the need and joy of gardening and passed that on to my mom, who then passed it on to me.

After his retirement from the auto factory, Grandfather's most challenging cause was to grow a record-breaking watermelon up North. Down South, anyone and everyone could grow watermelons with ease. He believed that it would happen if he did it right, but other neighbors and family members doubted him.

He would plant the watermelon in a hill of compost, surround it with a small fence to keep predators away, and as the vine grew, he pinched off small blossoms until he had two or three promising fruits. Then he fertilized and watered the heck out of the plant until he got a real melon. It took all summer, but he succeeded. He taught me the value of patience, perseverance, and attention to detail. And a love of The Melon—watermelon.

## DIGRESSION #2: THE MEDICAL SELF CARE KIOSK WILL OPEN AT BIG-BOX DISCOUNT STORES

Originally this was a joke of an idea. My staff and I in the Covert Medical Clinic, near South Haven, Michigan, thought it would be funny to just do drive-up medicine.

That idea would work just fine in our office, which was a converted bank with a drive-up teller window. Why not just have a menu board on the front that includes: a panel for people to punch in their symptoms or needs; a credit card chip reader for payment; a testing station where people can provide a urine sample or blood stick test; and a lane to drive up to the dispensing window for their medication and the return of their credit card?

That day is not too far in the future. By hooking into the AI supercomputer, it would be possible to provide basic care just like that. No need to hire Nurse Practitioners or open a mini-clinic; just have the kiosk.

Imagine a central station with six privacy kiosks. A person enters, slides in a credit card and ID, such as a driver's license, then they obtain access to the AI supercomputer function.

The AI supercomputer obtains a chief complaint, an HPI (History of the Present Illness) does an ROS (Review of Systems), all by an AI voice control whom we can call Tori. The patient can provide a urine sample, a finger for a micro venipuncture, maybe even a robotic-guided ultrasound in the private kiosk. X-rays and MRIs are not an option due to radiation shielding requirements and the size of an MRI. But this is just quick care, not a full diagnostic workup in a health clinic.

How does this happen? Simply because there is money to be made, a demand for quick service, a need for health care in low-income populations, and technology that allows implementation of all that I describe below in more detail, so you can recall how it works. Big institutions like Cleveland Clinic, Henry Ford Health System, and Mayo Health are not putting primary care clinics in low-income neighborhoods. Those folks all have low pay Medicaid and are non-compliant. That was the mantra I always heard whenever I challenged administration on this point in Detroit, South Haven, and Cleveland.

Then let Big-Box Discount Store, which has megacenters across America, figure out how to provide primary care and make money at it, too.

The shopper comes in, enters the AI supercomputer booth. He swipes his credit card. He picks from a list of symptoms and provides some time-related answers, such as when did it start, and how long does it last. He answers a basic list of questions: current meds, surgeries you have had, allergies. He gets a printout with the most probable conditions listed.

He is next able to seek care by selecting the "treat me" button. He picks the condition he thinks he has. More questions are given to him by the computer. If necessary, the machine will ask him to provide a urine sample or fingerstick for micro blood testing. In 20 minutes, he will get a printout with his most likely condition, the most reasonable differential diagnoses, a page full of legal boiler plate verbiage that protects the Big-Box Discount Store Med Bot from legal action, his treatment program and a prescription that has been sent electronically to the Big-Box Discount Store's pharmacy for pickup. He removes his credit card, gets a receipt for the transaction, and goes to the pharmacy for pick up.

The wealthy will have augmented physicians who will provide personalized high-priced, individualized care. The very poor will have the Big-Box Discount Store Med Bot Kiosk. What happens to the income group in-between is uncertain, but they will have access to people who are medically trained but not augmented, therefore less expensive, and who are able to accept government payment for health care.

The accuracy of this is probably low, but with machine learning and better AI interface technology, it will only get better. So, you see how there is no need to have physicians, nurse practitioners, or physician assistants in the loop. It is all free- flowing money into the megastore chain's pocket.

If there is the need for a medication refill, the request can be done online, like it is now with MyChart in hundreds of major health systems. Strep screens, blood sugars, blood pressures, and dozens of CLIA waived tests (Clinical Lab Improvement Amendments), and even some that are not CLIA waived, could be done at the kiosk.

My guess is that this scenario will be accurate enough for the general population with the low-hanging fruit diagnoses like cough, cold, UTIs, skin rashes, and if a way is found to bypass the liability issues, I am sure the Big-Box Discount Store will jump on this like white on rice.

Patients really want an answer. If they can possibly have treatment, too, they would pay cash for the privilege. A $25 fee would be affordable, and with high volume and low-overhead, the MSCK (Medical Self Care Kiosk) would be an up-and- running feature on the health horizon.

Someone will take this up and make it happen. They will probably need a boatload of lawyers to write the program protections so that their MSCK business does not get sued to death, but I am sure a big operation like the Big-Box Discount Stores or drugstore chains will find a way. If there is money to be made in American Health Care, the Big-Box Discount Stores will find it. Not only will the Big-Box Discount Stores and drugstore chains find this, but they will think about expansion of their low-fee, mass health care into as many other ancillary health areas as possible.

Think how the Big-Box Discount Stores could have the AI self-serve medical supercomputer, and have in-house optometry, dental, podiatry, physical therapy, and massage services. They would only have to hire a few physicians to oversee the treatment algorithm and serve as advisors to the program.

Oh, physician, where art thou?

WE'RE BACK . . .

### George Henry Hutchinson, Large and in Charge, June's Second Husband

Let us leave the gentle, bucolic life of Vela and Simpson Malone, and focus a bit on what trajectory my mom was taking. She lived with her parents, but still got around socially. But being alone, Black and female, and with a child, she knew she needed a man in her life. The goal for all women then was to have a man who would provide. The man was the source of money, protection, and social standing in the community. With one, you were somebody; without one, you were just a body.

Her second husband, George Henry Hutchinson, was mentally ill and ended up being confined to the mental hospital in Battle Creek, Michigan when it was still operated by the Veteran's Administration.

I recall their final meeting, watching them sit on a park bench and come to an arrangement where she got out from under his control. The man used to beat me with a rubber hose if he thought I was lying. He never believed what I said, and always sided with the live-in housekeeper. I recall her smiling as he beat me on my shoulders and back. My mother said that I must have done something to deserve it and never provided any comfort during those times when I was crying and hurting. I never realized that she, too, was crying and hurting as an equally-battered wife of this abusive man.

Mother met and married George Hutchinson on December 7$^{th}$, 1949, when I was just five years old, and they moved to a house on the east side of Detroit around 1950. I was six, and we lived at 3753 Fischer, just north of Mack Avenue. The side of Mack Avenue we lived on was north of Indian Village.

### My Life as a Child on Detroit's East Side

Indian Village was the ritzy-rich eastside neighborhood where the managers and relatives of the auto industry's families lived. The Fords, Fishers, Dodge Brothers, and such other giants of the industry lived in the fancy-schmancy suburban neighborhoods like Grosse Pointe.

You can always determine that rich people live in a neighborhood because there is an "e" at the end of a perfectly good word that does not need it.

The homes were gilded, gabled, gardened, huge structures, with carriage houses, porte-cochère (there goes the "e" again), marble, mahogany fittings and finishes, ballrooms, landscaped flower beds, and no Black people allowed, except as servants.

Our house on Fischer was in a wonderfully mixed neighborhood. Across the street was a VFW hall, and every weekend a function of some kind was happening there.

Sometimes there was even a fight causing the cops to show up with great regularity. One night, in the summer long ago, there was a wedding, and it was a mixed marriage. That meant, back in my childhood, one party was Italian and the other party was Polish. There was no love lost between the opposite members of the wedding celebration, and shortly after 1 AM, a fight broke out: people ran out of the VFW hall crying, screaming, shouting and cursing, flinging cups, bottles, chairs at each other, rolling and fighting on the ground and into the street, tearing off clothes, throwing knives, and shooting guns. People from each family streamed up and down Fischer, searching for a way to cause more mayhem, and one woman even came to our front door, banging on it, begging to be let in.

My mom definitely said no. The woman ran down the steps into the rest of the crowd just before the cops showed up and put it all to an end. That was frequently the way Saturdays went on my street. You see where I got my love of big parties; they seemed to be such a fun-laden community event.

On the corner of Mack and Fischer was a gas station, run by a fellow called "Spud." Just up from his shop was a three-unit apartment building with lots white people from somewhere in Appalachia. Next was a house with a family from somewhere in eastern Europe; they had two boys—and then there was us. Down the block was our unofficial leader, a Hispanic teenage boy.

Every morning we would gather at the corner by Spud's garage and plan our walk across Mack Avenue to our elementary school. There was no traffic light, so we had to watch right, watch left, and then run like the dickens to cross. Our school was Nichols Elementary—which still stands and is still used as I am writing this—on the corner of Burns and Goethe, just one block into Indian Village.

If you asked us for whom those streets were named, we would have been lost and unable to state the Scottish poet, Robert Burns, and the German statesman author, Johann Wolfgang von Goethe.

In fact, no one even knew how to say his German name; we all said "Go-thee," being unable to pronounce the German name correctly. But we were happy. We played together in the street, in each other's yards, in each other's homes, with never a thought of our superficial differences.

Poor, Black and white and brown, but happy together, we pressed on down the street to school after safely crossing the hazards of morning rush hour on Mack Avenue.

Imagine the fear we had, a rag tag, multicultural, noisy group of fourth graders walking down the street to our school. We knew we would be punished if we veered too close to the grass, or picked any flowers, so we moved quickly to our school. If you have seen the original movie *The Wizard of Oz* with Judy Garland, then you should recall the scene where she and her companions—Tin Man, Scarecrow, Lion, and Toto—walk through the forest and, at the end of the forest, gaze out over the field of poppies with Emerald City on the near horizon.

We had to make it to the Emerald City (our school) and not get stuck in the poppy fields (rich, white people's yards) or we would be punished.

That was the feeling we had as children going down the street in Indian Village, waiting, not for beautiful poppies, but rather for some angry disaster in the form of an outraged homeowner lady—what is called a "Karen" today—to come out and curse at us. School daze indeed.

Back at home, life with George Henry Hutchinson must have been difficult for my mom. I really do not recall what he did for a living, but he was making enough money for us to have a single-family home. My mom also worked, so we were making it OK.

George liked to fish, and I recall trips to Georgian Bay in Lake Huron for fishing trips. We would go with his friends on the long drive up to this Canadian parkland and have great times on the water.

George Hutchinson formally adopted me on October 26$^{th}$, 1953, and changed my middle name from June to Georgia. I found out that my birth name was Sylvia June Brown, then my adopted name was Sylvia Georgia Hutchinson. I picked my *nom de plume* at the TV station to become Sylvia Wayne, and earned my married name of Sylvia Mustonen. So that means I have been four different women, on paper, anyway. I lived in that house until Mom divorced Hutchinson, and met and married Warren Garner in 1960.

She was married to a man who was able to provide for her and a child, but she never stopped working. Maybe work was her escape from his abuse. Maybe she was just a workaholic. Maybe it was a little bit of both. She was independent to the bitter end, and I am sure I learned that from her. She made the wrong choice again for a partner with George, but made the right choice to protect her earning ability by never quitting what she loved and what she was good at. I'm sure I learned that from her, too.

**June and Her Career**

My Mom was a wonderful woman with boundless energy, an active imagination, and a cheery and fun-loving personality. She was also a hard-driving workaholic. Too bad she was Black and female, because any other combination would have made it possible for her to rule the world.

She grew up the youngest child of six; one sibling died young, so only the five of them made it to adulthood. She got an education, got a job, got married three times, got pregnant once with me, and got along in her life in a marvelous fashion.

Had she been born in another time or another place, she would have been a queen. She was a fun-loving, energetic, hard-working woman who was extremely competent in most everything she tried. Her first two marriages failed because the men were failures. Max was not suited for married life and fatherhood, and the responsibilities that attended them. He was a drinker and a gambler. George Hutchinson had severe mental illness, was a wife and child abuser, and would not have been a life-long partner who could provide what June needed.

I think she needed love, and someone to care for. She never had pets when we lived in the house with Vela and Simpson, so she wanted someone upon whom she could show tenderness and love. She probably got very little love being the youngest child growing up, Black, during the Depression and wartime in America, and she probably had me only because I was a mistake. There was no birth control for Black women in 1943 and 1944, so I showed up, and was not the object of her tender love. But motherhood alone probably made her realize that caring for someone required a lot of help.

She turned her attention to work and excelled at her job at the *Michigan Chronicle*. She was there from 1945 to 1974. She turned the classified advertising section into a powerhouse and had a staff of two other Black women who were almost as productive as she was. She had two women working with her, and they made money hand-over-fist for that newspaper every week that it published. June was the manager of the classified section, and was a friend to everyone who worked there.

She brought me to the newspaper office frequently, and I suspect it was because she did not have daycare. I remember being the gopher for the office staff. They would send me to White Castle to bring back lunch for everyone. I felt so important, coming back with bags of greasy burgers and hot, salty fries, giving the change back to the group, passing out the orders, setting up the table as we all joined in to eat lunch in the office.

She also gave me work to do, so that my being there was not viewed as just babysitting. I was assigned to clip ads out of the most recently published paper for reprinting in the next weekly edition, if the advertiser wanted to simply repeat what was being sold. Usually, it was homes for sale, and if the place did not sell, the owner of the house would want to run the ad again, so it was easy work for me to do.

I felt so at home with the crowd of Black people at that paper. All of them had such unique personalities, and all of them seemed happy to be productive and free, to be the voice of the Black community via the *Green Sheet,* as the *Michigan Chronicle* was called. It was published once a week on Tuesdays, and the front page was a light-colored, mint green.

The office building was a converted brick house on the eastside of Detroit, at 479 Ledyard, and the publishing office was Unique Printing, located in Hamtramck. I got to go with my mother on the nights before publication. I saw the linotype setters working at their machines, and I watched Mom talk with the printers about changes that were made from the "hot sheets."

I really enjoyed the sight and rhythmic noise and smell of hot lead and warm sheets of paper running through the printing press, piled up for packing and distribution. The printing press was a marvelous metallic monster of early twentieth century engineering, and it dominated the room. It was a one-story tall, black-iron, noisy contraption running high speed sheets of paper in, and pushing out the finished collated bundled newspapers.

I still recall the sound it made: *clank ata, clank ata, clank ata, clank ata, clank ata, clank ata, clank ata.* Try saying that as fast as you can to get the feel of the sound it made.

Sometimes we would be there until midnight making corrections and putting in additions of late breaking news events in Detroit's Black community.

My mother was also a party animal. She loved music, food, and dancing, and she was a wonderful hostess. She threw house parties that were the talk of the neighborhood. Her style was the mold for my style of party-hosting. Lots of music, lots of people, lots of fun. Pearl Mesta would have learned a thing or two from watching my mom be a hostess. She would find a way to get things done: parties, music collections, and travel. If she put her mind to it, it would get accomplished. Because she wanted to meet Fidel Castro when he first came into power, she wrangled and managed a dream trip to Cuba!

She had a collection of Frank Sinatra blues and jazz recordings that we listened to all the time. This was probably my inspiration for my record collection.

She never had a complete college education, being only able to attend Wayne State University for one year in 1941, but she had drive and ambition. She developed a newspaper column called *Other People's Business*. She would print anonymous articles filled with gossip about the infidelities and goings-on carried out by well-known figures in the Black community of Detroit. She never mentioned any names, but readers would be able to quickly narrow it down to the right person just by the descriptions of the activities she reported.

It quickly became the "other" society news in the *Michigan Chronicle*. If the church section talked about preachers and sermons, her column talked about the preacher's girlfriends and illegitimate children. If the society section talked about weddings, her column covered the nasty divorces and fights that high-profile Black couples had on the streets. She got newsy tidbits about the big-time pimps and players and gangsters in the city.

She also began to collect jokes that readers would send to her. Most of the jokes would be way off-color, and even more off-limits by today's standards, but the *Chronicle* was happy to have the readership, while the words "politically correct" were lightyears in the future. Many of the jokes started with some culturally insensitive pejorative, linking several ethnicities along the lines of, "A kike, a darkie, and a wop die and go to heaven . . . "

No way those would get past even the most liberal TV show today, and YouTube would probably dump it off the platform. But back then, everyone read the jokes and laughed.

Her career kept going upwards. She became the most popular person on the staff and the best known at the *Michigan Chronicle.* This was at a time in Detroit when there were two competing daily newspapers, *The Detroit News* and the *Detroit Free Press,* as well as a half dozen community papers, such as *The Jewish News, The Arab American News, The Italian Tribune,* and the *Michigan Chronicle,* among others. As I mentioned, the *Chronicle* was also known as the *Green Sheet* because the front page was printed in a light green color, so it stood out from other weekly ethnic publications.

A year later, Mom got a spot on a local TV station, hosting a talk show called *June Brown's Detroit,* that aired on WDIV/Channel 4. She used her married name, from the time she was married to Max Brown, so that people would not know she was married to Warren Garner, and therefore could maintain some kind of privacy. She interviewed various interesting people from Detroit's Black community, and had a good following. She gave a voice to Black leaders who were active in the realms of education, religion, politics, business, finance, and more.

She was also a member of the Lawrence Institute of Technology's Founders Society. LIT actually helped her write her book, *June Brown's Guide to Let's Read.* It was a supplemental study book for the Let's Read series that was a popular teaching method for young children. She used it to help your mother learn to read as a young child.

Her fame spread to the point that *The Detroit News*—the rich white people's paper—wanted to hire her to work for them, which meant she would have to leave the *Chronicle.* I think she would have preferred to go to the *Detroit Free Press*—the more liberal paper favored by working-class people of all races—if she could, but the *Freep* never expressed an interest. She left the *Chronicle* after the Detroit riot and took her column to *The Detroit News,* working there from 1974 to 1987. And I am sure *The News* gained readership because of her move.

I do know that the *Chronicle* began a slow decline after she left.

Whether it was because she left or because of other factors, I cannot say. I do know that many other writers left the paper for other work, or just plain retired.

For a short while, from 1990 to 1992, she returned to the *Michigan Chronicle* as a columnist. But the paper was never the same, and it became a sad mouthpiece for anyone who would give them a prepared handout. It no longer had the political caché and social fire that it had when it launched in 1936. The reporting on church news kept the paper alive, but the times were changing in Detroit, especially after the riot of 1967.

**June and Warren**

My mother took such good care of her third husband, Warren Garner. He was a real estate broker, and met her at the *Chronicle*. He was exactly what she needed and wanted.

They were instantly attracted to each other, and soon found a way to get together permanently about the time I was a senior in high school at Cass Tech from 1961 to 1962. They married, and she began to change his life. The first thing she changed was his drinking habit. Warren liked to have a little nip every now and then, more often "now" and less often "then." Because of her experience with Max and Vela, June made it plain that Warren had to give up the alcohol, or give up June.

*Kaboom!* The alcohol went away. That was a major turning point in his life. He realized how much it had been limiting his success and impacting his previous family life.

Warren had been previously married, but never had a child with his first wife. Instead, they adopted a son, Michael, but they were not able to stay together. When Warren was in the Army, he fought in Italy, and moved with the Army up into Germany. Eventually he was stationed in Darmstadt, Germany, and there he met and "married" a German woman and had a child, Josie, with her.

I was fortunate to meet Josie in 1964 when I traveled in Europe for a month- long university-sponsored trip. With 100 other Wayne

State University students, we flew to London, then hopped over to Paris. For one week, I stayed in youth hostels, traveled by train, hitchhiked, and found myself at a U.S. Army base. I had a scintillating day and night in the enlisted men's club. Eventually, I asked to leave and two soldiers took me to Josie's address and she took me in. We bonded immediately, and I stayed there for two weeks, learning to love rich German dark beer, brats, polka music and the woman whom I call my half-sister-in-law. Warren may not have really married her mother, and he was not my biological father, but Josie and I both knew and loved him because of his character and the protection he gave us both. We agreed, that was enough to make us sisters.

After the war, he came home, got a divorce, and never brought his family with him. Perhaps his drinking was a problem then. He never spoke about it, so we never knew.

## DIGRESSION #3: MEDICAL SCHOOL WILL BE OPEN TO ALL WHO CAN AFFORD IT

I want to share with you a list of my students who were in the Michigan State University College of Osteopathic Medicine (MSUCOM) in their first or second year; one or two of them were actually residents, but they all were people in medical school.

I am proud to say that the students I was gifted with teaching represented my college's commitment to diversity in the profession. My students were male, urban, female, rural, white, Black, Latinx, gay, older, Asian, and Indian. I have had others, but I have not retained their profiles, and so all their names are lost to me. But there was a cohort that I trained when I was in my office in Stanton, Michigan. I am honored to have had them under my guidance as well. I tried to show them all aspects of my life and work as a physician.

Not only did they follow me on patient visits in the office, but I also took them into the hospital, if I was called there during their sessions with me. I also made sure they spent one week with my business manager learning how to get paid for the good work they would be doing.

Here are their names and the places where I taught them.

When I worked for Visiting Physicians Association in Okemos, Michigan:

Jack Davis, February 27th, 2009
Heather Schmitz, October 24th, 2008

When I worked for MSUCOM in East Lansing, Michigan:

Joshua Drumm, January 8th, 2007
Lynn Coraci, July 27th, 2006
C. Luke Wilcox, April 2nd, 2006
Nurin Dashoush, August 2006
Swathi Pullela, August 2006

When I worked for MSUCOM and IRMC in Okemos, Michigan:

Jamie Wright, April 18th, 1998
Victoria Landolt, August 2nd, 1999
Alyse Ley, August 2nd, 1999
Jennifer Sommer, December 1st, 1998
Xuan Tran, December 1st, 1998

When I worked in Greenville, Michigan:

Jennifer Shirkey Paltzer, November 11th, 1997
Kimberly Bain, November 11th, 1997
Josie Muhhammad, July 29th, 1997
Sarah Nielsen, July 29th, 1997
Neelam Trivedi, August 1st, 1996
Judy Lynn Kirkwood, October 12th, 1995
Kristin L. Mcadden, July 28th, 1994
Katrina M. Cisaruk, August 5th, 1993 (Rakowsky, my most long-term connection)
Lynn E. Beals, December 23rd, 1992

Julie A. Burnham, March 3rd, 1992
Jennifer Ross, May 17th, 1991
Hallie Jo Wilson, January 23rd, 1991 (my oldest)
Catherine A. Kerschen, May 18th, 1990
Deborah Ondersma, February 14th, 1997
Sy Hoa Oang, November 24th, 1989
Roberto Baun Corales, November 10th, 1989 (my first)

When I had my office in Stanton, Michigan:
John Tower
Elsie Baccari
Gust Bills (I met his daughter at an OsteoCHAMPS session)

When I was retired:
Johnice Littlejohn
Harmant Grewal
OsteoCHAMPS classes

My students were all going to graduate with huge debt, so I thought knowing how to work their way out of debt would be important. They were all lucky to have found a way to afford medical school, even if huge debt was part of the deal.

But what if medical school were open to all who could afford it? Even before the COVID-19 pandemic of 2019 to 2021, medical schools (including Wayne State University in Detroit) were making changes by offering full-ride scholarships to students of color who qualified. Some offered free tuition to students of color in an attempt to rebalance the health disparities gap in the physician workforce. Some universities, like New York University, offered tuition-free education to all who matriculated.

Regarding the list of students I shared, what must they have done to get there? The financial sacrifice alone must have been daunting and onerous, and how long did it take for them to come up into the air of non-indebtedness, G.O.R.K.?

But if a person could afford it, would that be enough? We make people go through inordinate hoops of greater and greater complexity to get in. We demand intelligence, passage of several arcane tests, letters of recommendation, proof of determination to the altar of altruistic behavior.

What if all you needed was money? No screening exams, no MCAT. How would that work?

Class sizes would probably be huge in the first year, around 2,000, as opposed to the 200 to 300 that are enrolled now. But if a student were unable to pass all exams, he/she would be dropped from the enrolled list. That would be a great hurdle and would clear away those who did not have the academic rigor to learn and study for medical school. Sorry, dear grandchildren, but Dr. Google is really not enough to get a person through that first year and the anatomy lab will take out a lot of weak players.

The class would drop from 2,000 to 500, and the same standard would apply to those second-year students who are now tasked, not only with academic didactic work, but also with seeing live patients in real clinical settings. Their preceptors would wield a huge hammer, able to weed out any who cannot communicate. Lord knows I have seen some interns who have had top marks when it comes to taking a test on paper, but who failed like flies stuck in flypaper going down a toilet when it comes to talking to a person who is in patient-mode.

There is no test for empathy, the ability to understand someone else's feelings; either you have it or you do not, and a physician should have a boatload of it. The end of the second year will see a 50 percent drop in class size. The way we select for medical school now makes me doubt that empathy is a top characteristic. Some say empathy is a teachable skill. I think empathy is a talent, like art or music or mathematic acumen or dunking a basketball. Some of us have more of that talent than others.

By the third year, the class would be 250 students, and that is about right. The medical school will have made money from the tuition funds it garnered from people who thought they could

Google search their way through medical school and from people who thought that intelligence alone is enough to be a physician.

Is this too cruel? I do not know for sure; I am just making a suggestion—a thought experiment, if you will. I think my point is that we are selecting a certain kind of person to become a physician, and maybe we need to change the selection process, because of the bias that is built into the entire process. People who are smart and who have money will get in. But they may not be the best physicians, and we may have arbitrarily removed the pulse of empathy from the profession in favor of pure brain power.

I came to love and admire all the students on that list of names you saw. I do not know where they landed or how they did, but they are all members of my profession now, so that is OK with me. So I will say to all of them: "Hey, y'all, you dun good!"

The current situation of medical education removes a lot of talent who are good, smart people, who could not excel on a test on one particular day, or who did not interview well one particular day, or who were just one decimal point below an arbitrary cutoff one particular day. Where do they go and what do they do and how do they acclimate to the loss of this opportunity? I will never know. But I imagine it is crushing.

Why not give all who seek admission, admission? The only thing that would be a challenge would be tuition. But if a medical school, like my alma mater, gets 3,000 applications a year, why not admit them all? (In 2021, there were 8,000 applicants.)

The kicker here is that the physician being turned out in this strange future, is not at all like the ones being turned out today. A hundred years ago, a physician was a person, usually a white male, who was a competent surgeon, capable of doing an operation on any part of the body. But then, 100 years ago, we did not have the diagnostic or therapeutic interventions of today. But I predict that 100 years into the future, those interventions will be so sophisticated that a person could be outfitted with internalized devices that allow diagnostic interventions on one hand, and therapeutic interventions on the other hand, literally. That if a person were also fitted out with an internalized cerebral-to-digital interface with the AI medical supercomputer of 2118 as well, then the only thing lacking would be the ability to perform some kind of surgery.

Imagine the cost of producing that physician and the change in training for that person.

If 3,000 are admitted, then at the end of the first year, there are only 1,500 remaining; at the end of the second year, there are 750 remaining; at the end of the third year, there are 375; at the end of the fourth year, 188; and at the end of the fifth year, there are 100.

Yes, you would need five or six years to produce 100 Fully Augmented Physicians. These 100 have implants in the left hand that provide diagnostic information (blood tests), and implants in the right hand that provide therapeutic interventions (immune therapy, antibiotics), and these 100 have access to all the medical information via the AI supercomputer, so that differential diagnosis is obtained within minutes. There is no longer a need to separate the surgeon from the internist. With proper training, there is no need to have surgical sub-specialties. All physicians are like the physicians on the USS Enterprise in the television show *Star Trek.*

These 100 FAP will be trained in anatomy, physiology, immunology, genetics, and all the hands-on techniques of the time. In addition to all the surgical specialties, they will also know OMM, Acupuncture, Reiki, and all other complimentary medical approaches.

They will have five years of training, then in their last and sixth year, they have implants and digital interface applied and learn how to use and control their new augmentation. They practice on simulated patients to gain control. They move on to volunteer patients, and then they serve in underserved communities for the remainder of their sixth year. Then, they go to a one-year residency with another FAP. After six years of training and one year of residency, they are now ready for employment. Who can afford them? Obviously the very super-wealthy. The Silicon Valley multi-millionaires and leaders of nations will have a family physician who cares for all their needs.

So, now you ask, what happened to those other 2,900 who did not make it through the years of training? And what happens to the rest of humanity that cannot afford a FAP?

With the advent of the FAP and the Medical Self Care Kiosk, there is no longer a need for a mid-level anything. Opticians, chiropractors, audiologists, nurses, nurse practitioners, and physician assistants, will be marginalized. In those areas where there is no technology or money, they will find opportunities. Let us just be realistic before you shout out in hoarse criticism. The rich and famous and powerful always get the best of whatever there is, and they get it first. Then it trickles down to the rest of us as the innovation becomes more cost effective.

Examples? Indoor toilets, automobiles, electricity, televisions, cell phones, clothing, shoes, pretty much everything. The king had it first, then his family and friends, next the aristocrats, then the wealthy merchants, the up-and-coming, and then everybody else. The "thing" that started off as a one-of-a-kind wonder for the king, morphed into a bobble of delight for the wealthy, then moved over to become a necessity for the majority, before it became a right for everyone.

The remaining 2,900 will call themselves Health Professional Level 1, 2, 3 or 4 to indicate how many years of training they achieved. These HPLs can work with a FAP, or work independently. People will get what they need from whomever they can afford. The world's billionaires each have a pair of FAPs. The CEOs at smaller companies have HPLs 1 to 4, while the rest of us have the Medical Self Care Kiosk. Some of the HPLs will join some of the FAPs and perform important research. Pharmaceutical companies and the military will be looking for both HPLs and FAPs as usual and as always.

The licensing boards can struggle with all of this. So can the professional associations. Did I mention that the American Osteopathic Association (AOA) and the American Medical Association (AMA) will merge when medical schools' open enrollment happens, so that when you graduate, you are an MD DO, or a DO MD, depending on from which school you graduated? Perhaps trial lawyers will stop feeding off medicine and perform useful work somewhere for a change.

With access to the AI Medi-Supercomputer, the need for CME (Continuing Medical Education) and MOC (Maintenance of Certification) will evaporate into the wind. Continuing Medical Education is what the FAP will get when he/she plugs into The AI supercomputer at the end of the day. Maintenance of Certification will be seen for the monetary running lapdog of the greedy Professional Associations who promote it, and will be ignored or dropped as FAPs become more and more integrated into the population.

Large hospital corporations will hang on for a while, but eventually, the FAPs realize they do not need those cumbersome, overpriced conglomerations of ineptitude, but rather they just need a place to work, or a single employer, such as the Sultan of Wherever, the Premier of Someplace, or the CEO of Successful Startup, etc.

WE'RE BACK . . .

**Wayne State University and My Life on Campus**

Together, June and Warren worked his real estate business into a profitable enterprise. She was his Chief Financial Officer for all the years they worked in Detroit. She and Warren spent a lot of effort employing family members, myself included, and friends as workers in their real estate business. They opened an office in Southfield, which was becoming the new center of commerce in the Metro Detroit area. They still lived in Detroit, on Taylor Street. The nice thing about Warren being in real estate and being a broker was that, whenever he saw a house that he liked, he would move us into it instead of selling it to someone else.

We lived on Atkinson, which was near Joy Road, then out by the Dexter-Davidson area, and then on Taylor Street, near the old Detroit Northern High School on Woodward Avenue.

I lived with them in the house on Taylor Street, and from there began my college education at Wayne State University. It was a great place to study, and because it was located within the city of Detroit, it was very easy to get to. I took the bus to school and home. Eventually, I realized I wanted to be more independent. This happened when I was a freshman, going to major in journalism.

I met a really nice guy and we spent a lot of time talking politics, art, and life. One summer night, we stayed out past bar's closing time (2 AM) and went to the reflecting pool near one of the lecture halls on campus. We talked, we necked, we talked, we necked. Not much more than that happened because neither of us had a private place to live. Eventually, he drove me home. When we got to the house, I saw that lights were on upstairs. It was 5 AM. I told him good night, and a permanent goodbye, and said that he would probably not be able to take me out again once my parents knew who he was, and that no matter what I said had happened, my parents would make assumptions about what had happened, and I would never dissuade them from their opinion. And also, that he should quickly leave, right after I got out of the car, because my dad has a CCW permit, and a gun to go with it, and he will use it.

I was right. So, I asked Warren and June if I could live on campus. They said OK, and I moved into the dorm on campus, Helen De Roy Hall. It was hell. The bunkbed was small and narrow and hard, and I hated sharing the room with a non-Black person. There was also the matter of the 9 PM curfew Mondays to Thursdays, the midnight curfew on Fridays and Saturdays, and the 10 PM curfew on Sundays.

Warren, the real estate broker, came to the rescue. After one semester in the dorm, he asked if I wanted to live in a unit he owned on Fourth Street. It was a three-bedroom duplex tucked into the place where traffic from the eastbound Edsel Ford exited to the northbound John Lodge freeway. Out of the 20 buildings there, only one was family occupied, and all of the rentals were filled with students at WSU.

I told him I would be happy to live there and serve as the building manager. I moved in and found a roommate, Linda (not her real name). We found a second roommate, Shelley (not her real name).

Next door were three guys, none of whom we wanted for boyfriends. We were *Sex and the City* before it was a thought in a producer's mind.

Pretty much every weekend was a party weekend, unless it was midterm or final exam weeks. Then we had to study in order to pass. The rule was if you have a party, you must invite everyone on the street. That kept the peace because the party would usually go very late and involve a lot of drop-in guests so that there was a house crowd into the wee hours of the night.

My first roommate, Linda, was a most beautiful Black woman, who had a gorgeous voice and a body to match. I am sure I was in love with her.

This was an era of sexual freedom, but birth control pills were expensive. As a result, missed periods during a time when abortion was illegal often inspired searches amongst my friends for help from back-door purveyors of illegal abortifacients. Witnessing this, I became an advocate for freedom for women's reproductive rights. It was so wrong for women to suffer so much because they could not afford birth control.

We two had a third roommate, let's call her Patricia, who actually predated Linda. Patricia was from the Midwest. White and wealthy, she was one of the filthiest people I have ever known. She never cleaned herself or her room, never cleaned up the kitchen when it was her turn, or cleaned her items in the shared bathroom. The final straw was when she bought a puppy, but never cleaned up the poop. As the house became a smelly cesspool, Linda and I banded together and told Patricia she had to go.

It took us two weeks to clean it up and deodorize the place.

It was while I was living on Fourth Street that I met Arney Mustonen. More on him later. Now back to Warren and June.

### Warren and June, and the G2 Ranch

After the Detroit riot of 1967, they bought property in Holly, Michigan, and I recall going there to hunt with Warren before the riot. He bought a .410 shotgun for me and taught me to use it while we hunted on the undeveloped land. The first thing I killed was a small squirrel. It made me so sad to see the dead animal torn to bits by my gunshot, but I was proud that I was able to hit the target.

Warren loved that property and decided to purchase it. It was on a lake and was very secluded. They made plans to sell the house on Taylor and move to Holly. This would require an hour-long drive to Southfield going down I-75, but they did not mind the commute. They had good cars, and the highway was well maintained. They spent the time talking and planning their business on the way into work, and talking and planning the ranch on their way home.

They started with an airstream trailer and lived there while their home was being constructed. Then, Warren wanted a barn because he wanted to have some horses. June thought that was a good idea, and so they launched into horse ranching and built the barn. Warren bought more land so he could grow hay to feed the horses. Then he bought more equipment, so he could harvest the hay. Then he constructed more storage units for storing the hay and the farm equipment, which included the big truck for hauling, the pick-up truck, and the hay wagon. Then, June decided they should get more horses and rent them out as a riding stable. Warren thought that was a good idea, and away they went. They even bought a horse for me, named Flicka. I never wanted a horse, or asked for it, and so I made sure the animal stayed at their ranch. They eventually had a full stable of more than a dozen animals.

My cousin Keith Ledbetter and, before him, my cousin Wade Kirksey, both came to live at the ranch and helped take care of the horses. They became accomplished riders and ranch hands, and worked the riding stable for Warren and June. Warren and June made each of those young men understand the value of honest, hard work, and shaped them into the men they would become.

My mom then decided that Black singles in Detroit needed a social outlet of a wholesome nature, where they could meet each other. Thus was born the G2 Ranch and the Bachelor's Book. It was a list of eligible single men and women who would have membership at the G2 Ranch, and come up for weekends of horseback riding, picnics, swimming at the lake, and, in general, hooking up.

In addition to developing the G2 Ranch and Bachelor's Book club, she dove into Warren's family activities and made herself part of his family as much as she could. He had several siblings and they all had lots of kids. One of his nephews was Dennis Archer, the former mayor of Detroit.

Dennis initially wanted to become a pharmacist and entered the program at Ferris State University. I recall him coming to visit us one day and talking to Warren about how unfulfilled and unhappy he was with the demands of learning pharmacy. They talked all day, from mid-morning till past dinner. We had pork chops and mashed potatoes, and they talked and talked. They went to the basement and played ping pong—Dennis was good and Warren was even better, so the game was hot and loud and a long evening of fun. And they continued to talk and talk. At the end of that day-long session, Dennis had been given clarification on what was expected of him as a member of his family, his race, and as a man. Warren probably saved him.

Warren and Dennis were so close because Dennis' father was out of the picture, so Warren was the *de facto* father figure. Warren enjoyed that role as uncle and father stand-in, and he spent the rest of the day advising and guiding Dennis. Dennis eventually dropped out of Ferris, transferred to Wayne State Law School, and became a successful attorney and, later, Mayor of Detroit.

If you ask any of the young men that Warren mentored, sheltered, worked with, or hired, they would all probably agree that he was a superhero person. The superpower that Warren Garner had was that he could transform any young man or woman who was troubled, lost, uncertain, insecure, etc., into a self-actuated confident human, willing and able to identify and express all the God-given potential within them.

He was that way with every male he ever knew, and I know he was that way with me, as his daughter, not by blood or adoption, but by a loving, mutual agreement.

## DIGRESSION #4: CUSTOMER VERSUS PATIENT

How do you know if you are a customer or a patient?

In the world of corporate medicine, patients have become downgraded to consumers/customers, and physicians are downgraded to employees. Recall how THEY changed the names of what doctors were; physicians became providers and patients became covered lives. In some places, all medical personnel have name tags that call them a "Health Care Team Member." This piece of corporate BS terminology completes the blurring between professional training and all the differences that matter.

The place you go to for health care may look like it is a medical office, but in reality, think of it as just being in a "store" where health-like activities are sold to you.

If your health care adventure feels like a trip to a discount department store, then you are a customer. Look for a large parking lot filled with cars, a large office filled with artificially busy employees, throngs of customers in a crowded waiting room, lots of shopping options marked with confusing prices, or no visible prices, long wait lines, security cameras inside and outside, noise and smells. In health care, you do not even know the price, but if you have insurance, you pay very little out of pocket.

You have no idea who is in charge; there are forced smiles on the faces of workers, but no eye contact with them because they must stare at a computer screen. The cleanliness is dubious in the facility, and you know that you are being watched by the store security team to prevent shoplifting. And just like the Eagles' song about a hotel in California, you can check out, but you can never escape the merry-go-round of health care activities—because you are just a customer.

Physicians are being encouraged to give up their autonomy and to sign with a hospital or health system as an employee. They are told that life will be so much easier for them because they will only have to see patients, and not ever worry about all the administrative chores ever again.

In truth, physicians and nurses are hampered and then hammered by administrative constraints and demands that they cannot ever change. Furthermore, the government and the health system they work for will change the rules every year, thus requiring more time away from patients, learning the new compliance rules, which have no impact on making you well.

The physician does not participate in decision making and has no voice in the organization. The Health Care Organization must enlarge itself (Grow or Die Philosophy) and engage in mergers and acquisitions on a regular basis, causing disruption, chaos, and fear among employees, plus shifting patients/customers in and out of their circle of care based on arbitrary agreements with health insurance companies.

Advertising replaces information. If they are spending money on billboards and TV ads telling you how great their System is, rest assured that you are getting short-changed somewhere else. Deals are done between the HCO, pharmaceutical companies, and health insurance companies. The national overseer, Medicare, and its state-level avatar, Medicaid, promote rule after rule in a futile attempt to cut costs. Lawyers swarm at the edges of this conglomeration, seeking ways to suck out health care dollars if physicians deviate from some rule, whether or not there was significant injury to a person.

Here is the rundown of the major differences between consumer and patient experiences. Pay attention, so you will know which one you are:

- Customers wait in line, regardless of the urgency of their need.
- Patients are seen when they have a need.
- Customers experience continuous turnover of employee staffing.
- Patients see the same physician consistently.
- Customers never see the owner.
- Patients can speak to the physician who owns the clinic.
- Customers are valued only if they have money.
- Patients are valued all the time.

- Customers are encouraged to keep coming back for more treatment.
- Patients are treated until they are well and only need to return as needed.
- Customers receive advertising about how great the organization is.
- Patients receive information about what is important to their health.
- Customers can only afford what their pocketbook can support.
- Patients can afford their health care needs.
- Customers are shifted from one owner to another whenever there is a merger.
- Patients remain with the physician of their choice.
- Customers face frustrating automated service whenever possible.
- Patients can speak to a real person whenever they need to.
- Customers deal with employees who must be paid to care.
- Patients are treated by physicians who care.
- Customers encounter employees who do not do more than scheduled.
- Patients have physicians who provide regular and open access.
- Customers deal with employees in similar uniforms and obscure name tags.
- Patients have physicians who are easily recognized.
- Customers are saddled with employees who shirk from responsibility.
- Patients have physicians who take responsibility as a part of the relationship.
- Customers deal with employees who give what they want customers to have.
- Patients have physicians who give you what you need.
- Customers are asked to give high scores on employee satisfaction surveys.
- Patients receive high levels of satisfactory interaction with their physician.
- Customers interact with employees who follow rule books and compliance charts.

- Patients have physicians who use skills, training, art, and science.
- Customers deal with employees who do not look at or listen to them.
- Patients and physicians look at each other and have true dialogue.
- Customers have limited time for interaction with employees.
- Patients have realistic and meaningful time for interaction with their physician.
- Customers are dropped when they lack money/insurance.
- Patients are kept and ways are found to make payment less of a barrier to care.
- Customers are limited to one item of health consumption at a time.
- Patients can discuss many health concerns at any time.
- Customers deal with employees who must be trained to be honest with them.
- Patients have honest physicians who give honest answers.
- Customers are ignored by employees in many ways.
- Patients are not ignored by their physicians.
- Customers' choices are limited to proprietary items.
- Patients have choices that return the best results.
- Customers hope the employees follow the rules, even if they are not being watched.
- Patients know physicians watch themselves and follow compassionate rules.
- Customer frustrations are channeled to a professional but uncaring soother.
- Patient frustrations are discussed directly with the physician.
- Customer records are lost in the computer; computers fail, and are then replaced.
- Patient records are kept up to date, securely held, and open to the patient.
- Customers deal with employees who are just doing a job for a paycheck.
- Patients deal with physicians who provide healing and work in the patient's best interest.
- Customers cannot leave the system without repercussions.
- Patients can always exercise their choice of physicians.

Use this as a check list and take it with you to your next medical appointment. See how much of the Customer status applies to you.

There are 28 items on the list. If you have 10 to 15, you are an average customer; 16 to 20, you are a captive customer; 21 to 28, you are a slave to the system.

If you want to get out and become a valued patient, find a physician who is a DPC—Direct Primary Care provider—and go there. The difference will be astounding, rewarding, affordable, and you will actually get answers and get better while getting better care.

That list above, my dears, was a WIIIFY—What Is In It For You. I will have more for you as we go along.

WE'RE BACK . . .

**Warren and June in Virginia**

The Garner family was quite large with its roots in Virginia. We took a trip there for a family reunion in the late 1990s.

The gathering was held at the county fairgrounds just outside Bluefield, Virginia, which, interestingly, is just across the state line from Bluefield, West Virginia. Seems like, in the South, when you have a name you like, you can use it as many times as you want, and wherever you want.

I drove there with Arney, Ophelia, and of course, June and Warren. We stopped in a Shoney's restaurant, which is called an Elias Brothers Big Boy in Michigan, and had a country breakfast. It was my first experience with biscuits and gravy, Southern style.

I never met a calorie I didn't like, so I tried it, just once. I will not, and have not, tried it again. The buffet had a large bucket of white, thick, hot paste, peppered with tiny dark chunks of matter that could have been flies or sausage bits—it was indeterminate which meat prevailed. There were biscuits, formerly hot, but now just better than room temperature, reclining lazily against each other under the infrared lights. Cold, scrambled, overly-yellow, dry pebbles of egg-like substance lollygagged in a warming tray across from packaged condiments—salt, pepper, butter, syrup, and sugar—completed our morning repast choices. I really did try to like the gravy, but I just could not find a way to convince my tongue that my eyes were not lying about it being actual food. I think I found the calorie I did not like, right then and there.

After that exhilarating country breakfast, we had to find the fairgrounds, so we asked one of the locals who was in the restaurant for directions. He said we should take the interstate going south and get off at Exit 25.

We thanked him and piled into the car. Arney was driving, and he got on the interstate and started down the road. The exits are numbered, and the first one we saw was Exit 345, the next was Exit 333, and the next one was Exit 329. Arney was convinced that we would be in the next county, or the next state, before we ever got to Exit 25, but Warren suddenly shouted, "Take the next exit! Take the next one!"

Arney did as Warren asked, and when Warren began to laugh, we asked what was so funny. Warren pointed to the speed limit sign on the exit, which read "Exit 25 mph," and said that is what the local man was referring to, not the interstate exit number, but the speed limit sign, which he thought WAS the number of the exit. Soon, we saw the sign directing us to the county fairgrounds and we were happy to join the family.

Oh, you gotta love those country ways.

There must have been 150 people. I am not sure that I recall the names of any of them, but they were all just like Warren—looked like him and talked like him, and they were even more friendly. And they had come from all over the USA, as relatives from New York, Michigan, Indiana, Virginia, and West Virginia gathered. The party lasted into the evening and was a smash hit with all of us. Interestingly enough, Warren's name was a combination of the three family names that united his people: the Warrens, the Carrolls, and the Garners. So, we met the Carroll branch, the Garner branch, and the Warren branch, and connected with lots of stories of who is related to whom, and how far back can you trace the connection.

Naturally they found out I was a physician and I got surrounded by a lot of people who started asking questions. Actually, they were looking for medical help, because most of them had such piss-poor medical care in the South, that their concerns were unmet. I did my best not to incriminate myself or give bad advice, or appear to be working for free, but it was hard not to want to try to help.

Fate intervened and I actually got the chance to help. It was a party with drinks, food, old people, and hard-surfaced, and wet-slippery floors. *Bang!* The frail, elderly relative from New York went down on her outstretched hand, and she had a fracture in the wrist—a Colles fracture, non-displaced.

Naturally, I came to look at her as the family crowded around. I said that she needed to go to the hospital, so I piled into the car with her, Warren, and another relative of hers. We arrived at the local hospital, where they got an X-ray and called the physician to come in to see her.

Somehow, he did not inspire confidence in me. He looked slovenly with a Richard Nixon five o'clock shadow. I knew it was late, but he did not have on a white coat or a name tag. My not-quite-related-to-me-in-law, sweet, aging, frail old Black lady, looked at him, looked at me, and looked at him, and looked at me again, and said, "What should I do?"

What he wanted to do was surgery that night. He was white, we were all Black, and my in-law relative was from New York, with good Medicare insurance in this small-town hospital in the backwater part of the South.

I knew she would need casting and surgery, a long time for recovery, and pain management. I also distrusted his motives, fearing that he saw easy, quick payment and a patient who would soon be gone. I saw a place that had no real trauma level, that was not well staffed, and had uncertain infection control policies. My in-law relative would be abandoned here at the mercy of the South. We respectfully declined surgery, got the arm casted, and made certain she was on the plane back to a New York Orthopedist the next day.

The next day, we had a chance to tour the family graveyard and other local sites. After that, Mom took it upon herself to make a collection of the family ancestry and did a prodigious amount of work tracing who married whom and where people came from.

On the way home, Warren and my mother were busy discussing retirement. That had never been on their radar until two things occurred. The first thing was attending the family reunion, and the second was that Warren had a heart attack.

When it happened, I was practicing in Greenville, Michigan (from 1988 to 1997), when I got a phone call from my mother that Warren was in the hospital in Flint, Michigan, and was going to have a heart procedure that day. It was summer of 1996.

Could I come? Of course, I could! I cancelled my office visits for the rest of the day and drove like a bat out of Hell to get there. I was so thankful that patients understood my needs and were willing to wait for me to return. And I was so thankful for my staff who helped my covering physicians take care of business for me.

I drove to the hospital in Flint and arrived just after Warren had his heart catheterization. I am not sure if he had a stent placed, but he was decidedly better.

Mom devoted her days to his care and was his advocate for all health-related actions. She made sure he never saw another molecule of cholesterol, and that he took his coumadin blood thinner like clockwork.

She made sure he had a low/no cholesterol, no/low fat, low calorie, high fiber, vitamin enriched diet, with regular trips to the cardiac rehabilitation center. She set his watch with a timer to alarm him when it was time to take his medicine.

One of the things Warren did for me as a young person was teach me to play golf. He gave me a driver, a 5-iron, and a putter, and we went to the public link in Detroit.

He said, "When you are good, those are the only clubs you need. When you are bad, those are the only clubs you can handle."

I loved the game, and he and I made sure that at least once a year, the two of us would have a Daddy-Daughter summer game.

After his heart attack, I made sure I had a chance to play golf with him, just the two of us on the course. I recall we made the turn at nine, and he got a call from June on the cellular, reminding him to take his heart pill. I watched as he pulled a cylindrical container on a chain from underneath his golf shirt, popped open the top, and took his coumadin. I asked where he had gotten the container, and he said June had found it in one of the houses he managed for the VA (Veterans Affairs).

I laughed and asked him if he knew what it was. He said no, and I said it was a coke tube, usually owned by big-time drug dealers. Dealers would wear the item as a piece of jewelry, and it was designed to hold a line of cocaine!

"People are going to get the wrong opinion of you!" I told him.

"In the neighborhoods where I have houses that I manage," he said, "that would not be all bad, and people might give me more respect and privacy!"

I have no idea if my mom knew what it was, but Warren loved it once he knew, and I am sure he loved June all the more for giving it to him. How fun he was!

After Warren's heart attack in 1996, he and Mom decided that it was time to launch into true retirement. They had probably planned to work forever. Warren's hobby was golf, and June's hobby was Warren. They were completely self-contained as a couple, and would have been happy to carry on like that forever. But the health scare changed their trajectory.

Warren was the first Black real estate broker to ever get a VA contract to manage its properties in Detroit. He hired people to fix up the homes for rent or sale. The work kept him so busy, he did not do any other real estate brokering work. Over time, he accumulated a large number of properties that he was managing as the broker for the VA housing agency in Detroit. After the heart attack, he had to unload 150 properties in less than a year. They managed to do that fairly rapidly, and they sold the G2 Ranch in Holly, Michigan, and bought a place in Tazewell, Virginia, near the Garner family origins.

The place was solid. It was a well-built, two-bedroom brick ranch with a finished basement and a parking ramada in a good part of town. June loved Warren so much, she gave up her work life to be with him.

She and Warren moved there and settled in. Because they had money and a large family, they were rapidly assimilated into the community. They found a church to attend and were doing great. During the family reunion, I had a chance to play golf with Warren at his new local course. He called it "goat hills," and it truly was. Each hole was a 30 degree slope up or down; remember we were playing in Appalachia, so there are lots of hills. But never mind the hills. We had fun as usual.

One night in February 1997, he started having seizures, and June woke up to find him gurgling and choking. He died in bed before the 911 ambulance picked him up. He had suffered another heart attack and died during that seizure. He was buried with his family in Tazewell, Virginia.

## DIGRESSION #5: THE BIOPHYSICAL BASIS FOR OMT WILL BE IDENTIFIED, QUANTIFIED, AND APPLIED

One of the main reasons I became a DO and not an MD was because DO doctors were given training in OMT, Osteopathic Manipulative Therapy—which is now called OMM, or Osteopathic Manual Medicine. It means we are trained to place our hands on you to make a structural diagnosis, and then using our hands, fix what is wrong. Those things can be simple, such as TMJ pain; complex, such as vertigo; and common, such as post-partum pain or post-operative pain.

Our Founder, Andrew Taylor Still, was an MD in the Union Army during the Civil War, and the son of a Methodist minister. He had God and medicine coursing through him all his life. He was very, very observant of life around him, and decided that the current medical therapies of the day—surgery, opium, and alcohol—were useless for treating the real maladies that he encountered.

Today we are just barely better. We still have surgery. We also have chemotherapy, which should rightly be called poison control; we have immunotherapy, which is on the right path toward letting the body fix the body; and we have pharmacology, which is more poison control. If you read the PDR—the *Physician's Desk Reference* of drugs—you will see, under the section "Method of Action," many of those sections begin with, "While the exact mechanism of action is unknown, it is currently thought that . . . " This means they haven't got a piss-pot of an idea of how the stuff actually does what it does, but they know it won't kill you, and that is good enough for the FDA to let them sell it.

I applaud the industry for all the good that it has done, but it still does not know what the fuck it is doing to most of us, most of the time. The list of side effects for most drugs is more frightening than the actual disease itself. A.T. Still understood this.

He also encountered lots of distrust, misfortune, opposition, and social isolation because of his medical belief. He was even thrown out of his church because he was laying on hands to cure people as if he were Jesus Christ, or so they accused him.

But he persevered. He said the "rule of the artery is supreme," and he meant that if a tissue does not have adequate blood supply, then it will generate pain, begin to malfunction, or die. He was right. He said the treatment we give with our hands is designed to restore that flow of blood.

He was popular with patients, opposed by the MDs of the day, and had his ideas stolen from him by the founder of the Palmer College of Chiropractic, John Palmer. But people like me, who read about him and experienced treatment by his students, really do understand how much he was correct in his observations and philosophy.

The problem is that, even as I write this, most folks outside of the DO profession have no idea how what we do with our hands works. They do not believe it will work unless they have experienced it themselves. I get tired of seeing articles talking about low back pain and how manipulation is useless. All of these articles are written by people who are not DOs, have not had OMM given to them, or seen it, done or listened to the hundreds and thousands of low back pain patients who have had recovery by the application of OMM.

The other problem is that we DOs do not yet really have a true scientific basis to explain how it works either. There is a need for rigorous science that explains why pain goes away when blood flow is restored to tissue that has been devoid of circulation for a short term, or only has had limited flow for a long period of time.

I think there may be an answer in the realm of tissue signaling. Meaning there are some substances, which we cannot yet identify, that are released by the application of OMM that travel through the body, triggering responses in the neurologic, hematologic, musculoskeletal, and lymphatic systems that interconnect all four of these systems and make pain go away.

It is not only the removal of pain that OMM addresses. Restoration of nasal function for people with sinus infections or allergy-sufferers is a known application of OMM. Treatment of uncomplicated pneumonia, bronchitis, and ear infection in infants are known applications of OMM. Treatment to restore cardiac function after cardiac surgery is a known application of OMM. The list goes on as the research goes on.

If tissue signaling is a valid pathway, I hope it becomes a research goal.

How we find it, I do not know, because I am not that researcher. When we might find it, I do not know, because those researchers have not yet started this journey. But if it is found, my profession will rise up to the top of the heap in the field of medicine, and all MDs will want to become DOs. Or at least they should be so lucky.

WE'RE BACK . . .

**June the Widow**

Now June is a widow. But she is still June. Loud, proud, and needing to be in charge. She barged into the life of the Tazewell Black church community with her Northern ways, her flashy expensive clothes and costume jewelry, and she was quickly shut out by the women of the church in a decisive and defensive way, like a top NFL cornerback shuts down a weak wide receiver. She left that church and found another one, run by a white minister and filled with white people. She also developed a friendship with two local white women, Miss J and Miss B (not their real names), both of whom attended that church.

She was getting monthly money via a land contract for the sale of the property in Holly, widow's social security payments, and whatever other income she may have had. By all definitions, $3,000 a month made her the equivalent of a millionaire in the back hills of Tazewell. She used her money to buy happiness and love from the church, and from Miss J and Miss B.

I have a nice recollection of Miss B. She helped my mom, and never asked for anything. My recollection of Miss J is that she was a leech.

Miss J was a person who hung on to Mom and "looked" after her. When we left Tazewell, on the day she was placed into rehabilitation, Miss J was a person with whom I could communicate, and someone I thought I could trust to take care of Mom's needs.

But Miss J had her own set of problems with a mother who was physically and mentally ill, and who kept wanting to move into some isolated shack away from everywhere and everyone, and just be there with Miss J. Miss J resisted that, and having June to take care of, gave Miss J an excuse to stay in town.

Miss J, however, was no angel. She was always in need of cash for one thing or another, or for one person or another. June was dependent on her, isolated, and probably frightened of her own disabilities. She was open-handed with Miss J, and never hesitated to give her a hundred dollars here or there whenever Miss J asked for it.

Around 2003, I decided that my mom could no longer live alone in Tazewell and that she needed to move in with us. "US" was Arney and me, and soon to be Ophelia.

The only way to get Mom from there to us in Prairie du Chien, Wisconsin was to charter a private plane and fly her in. There is no airport in Tazewell, and the airport near our home could only handle small propeller planes.

Veronica and her husband helped a lot with ideas and support of all kinds. We sold off a lot of Warren's left-over equipment and June's household items, and donated as much as we could to whoever needed it. Then we got her on the plane and flew her to Wisconsin.

Miss J was not dismayed or dissuaded from seeking ready cash just because June was 700 miles away. She would call June with a sad story, and one of the most popular ones was that a cousin had just died, and could June send some money to help with the funeral?

It seemed that this went on every two to three months. June never failed to respond with cash or a check in the mail. I figured that Miss J had either: one, a family large enough to fill a basketball stadium, and they were all in such ill health that they were dying off like flies; or two, she was just lying to bilk my mother out of money. I went with option two.

One day, she sent a letter with a note about an uncle who had recently passed away. I never let June see that letter. Instead, I sent a note that said, "My mom is in reduced circumstances now and sends you her love and condolences, but she has no more money to give for your ill and dying relatives now, or in the future. God bless you."

I never heard from Miss J again. Mission accomplished.

June must have been terribly lonely, unfulfilled, bored, and depressed. The last time she was in good enough health to visit was during the summer of 2001, when she came to visit me in Prairie du Chien, Wisconsin. She had a most unusual condition that took her down, and it started during the week of 9/11 that year.

Two days before the airplanes crashed into the twin towers in New York City on September 11th, 2001, she was admitted to the hospital in Tazewell with a strange elevation of her CPK. This is a muscle enzyme that is released when there is damage to the heart, or when there is a connective tissue disorder that causes skeletal muscles to self-destruct. The country doctors treated her for a heart attack, but when her CPK numbers did not come down and her EKGs remained normal, they were at a loss for what was wrong with her.

I literally called and talked with the internist and discussed her case, and suggested he consider a connective tissue disorder. It turned out to be dermatomyositis, a rare disease-causing skin rash and muscle weakness that pretty much incapacitated her. They put her on high-dose steroids, and she lost total control of most of her musculature due to the disease and the long-term steroids. She was bedridden, incontinent, and alone.

She needed to be in rehabilitation. Arney and I were living in Wisconsin. She called us and said they were sending her home on September 13th, and we needed to come help her. Because Warren's family had ostracized her, she had no one locally willing to help.

Arney and I had to drive, because no planes were allowed to fly for days after the attack. We drove from Prairie du Chien to Tazewell, Virginia in 36 hours, and arrived at her house in the dead of night.

On our way there, we made it to Chicago by the evening of the first day of our trip and booked a room not too far from O'Hare airport. The night was so eerily quiet because there were no planes in the air. The highway was dark and quiet, because no one was going to or coming from the airport. It was truly spooky.

The next morning, we drove down to Kentucky, and rode across that state. I marveled at the enveloping, copious loops and drapes of kudzu on the trees, and the unnatural green canopy that kudzu made in the forest and over the roads.

In the late evening, about one hour away from June's house, we approached a strange greenish-yellow light that was low, lying on the side of the highway, and as we got close enough to see, it was the opening to a coal mine. They had constructed a dome over the mine's entryway and lit it so that workers could come in and out, to keep the mine open for 24 hours. It was something that reminded me of *The Twilight Zone* TV show, because of its unearthly appearance. Those who go down into mines are incredibly brave.

It was around 1 AM when we got to her house and knocked on the door. There was no answer, but the door was open, so we went in. She was in a hospital bed, in adult diapers, soaked in urine. I cried to see my mother in such a weakened condition, but I realized that tears were not going to help. We let her know we were here and we bunked down in the basement.

The next day we got up and got going on what to do with her. We got the place inventoried, gathered everything that was valuable, and made phone calls to her treating physicians. We set up home nursing visits until she could be taken to rehabilitation, and we cleaned her up, and her place, too.

Miss J and Miss B were a lot of help and provided information to help me locate a rehab center. I placed her in it, and Arney and I drove back home. June stayed in rehab for a month and returned home, still weak and needing assistance with all her Activities of Daily Living (ADLs). She found a helper who did a pretty good job, and only stole a small portion of money from her.

But I knew that June could not exist on her own, alone in that condition, in that town. I marshalled the family and we found a way to fly her to Wisconsin, put her house up for sale, and moved her personal items to the assisted living facility in Prairie du Chien, and started her new life.

She was a totally different person.

No longer sunny and happy, she was despondent, depressed, by turns angry or demanding. She had developed a borderline personality disorder, and her dermatomyositis was part of her CREST syndrome. Calcinosis, Raynaud's, Esophageal dysmotility, Sclerodactyly, and Telangiectasias. In plain words, calcium deposits in the skin, spasms of arteries in response to cold, difficulty swallowing, tightening of the skin in the hands and fingers, and dilated small blood vessels on the surface of the skin. In addition, she had heart disease, diabetes, hypertension and much more.

Her life was miserable; she was 85 percent chair-bound, and totally dependent on others for care. She became a mistress of manipulation—lying, demanding and causing pain in the lives of others for her own entertainment. She was also incontinent of urine, and due to the chronic problem with skin breakdown and the danger of bedsores, she agreed to see a urologist who recommended placement of an indwelling catheter. What a relief it was to her and to my peace of mind when they inserted it. Nurses came every three weeks to change the catheter, and Medicare covered it!

We first lived in Wisconsin, and I placed Mom in a senior living facility/assisted living place close to the hospital. She was just a short walk away from where I lived. We tried to visit every other day, and Arney was so helpful with getting her TV and other electronic gear set up. She quickly figured out how to disable her computer so that he would have to come over and "fix" it. Attention is what she craved, and manipulation was how she got it.

I found employment back in Michigan at Michigan State University in 2006, and moved everybody with me. At the time, Ophelia, Arney, and June were all in Wisconsin, so we needed a multi-faceted plan. I wanted a house big enough for each of us to have our own bedrooms, plus room for an office, and a large garden. Eventually, I realized that June would be best located in an assisted living facility, so we adjusted the plan to locate a place for her.

We found one in East Lansing—an excellent, high quality, large, well-maintained facility—and put her there. The three of us moved to Okemos, Michigan, because it was close to the university where I was now working.

June began to follow a decidedly downward spiral. She consistently called us to complain about one or another of the workers who took care of her in the facility. She also called to complain about various items that were on the fritz or broken in some fashion—TV, radio, adjustable bed—always something. It turned out that she was sabotaging the items and lying about the behavior of the people who were caring for her.

She insisted on moving to her own apartment, and so we did as she wanted.

Once she got to her own apartment, she insisted on having a scooter. She saw those ads on TV and was hellbent for leather to have one. She wanted a candy apple red model, and there was nothing else that would do. I realized that she could actually walk, and that if she would do any kind of physical therapy, she would maintain mobility and better health over time, but she was adamant about wanting a scooter. I took her to the medical supply store to let her try a scooter. She could barely get into the seat and needed help to get out. That demonstration of her own inability to use the scooter convinced her that we should scotch that plan.

I decided that she could have a power wheelchair, and I found out that the aftermarket for used power vehicles was huge.

People who do not walk, do not live as long as those who do. That is a fact. So, all those folks who bought scooters were actually shortening their lives, and the scooters were going to the used market. They are remarkably well-built and, because the majority of them are used indoors, they last a long time. I found a used power wheelchair, and she was actually quite happy with it.

Even with the power wheel chair, she required daily in-home help because she was on her own, no longer in the assisted living facility. I must have gone through a half dozen in-home helpers, each one more docile than the previous one, and each one castigated and verbally punished more violently by June for some made up or imagined insult or incompetency, all of which were factitious. June lied about them and was absolutely horrible to care for.

Due to other circumstances, I got another job in 2007 in South Haven, Michigan, and decided to take June with me, while leaving Arney and Ophelia to fend for themselves in the house in Okemos. Suffice it to say that I was truly distressed due to being in a home with people who were needy. More on them and me later.

I bought a house in South Haven on Compton Avenue, and placed June in an Adult Foster Care home that was run by Grace, the aunt of a lady who later became my medical assistant in the office where I worked in Covert, Michigan.

I remember preparing to give Grace a list of June's diagnosis, but I heard her say that she could handle most anything, except people who had borderline personality disorder. I quickly edited that list and gave her another one without that diagnosis on it. As time went on, it became obvious that June was going downhill mentally, physically, and emotionally. She and I discussed guardianship, so I filed to become her guardian, which gave me the ability to make decisions for her and stave off a lot of problems that would have occurred with those who were caring for her. But true to her now-bad personality, June decided to sue me for being a bad guardian. She found a friend in Detroit, a former judge, who hooked her up with a lady lawyer, who told me what June planned for me in the suit.

I spent a lot of time with June's attorney and, finally, we reached an understanding after the lawyer met with June in the AFC facility, and had a chance to hear from the owner of the AFC and the other residents. The case went away. I remained guardian. I really was ready to stop being guardian and let June go her own way. That is how burned out I was with my sicko mom's mental health circus.

I came over to the group home and had a private session with my mom, as they say, A Come to Jesus Meeting. I told her I would resign as guardian and never see her again if her lawsuit against me persisted.

I told her she would be responsible for paying her bills and handling her life all on her own. She would have to get her own medications delivered, handle her accounting, and arrange transportation back and forth to doctors and clinics. Somewhere in the back of June's rational mind, the light broke through and she decided that it was OK for me to continue as guardian.

Nonetheless, June continued her bad behavior and was eventually kicked out of the AFC home.

I found an apartment for her and, again, hired in-home helpers to come by each day. Plus, I got smart and had a home health agency send aides and nurses on a regular basis.

She declined physically and ended up in the hospital with severe heart failure. She was so weak and incapacitated, she thought she was going to die. She had signed papers, as part of the guardianship, which allowed me to also make her medical decisions. From the hospital, she was transferred to the extended care facility.

Those places never have been, are not now, and never will be well-run as long as mentally and physically helpless people depend on poorly trained, poorly paid, poorly motivated, poorly educated, disempowered women for care. They did the best they could with what they had, and I was forced to put my mom into their care.

She hated the place, I am sure. I tried to make her life better. She wanted a garden, so I found a carpenter who constructed a raised garden bed that was wheelchair height. She never used it. I visited her three times a week. She never said thanks or gave any sign that she was glad to see me.

One day, I got a call on a Sunday from the facility saying that she had suffered a stroke. I came over and saw her, and she was now unable to speak, where previously she had just refused to speak to me. I felt so sad, but also so angry at the same time. Shame on me.

## DIGRESSION #6: THE AI NURSE-BOT IS COMING

My friend Anita, who is now deceased, was one of the best bridge players I have met. She and her husband Ron were a great couple at the bridge table. She was the master player, he was the student player, and they were a delightful couple. He died early in 2017, and she carried on with the pieces of her life, but still played bridge. I think it was all she had because they had no children and no younger relatives.

One month, we bridge players at the Senior Center remarked to each other that we had not seen Anita for a while. We found out that she was in rehabilitation after a slip and fall accident in a mall store during which she sustained a fractured femur. She was going to be laid up for eight weeks.

Two of my lady bridge player friends and I met at the rehab facility to play bridge with Anita on Labor Day in 2019. We had nothing else to do, and she was certainly available for a game. She was confined to a wheelchair and required attendance to transfer because she was not allowed to put any weight on her newly pinned right femur.

Between deals, she raised her hand to get the attention from a group of three workers sitting at a table by the hallway. She needed to go to the bathroom. We knew we were not allowed to help her with that, so we waited for the attendants to come over.

All three of them turned their backs, two stood up and moved into the hallway, while one remained at the table focused on her phone. Time passed. I finally got up and walked over to the group and asked them if they could help Anita.

One of them said to me, rather sharply, "We know. We are going on a shift change now. We'll get to her."

This was getting me pissed off. Anita was white; the attendants were all Black. So, maybe it was reverse racism. I did not care; it was wrong, whatever the fuck it was.

I walked back to Anita, took out my cell phone, and turned on the camera. The attendants must have seen the camera come out, because one of them came over and began to wheel Anita to the bathroom. As Anita was being rolled out, I walked beside her and recorded her on my phone, and said we would wait to deal the hand until she returned. I went back to my seat.

She was wheeled back, and we resumed our game. About five minutes later, two white male supervisors showed up, and asked me to step into the hallway with them. One of them told me that there was a policy that prevented any photography of staff in the facility. I asked where that was posted so that a visitor would know and see it. They had no answer for that. I told them I had deleted the video anyway and went back to my game.

All the workers, except for one, were youngish, Black, and women. These jobs are dead-end, low-pay, boring, physically demanding, bereft of training, and not at all appreciated by the supervisors who are uniformly older, male, and white. Nor do the families of the patients, or those patients who are demented, understand the onerous burden of working in these places.

This is the perfect storm leading to the automation of extended care facilities. I have read reports about how nursing home aides are overworked and underpaid in understaffed facilities amidst conditions that put them at high risk for work-related injuries that disable them from working at all. They are also mostly women. They are not unionized, not recognized, and not promoted or trained. In 2022, the turnover rate for CNAs (Certified Nursing Assistants) was 54.8 percent[1] nationwide.

Those facilities that employ special lifting units have the lowest work-related injury rates, and the highest worker retention rates. Seems to me that it is time to take advantage of technology.

There are robotic devices in factories, in offices, in warehouses, on garbage trucks, in your living room, and in so many parts of our lives. Why not bring robotics to the bedside, in not only nursing homes, but also as home health aides, and in hospitals, as well?

Robotic aides can be monitored by a human overseer. They can be programmed to deliver medications, water, and food, and assist with bathing, toileting, and walking. They can be programmed to provide turning to prevent bedsores. They can stand at a bedside and prevent falls. They can provide restraint for the agitated patient without harm to a human who would have to provide restraint. They can be fitted with entertainment and interactive capabilities, to engage the person in their care on a PRN basis.

Imagine a facility where each person has a robotic attendant, available 24/7. The AI Nurse-Bots will provide water to drink, nebulizer treatments for the COPD patient, oxygen for the emphysematous, insulin for the diabetic. They could check blood sugars, oxygen levels, heart rates, blood pressures, and respirations. The AI Nurse-Bot will provide transportation, monitor vitals, provide entertainment, and serve as a communication link with the human directors.

The specialized heavy duty AI Nurse-Bot will lift patients who need to transfer from bed to chair, chair to toilet, and back again, so that a human will never have a work-related back injury. Medications will be programed into the AI Nurse-Bot and dispensed to the patient on time, on schedule, in the right amount. Only those patients who cannot cooperate with the AI NB will need a human to administer meds. The patients will get turned so that bedsores do not happen, get toileted so that UTIs do not occur, and get monitored so that health emergencies are prevented, or at least reduced.

The AI Nurse-Bot can monitor a single lead EKG strip, oxygen levels, respirations, and temperatures of sleeping patients, as well as provide alerts when any of those values become problematic. The AI Nurse-Bot can assist the patient with ambulation on any level surface.

The device can hold a pair of headphones that connect with all libraries, so that a patient can access audiobooks or music files from hundreds of streaming services, or hear a message broadcast to the entire facility from the staff, or a private message from a human attendant specifically for that one patient. It can be fitted with a Virtual Reality (VR) headset so that the patient can also have video experiences, including movies, television, virtual museum tours, games, and more.

If the patient is a fall risk, the bed is placed on hydraulics. At night, the bed is lowered to floor-level, and the AI Nurse-Bot is stationed by the bed, ready to raise it up, so the patient can get up and out of the bed with a simple grasp of the handle on the AI Nurse-Bot for stability, and be able to walk. There is a Bluetooth connection, so that each patient has a dedicated AI Nurse-Bot who is coded to the identification band on the patient's wrist. The AI Bot has a powerful LED light source, for use in the dark. The AI Bot is able to dial 911 if the parameters for vitals fall into a critical and dangerous range.

There are video cameras all through the facility, so that the staff monitoring the activity has full visualization of all patients and their attendant AI Nurse-Bots.

One human director for each section of the extended care unit can be in charge of up to 10 AI Nurse-Bots. Each AI Nurse-Bot can be programed to manage five patients. A well-designed extended care facility can have 200 patients, 40 AI Nurse-Bots, and four human directors per shift. There could even be four, six-hour shifts a day, and savings would still be realized, because a facility would drop from 80 to 100 employees in a 24-hour day to 16 to 20. It might be possible to let some employees work from home.

Yes, the initial cost to purchase the AI Nurse-Bot staff will be huge, but the cost savings will gradually catch up so that facilities will operate with fewer and fewer human employees.

Someone has to make the robotic unit, and make it adaptable to the nursing home environment, as well as flexible enough for the private home environment. The engineering, programing, and medical monitoring functions will be a tremendous hurdle. But once these are overcome, then they will find their market.

If the average pay currently in Ohio for a nursing home aide is $13.50 per hour—round up to $14 and a full-time, 40-hour week—it would add up to a yearly cost of a little over $26,000. Be generous and call it $30,000 a year, without benefits, for a full-time employee. The Robotic Home Health Aide might cost $150,000, which is the cost of five full-time aides. In two years, the owner has made back that amount because there are five less people to hire and pay for the work that the Robotic Home Health Aide will be doing.

The AI Nurse-Bot works 24/7, perfectly according to whoever writes the program. Each program is individualized for each patient's needs. The savings in salaries, benefits, time off, injuries, mistakes, policy breeches, and medication errors, not to mention the elimination of human interactions of a negative nature—arguments, fights, sexual entanglements on the job, harassment, etc.—will make the AI Nurse-Bot the preferred method of care.

The AI Nurse-Bot will move out of the extended care facilities and move into the home-based care arena in a short time. Conceivably, the transition may actually begin in the home-care field and move to the extended care facilities. The point is the AI Nurse-Bot is on the horizon.

Robots already build the majority of automobiles and have replaced thousands of workers in those factories. Robots work in industries and factories, and are now replacing unskilled labor, and the trend is relentless and growing. AI portfolio managers now are invading Wall Street. Computers using AI programs are already in your house in the form of Alexa, on your phone in the form of Siri, and everywhere in between.

Look at the benefits to the patient. No fear of neglect or incompetence at the hands of emotionally overwhelmed, physically exhausted people taking care of you. No one will molest you, give you the wrong drug at the wrong time, give you a bad attitude, or just fail to show up when you have a need.

"But," you say, "where is the human touch?"

The human touch is infrequently provided in nursing homes now, and there is limited time when it is provided. Human touch can be provided when there is increased opportunity for true interaction with other staff consisting of people in the nursing homes who are relieved of routine assignments by the AI Nurse-Bot.

Properly designed and arranged facilities can have a huge central common gathering area with functions in multiple domains—dining, games, visual presentations, sing-alongs, parties, family visits, Wii bowling, pet therapy, crafts, and even outdoor activities can be part of the interaction.

It takes so much time to just complete care on one person by one human Home Health Agency (HHA) that there is scant time for interaction. The aides will tell you they do not have time to sit and chat with their patients, because they are constantly running from one room to the next, trying to keep up with the demand of the pace of work.

Look at the benefits to the owners of home health facilities. There is no need to do background checks, drug screenings, or on-boarding trainings. The RHHA needs a power source and a human monitor/operator, plus a hardware, software, and mechanical team. Costs for workers compensation insurance go way down. Drug diversion is reduced, if for no other reason than the numbers of humans on site are reduced. The RHHA will show up sober on time every day, with no need for lunch time, break time, smoke time, pee time, union meetings, personal days, sick days, vacation days, benefits of any kind. There is no need for employee chart keeping, reprimands, warnings, and performance reviews. Your HR department shrinks along with its budget.

Imagine you have a senior relative at home, perhaps living with you, or perhaps alone. How nice to know there is the robotic aide who can provide auditory and visual monitoring, take a temperature, blood pressure, heart rate, single lead EKG strip, $O^2$ sat reading, weight, respiratory rate. The robotic unit can get your relative up to the toilet without fear of a slip and fall, day or night. The unit stands guard at night for not only medical situations, but also for intruders into the home with a built-in 911 call feature. The unit also has an AED function and a sleep apnea monitor, with ability to provide oxygen and nebulized aerosol treatments for those with respiratory impairments.

All these pieces exist now in small enough packages that individuals can afford them. Home sleep studies are very complex investigations that incorporate $O^2$ levels, EEG, EKG, and video recordings. If we can do complexity like that of a sleep study, then I think we are not that far away from a Robotic HHA.

As usual, the wealthy will obtain this functionality first, but once the engineering and development tools become more sophisticated, the price to produce the devices will come down and the demand will climb. We are all aging—our cities, states, nations, worldwide—at home, in nursing homes, and just about everywhere. This robotic feature will provide safety and comfort for patients, while reducing the injury that occurs to those who work in the home health and nursing home industry.

Again, let us not forget, here is a workforce composed mostly of women, who are exploited, underpaid, and tossed aside if they are damaged. The robotic home health aide is a liberating piece of feminist power if used properly.

If there is money to be made by developing an AI Nurse-Bot, and money to be saved by using an AI Nurse Bot, then it will happen, and it will happen in America.

WE'RE BACK . . .

**June Dies**

I visited my mom and tried to apologize for any of the harsh words that we spoke to each other. She just looked at me and never said a word. I got the silent treatment day after day. Eventually she died on Tuesday the 13th of September, 2011, a few weeks after being admitted there. I donated her body to MSU's Anatomy Department, where she served for three years teaching anatomy to medical students.

For all of those three years, I thought I hated her.

I never spoke about her until after I attended an Al-Anon meeting and heard a speaker who reached the spot in my heart that had become a lump of emotionless, brittle obsidian, and changed it into warm love for my mother, and also, amazingly enough, for my dad, Max Brown.

I realized that they were unschooled in the art and science of child-raising, that both of them were beaten and damaged by, not only their family, but also by society and racism in America, and lived in fear and privation all the days of their lives, either in fact or in the recesses of fear in their minds. The fact that they had me and gave me whatever love they had was what I needed to focus on and celebrate and cherish.

After that moment, I was able to reconcile with my mom.

And after that, any time I went to East Lansing, I would take a moment to visit her memorial gravesite at East Lawn Memorial Gardens in Okemos.

I recall the day that the MSU Anatomy Department held its memorial service for all those who were donated to the anatomy lab. I was there with my good friend, Alice Raynesfield Shanaver, DO, who was also my classmate at MSUCOM. The service was unremarkable, but moving in its sincere simplicity. The speakers were all current medical students from both the MD and DO programs. I was moved to tears and thankful that Alice was there to comfort me.

That was the day of reconciliation with June, who remains my mom and best friend. Trust me when I say that I still speak to my mother on a regular basis in my own special way. I make sure she knows what you two have accomplished, and how you are progressing in this life in these times. She is pleased with you both.

## DIGRESSION #7: MEDICARE FOR ALL

It is 2020, and there will be an election in November, as I write this, when Donald Trump will face Joe Biden.

Mr. Biden has a plan for health care, as did all the democratic candidates. The one that most people seemed to like was the one that stated Medicare for All. That was actually one of the main platform planks in the Bernie Sanders 2016 campaign, and in 2020, all the other candidates co-opted pieces of it.

It is a good idea and it is a bad idea at the same time.

Medicare for All would be run by the same government that gave you the personal income tax by way of an amendment to the Constitution, a military budget that dwarfs the GDP of a dozen nations, and the failed anti-communist policy known as The War in Vietnam. They run Medicare now as if they are blind billionaires who completely trust the seeing eye dog that begs for bacon every day, but poops in their shoes every night.

They have devised a system of payment that rewards waiting to fix what is broken, and ignores preventing things/people from becoming broken. Doing something to a patient—like an imaging study, surgery, or invasive procedure—pays so much more than spending time talking, counseling, and advising people on how to stop doing the things that are killing them. The Center for Medicare and Medicaid Services is one of the largest bureaucracies in the government, and it only handles some of us now. Imagine how large it would grow if it had to expand to serve us all.

That would be a bad thing.

Once everyone is covered by Medicare for All, Medicaid will go away. That could be good for state governments who have to run and administer the program, but it would be bad for all the people who work in that field. Where do they go and what do they do? My suggestion is to make them the advocates for people who cannot handle the digital requirements and other tasks necessary to interface with government health care. Keeping them employed is important to us all.

This might be a good thing.

Once everyone is covered by Medicare for All, private health insurance will shrink. No employer will want to keep private insurance for his employees when there is Medicare waiting for everybody. The cost savings would be huge. Maybe employers would keep private health care for just top people as an inducement to get the best employees for key positions.

I am not sure if that is good or bad, so I am not going to make any ethical judgements on it; I will only say it will probably happen.

Once we have Medicare for All, there must be some adjustment for the Indigenous peoples who live on the reservations. They should be eligible for this if they are not living on their own lands. As long as they are on their own lands, they are covered by their own "Indigenous Nations Insurance," but even that is tangled up now with Medicaid, so it is a mess. How that would change with Medicare for All is hard to imagine, but I think it could be worse than it is now.

That would be bad for Indigenous peoples.

Once we have Medicare for All, prisons will have to consider how best to provide care under new payment rules. The privatization of prisons has made health care a lower-ranked budget item than food in prisons. But if Medicare for All applies to incarcerated people, then they have what you and I would have for services and care, because the payment model is the same. Prison health care costs are sent to the federal government known as Uncle Open Hands Deep Pockets, instead of money requested from a state's limited budget channeled to a for-profit company.

This might be a good thing.

Once we have Medicare for All, how does that impact the VA? The VA is like the Borg ship on the television show, *Star Trek Next Generation*; impossible to escape from it, totally incomprehensible, magnificently huge and powerful beyond belief. Resistance is futile with the VA. The VA will not go away.

That is good and bad.

Once we have Medicare for All, would it cover situations like my mother's stay in the extended care facility? At that time, Medicare paid for 100 days of care, then she had to go on Medicaid for payment of the rest of the bills. People who go into extended care facility nursing homes must divest themselves of all wealth or possessions, generally speaking, so that they can prove they are too poor to pay for their care themselves. Then, the state picks up the tab till they die. Will Medicare for All do that?

If they did, the cost would be huge and that would be a bad thing.

Mostly I am happy that I do not have to solve this problem. Most of the remainder of the civilized world laughs at, and alternatively, pities us because we lack any kind of national health system that includes everyone. Those socialized nations pay a smaller portion of their budget for health care than we do, and they get better return on their investment by way of lower rates of maternal infant mortality, longer life span, and lower prison incarceration, because drug use is treated not punished, and on, and on, and on.

We need smart minds from all parts of our nation to solve this problem. Researchers, clinicians, policy experts, patients, and all segments of U.S. life need to meet at some giant round table and come up with a solution. Certainly, I do not trust politicians to fix it. Do you?

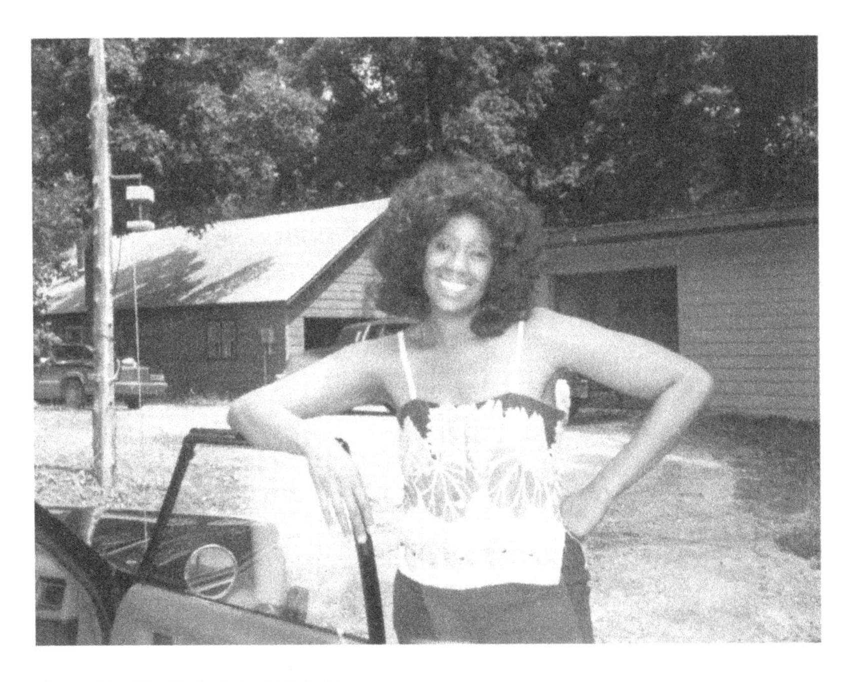

# SECTION TWO
# MY PAST: SOME OFF-THE-TRACK-OF-TIME INTERMINGLED MEMORIES AND MOMENTS

**I Revisit the East Side of Detroit**

In October of 2017, I had an opportunity to revisit all those places of my childhood.

I was hired by Michigan State University on September 1st, 2017, as a clinical faculty member to substitute for Derrick Williamson, DO. Dr. Williamson was the program director of the family medicine residency run by MSUCOM, and the Detroit Wayne County Health Authority Graduate Medical Education program. The clinic on 10809 Mack Avenue was started by Michael Popoff, DO, who was an MSU alumnus and long-time east-sider. He treated the residents who were originally from Poland and Russia, and continued to provide great care, even as the neighborhood changed demographically to Black people from the South.

After he died, his wife donated the MSUCOM building, and it was turned into a training facility for family medicine residents. The Dean, William Strampel, DO, told me that originally the plan was to sell the building and create a scholarship in Dr. Popoff's name, but his wife pressed to have the clinic remain open to continue serving the people there. The Dean said he thought it would be a good idea, and got immediate approval from Lou Anna Simon, president of MSU.

Initially, the Dean thought it would be easy to just paint, clean, and fix up, but he found out that the building was previously a dry cleaning shop and, as such, had to get cleared by the Environmental Protection Agency for chemical toxic waste. Sure enough, there was plenty of toxic material in the soil and the Dean said the clean-up was like the Tom Hanks movie, *The Money Pit*—over budget and nowhere near on time, but eventually they got it done and opened it up in January 2017. I spent my first week there from October 8th to the 13th in 2017 getting to know the residents, the patients, the Athena EHR (the electronic health record medical software that manages patients' information and billing), and the office staff. I also got a chance to visit my old homes on Fischer and Trowbridge.

Understand that the east side was always the poor side of town, but it was intact and had business and commerce along Mack Avenue. Real neighborhoods existed, and culturally and racially-mixed people of all kinds were living together very well when I was a child.

As a mature 70-ish person, it was shocking to see what had transpired in the area. Houses were gone in large swatches of land. Sometimes an entire city block had been razed by the city due to decay and drugs, so these places were condemned. I drove by the Dom Polski Community Center on Warren each day going to work at the clinic. It stands alone surrounded by grassy, tree-dotted, weed-filled blocks. Every once in a while, a dilapidated house or two stands along Warren. Mack Avenue is a road of churches. There are a couple of gas stations, a school, a funeral home, a store that sells some groceries in between, a store called Liquor Lotto Beer, and a place called Dairy. Not sure if it is Dairy Queen, Dairy King, or dairy drag queen, because it is no longer a chain, but has been taken over by a local owner.

The churches are well-kept, enclosed with gates and fences, and in good repair. They seem to thrive in places where Black people are in the most jeopardy, languishing under brutal economic privation and institutional racism. They do not seem to be hurt, no matter how badly their parishioners are hurting. And there was no Catholic church. That would have been a saving grace for the area, but I am guessing that once the Polish and Russian ethnic communities' second and third generations disbanded and decamped to the white suburbs, there was no way to support a Catholic church.

There is not one national fast food chain outlet on Mack, from Woodward to Connor, except for a local chili dog place. There is not one active bar in the same stretch. If you don't have fast food places, taverns, or bars, then you have no working people with disposable income. If you have three dozen churches, then you have dreadful poverty. If you have destroyed housing, then you have a huge drug problem. That is what I think I saw that week.

My house on Fischer was gone, but replaced with a new structure that looked like Habitat for Humanity had been there. The

VFW Hall was gone. Spud's place is still an automotive shop of some kind, and Nichols Elementary remains active in Indian Village. Trowbridge, where my grandparents lived, is a scene of devastation; missing houses on the block where I lived mimic the missing teeth in a meth addict's mouth. The Utley and McGregor libraries on Woodward are boarded up. Stores, shops, and movie theaters that I recall visiting as a child are all gone and have not been replaced with any kind of commerce.

Detroit's leadership boasted that the city is making a comeback. That may be true, but only for the downtown area. Downtown is thriving, thanks to the sports stadiums, hotels, and government and financial activity.

There is the Wayne State University area, which is called Midtown, and the New Center Area at the site of the old General Motors headquarters building. The flashy shopping area along Woodward, from Piquette to the Boulevard, is filled with closed shops. It just gets worse as you go up Woodward. The public golf course is closed. Eight Mile—the rapper Eminem's old stomping ground—and Livernois is the zone for legal marijuana sales and activities, interspersed with hardy but struggling small businesses. The car dealers that used to be the hallmark of Livernois are gone. Once I crossed onto Eight Mile and headed west to Telegraph, commerce and residential improvement came on like gangbusters. There is just not any of this in Detroit, outside of a few protected zones.

## DIGRESSION #8: THE NEW FQHC

Many communities have a Federal Qualified Health Center which functions like a regular fee for services at doctors' offices, but are few and far between. They serve the Medicaid and uninsured population, and do a great job, but they are chronically understaffed and are few and far between.

How might they be better?

If medical graduates completing residency were given the option of working for a FQHC, with the attraction of loan forgiveness, guaranteed income, and great work-life balance, this could be a major boon for underinsured, or non-insured, and poor populations. These populations are not just in urban areas; they are in rural areas as well. So, this is a national option.

Here is how it might work for places like Mack Avenue, on the east side of Detroit, or Kinsman Avenue, on the east side of Cleveland, both areas filled with an economically underserved population.

Let us start with six family physicians, three OB/GYNs, three pediatricians, and two surgeons in each FQHC. These centers are open from 9 AM to 9 PM, seven days a week. Patients pay $1 per visit. I like to make sure that everyone has some skin in the game. Even if it is just nominal, it does represent payment for service. Each physician earns $100,000 a year, and has a year of loan forgiveness for each fully completed year of service in the FQHC. When all the loans are paid off, the physician has the option of remaining at a salary of $200,000 per year.

All patients' visits are either 30 minutes or 60 minutes. Physician's work schedule allows for each family doctor to have two, three, or four days off. Additionally, we will rotate the schedule so that night call is shared, and house calls and office days are rotated. Patients have access to a doctor in the clinic, a house call visit, or after hours care every day, and advice that is also video enabled.

The spectrum of primary care is covered by having family physicians, pediatricians, OB/GYNs, and general surgeons in the same space. Patients will have care for all age groups for 95 percent of non-emergent conditions.

The 2020 election chatter from the Democratic candidates and health care reform continues to revolve around our headlines and talk shows. Each of the 24 candidates had some take on health care. Keep it, junk it, change it, upgrade it. I think they were on the right track, but were clueless about what to do.

Whatever is done, there should be a plan to have multiple national demonstration projects to test all the cockamamie theories that are out there for testing. It would be horrible to scrap Medicaid, only to find out that millions of people are dying and suffering because of some administration misstep.

I certainly have my own theories. One that I like is to give each American a piece of the national health care expenditure federal budget. Apportion it all equally to each of us. Then require each person to spend their share as follows:

- A certain percentage must be spent on acquiring catastrophic care insurance premium. This lets the insurance companies compete for customers and allows patients to customize what they need for coverage.
- Another percentage must be put into a national patient compensation injury fund. This allows for compensation for injuries and reduces the need for trials to sue doctors who may or may not have caused an injury.
- Another percentage must be put into a health advocates fund. Advocates are hired to provide health services to those who cannot do so on their own—the mentally handicapped, homeless, orphans. Advocates may come from the ranks of social service workers who used to be in the Medicaid system.
- Another percentage is placed into the fund for national hospice.

But there is one remaining obligation/caveat about that spending, and that is each person must have a general yearly physical exam, and complete a list of age and gender specific screening tests. Also, each person must complete and update his/her personal health history form that is kept in a secure online, cloud-based storage system. Government provides the cloud storage; the patient keeps track of all the information. When the person is being seen by any health care provider, access to their information is allowed so the doctor, nurse, etc. can see what has transpired and can also add information to the "chart" for ongoing care.

We also allow a patient to order his/her own labs and X-rays, and schedule visits with any doctor anywhere, and have money to pay for the visit. Since doctors will be in large, corporate, self-owned groups, they will have their own labs and surgical centers to cut down costs. Hospitals function for high-level trauma and tertiary care services, and are paid by the person's catastrophic care policy.

The market for used medical equipment will open up once the government stops paying for durable medical equipment. Remember, lift chairs and the Scooter Store items were paid for by Medicaid. Fortunately, someone figured out that millions of federal dollars were being wasted on shiny new health toys for people who did not need them. Beds, wheelchairs, scooters, walkers, braces, all last as long as a good model car and, like a car, can be resold in the used item market.

I can practically hear money being saved by this! Affordable health care, available primary care, physicians not stressed by loan repayment, and patient choice.

WOW.

WE'RE BACK . . .

**Max Brown is Alive and I Finally Meet Him**

Max Brown was an interesting man who also happened to be a shucking jivester, and my biological father.

He met Mom, generated me, and was gone into the wind. He told her he was in the Navy, but he never was. He promised a lot and delivered nothing. He left her when I was three months old, in March 1945. He disappeared from my young life and remained absent during my married life. But we did reconnect years later.

I recall getting a phone call from him when Mom and I lived upstairs on Trowbridge. He called me to say hello; Mom thrust the phone into my hand and I heard him call me "little pudding." I had no idea of who he was. I never understood the reason for this call until after he died.

For years, as I grew up, I thought of him as being not only gone but also dead. My cousin Sydney Rivers Swann and I were fairly close in the late 1980s. She was the child of Bea Rivers, Max Brown's sister. I recall speaking with her in the winter holiday season of 1991-92, and I commented, "It's too bad that my dad is dead."

"He's not dead," she said. "He is alive and living in Detroit, in a retirement community on Woodward."

## DIGRESSION #9: WHY THE ELECTRONIC MEDICAL RECORD SUCKS

Anyone who has to use one will tell you the same thing: that it sucks. It is just a device to facilitate billing. Its creation was foisted on health care by people who used it for engineering and business activities. Somehow, they figured it would work just as well for health care as it did for accounting.

Certainly, there may have been good intention by the planners, but as usual, money got in the way, and those who were in charge of getting money (the insurance companies) teamed up with those who are in charge of paying money (the government) and they let this monster medical blob ooze all over medical life.

When the Affordable Health Care Act (Obamacare) was passed, the EMR was an integral part of its workings. Physicians were first promised a reward if they had one, then later threatened with punishment if they did not, by giving small amounts of reward money or imposing small withholdings of payment. Those withholdings increased over time for each unit of time that a physician failed to install an EMR that met government requirements.

The next step toward insanity was the decision to use the EMR to keep track of quality in health care. Various programs and formulas were devised for the EMR so that physicians had to click many buttons and make the document say certain things so that payment would occur, no fines would be imposed, and actuarial masters could determine if a patient actually got a quality service.

WTF is quality? You know it when you see it, but can you define it, really? The difference between a BMW and a Pinto is pretty obvious when you place them side by side, or compare details of the engine and interior and when you ride in one compared to riding in the other. But both of them will get you from your house, across town and back. So, functionally, they are the same—right? Maybe the Pinto is a quality vehicle, just not as much quality as the BMW. Who decides which one has the best quality? Maybe quality is proof of regular service on the vehicle, meaning that as long as it has been serviced, and the records show the service details, then it has met quality standards. Hang on to that thought.

I think that the decision about quality should be made by the patient, who has to pay. Most folks want quality, but must settle for what they can afford. The champagne-taste and beer-budget conundrum applies to cars and health care, too.

Health care made the EMR follow this false comparison. Care at one clinic (Pinto) is just the same as care at another clinic (BMW), provided the EMR documentation (service record) was the same. Poor or little documentation is proof of poor quality, and therefore more documentation is proof of better quality. False, false, false!

Here is a copy of my EMR record from a visit I had on August 21st, 2019.

I circled the failures and numbered them to show you what is wrong with the EMR.

Number one: the documentation does not actually say what I said to my Nurse Practitioner (NP). I told her that I was concerned that my blood pressure was not well-controlled, and that I could not get an accurate reading with my home BP monitor. I told her I was so anxious about it that I went to urgent care to have it checked, and later visited two local fire departments over the next two days to get it checked.

This statement is called the chief complaint, and because my NP was in a hurry, she did not document any of it.

She copied the list of blood pressures I had obtained from those three visits.

Number two: all those blood pressure measurements were done by an automated machine. It would have been very easy to mess up those numbers by crossing my legs, by moving in my chair, by standing up, and no one would know because no one was in the room with me while those readings were being taken. And the NP did not actually check my pressure herself when she came back to review the readings.

Numbers three, four, five, six, seven, and eight are all lies. She never listened to my neck or felt my abdomen (I was sitting down at the time), never felt my pulses, felt my joints, or checked my gait or sensation. So why did she write this? She didn't; the EMR did. These statements about my physical exam are called macros. Macros are bits of statements that she can automatically add to the EMR documentation.

Why does she do it? She does it because, in order to get paid, she has to document a certain number of body parts/zones that she has examined.

The assessment plan is basically a summation of what we decided. I already knew that I wanted a nurse visit to check my blood pressure and a 24-hour ambulatory BP monitor test. The NP came to those conclusions on her own, thank goodness, and so they got added to the plan.

This was probably coded out as a 2213, which would be a regular office visit, established patient, moderate to low decision-making difficulty. My time in the office exam room was about 20 minutes, six of which were spent with her.

And here is another "semi-false" office visit note from a patient I sent to a rheumatologist, when I was working in Fort Wayne, Indiana:

***Physical Exam***

Constitutional: Alert and in no acute distress.

Eyes: The sclera and conjunctiva were normal and extraocular movements were intact.

ENT: The ears and nose were normal in appearance and the lips and gums were normal. The oropharynx was normal.

Vascular: There was no peripheral edema.

Musculoskeletal: Normal gait, no clubbing or cyanosis of the fingernails, no joint swelling seen, normal movements of all extremities, there was no joint instability noted and muscle strength and tone were normal.

Skin: No rash.

Psychiatric: Insight and judgment were intact and the affect was normal.

***Assessment***

Symmetric Polyarticular Inflammation 714.9

Taking OTC NSAIDs for a long time V58.64

***Plan***

Follow-up visit in two months, evaluation and treatment follow-up done: 04 June 2013.

C reactive protein, quant requested for 04 June 2013.

CBC without diff requested for 04 June 2013.

*Comprehensive metabolic panel requested for 04 June 2013.*

*Westergren sed rate requested for 04 June 2013.*

*A long discussion with patient regarding prognosis and intercourse. At this time, 2 we do not have any significant diagnosis. I do believe that affected yesterday patient maybe working on a mild report for several patient not involving the MCP joints the hands were difficult to color and forth worse at this time. Patient having some improvement in her overall joint symptoms so with a molluscan her to ibuprofen. Patients does persistently have pain. She worries about her long-term prognosis. And this was discussed with patient with the more than 50% spent in counseling with 30 minutes total while face to face time.*

This record makes me sad. I hope you read it carefully. I am sure the writer did not read it or say much of this, but his macro generating AI filled in a lot of it or his voice recorder, Dragon Speaking Naturally, mistyped what he said.

In the old days, when I first started, this note would have been handwritten. OK, so it would have been poorly legible and subject to degradation over time as the ink faded and the paper crumbled. But later, in the not-so-old times, this record would have been dictated to a human transcriptionist.

That human would have typed, with no errors, and made notations wherever there was a problem with syntax or comprehension. Then the physician would have received a preliminary copy to edit. The editing would occur, and the record would be clean, legible, and accurate.

By the way, I suspect that the first part called "physical exam" probably never happened. Or if it did happen, the method was strictly by observation, and that no physician's hands ever touched this patient.

Some insurance company paid a lot of money to this specialist for this piece of crap. This continues to occur day after day, in office after office, in hospital after hospital, because we physicians let it happen, and you patients are being hoodwinked into thinking you are getting medical care.

It would be a much different experience if the encounter were on video.

Just to illustrate how the EMR is a La Brea Tar Pit time sink, I made a notation of my exam with a patient who came to see me in Fort Wayne:

6:40 AM to 6:50 AM

Patient is with front staff, getting signed in and filling out paperwork. Then she is taken to the exam room, has a set of vitals taken, and the staff-person retreats somewhere to enter the information in the computer. The staff-person then signals me that the patient is ready by hollering down the hall, "She's in room two, Doc."

6:50 AM to 7:05 AM

I see the patient. We talk. I examine her, and figure out why she has a sore throat, and what I will be getting for her from the sample med locker. We give out meds on site at this clinic.

The patient and I cover a lot of other ground about other questions she had, because everybody gets a 20- or 40-minute visit. She only needed 15 of that 20, and because she was well known to me, I only needed five minutes to figure out what to do for her. But we used the time productively to enhance aspects of her past medical history. By taking time to do that, I made it possible to improve our next visit. History is a key component to any diagnosis and it takes time to obtain a good history.

7:05 to 7:20 AM

I spend this time gathering her meds for her, then retreat to another exam room—they did not provide a private work office for the physician staff—to chart in the EMR. I am a fast typist, but I still have to work with a slow AI.

The EMR tried to block my ability to smoothly and quickly enter the information, but I overcame it and made the note look really good. This is how doctors get paid. Remember, the difference between a Ford Pinto and the BMW is an example of quality. How payment occurs is a very sad intersection of lack of time and quality in American health care.

If health care is going to automate the charting process, then please be sure the AI does not have a hearing problem.

I might offer a suggestion on how to prevent the EMR from controlling the narrative, to help the physician and help yourself. Every patient should come to the office visit prepared in the same fashion as a person prepares to come to a meeting or other important professional transaction. You are prepared when you try to obtain a loan, renew your driver's license, or purchase a home. So here is how you can be equally prepared for your office visit.

Make a list and include the following items on it: all your

prescription medications that you are currently taking; all your supplements and over-the-counter medications; all your allergies and sensitivities; medications you are no longer taking; all the diagnoses which have been confirmed by some clinician; all your surgeries, invasive procedures, and diagnostics with dates; all of your immunizations, as well as the name of your providers, hospitals, and your medical record number if you are part of a health system.

Update that list every six months and take it with you when you are going to be seen in the clinic, going to the ER, or heading out for some tests. I put a copy on the front of my refrigerator, held in place with a magnet, in case I got picked up by the ambulance and needed to have it.

Then write out your concerns, questions, and symptoms prior to going to that office visit, and make two copies of the note. Give one to your doctor and keep the other, so that you can make notes on it and bring it home.

Please don't be unprepared for your visit. You must not be like sheep walking in to be shorn of your dignity, fleeced out of your money, and soothed into false security about your health. That is another WIIIFY moment.

WE'RE BACK . . .

**Meeting Max Brown: Face-to-Face with My Biological Dad**

I was stunned. Max. Alive. I asked if Cousin Sydney had any contact information, and she gave me his address and phone number. I wrote him a letter and asked if it would be OK to contact him. I was divorced at the time and dating a fellow who lived near the Greenville area. I called Max and asked if I could drive down to see him. He was absolutely happy to have me come, and so the man I was dating and I drove down to Detroit to make the visit.

Max lived in a nine-story apartment building full of retirees, and I went up to his floor. Nervous and filled with apprehension and curiosity, I knocked, he opened the door and I saw my dad for the first time with my adult eyes. He was very dark, with smooth skin of a color that was the purest mahogany brown, blue-rimmed eyes, bald, short, and smiling.

He invited me and my date into his studio apartment. It was small but well-appointed. He remarked at how proud he was to have created such a fine-looking person. He then began boasting about his life. I recall that he mentioned he had women and children scattered around Michigan and Ohio, but never married anyone but June, and said he only really loved her.

I never asked why he left us. I did not want to force him to justify a decision he made 50 years ago. I knew the answer.

He was not mature, not employed, not ready for a family, and not able to deal with Vela the harridan mother-in-law, or Simpson's silent disapproval of him. But then, what Black person was ready for life back then?

Recall when they met, just at the end of World War II, both had been children raised in the privation and hunger of the Great Depression, facing Jim Crow, living through Detroit's race riots, hearing of and fearing lynching by the KKK—which were still major events in their lives.

No Black person could have a job if a white person wanted it first. Detroit was still segregated, and unless you were in with the church crowd, there was not much for you to do socially. Even gang warfare was primarily white-controlled. Detroit was home to the Purple Gang, and was a major rum-running location in Prohibition times.

Black lives truly did not matter then, and Max was just not into being a criminal, nor was he able to be a family man. He left and drifted through life, smoking, drinking, womanizing, until he could not do any of them anymore. He had severe diabetes-related problems, peripheral arterial disease, COPD, and all the problems left over from drinking and gambling habits. But he still had family; plenty of them on his side still lived in Detroit. I met them after he died.

I recall being so disappointed in him. He had every bad habit I never wanted to see in a man, and felt so disconnected from him. At the time, I was really glad that Mom elected to divorce him, and glad that he left. I regret that I never knew any of my half-siblings, assuming he really did have other children scattered around Michigan and Ohio. My date and I drove back home to Greenville, discussing my reunion.

Sometime later, I got a call from Max. He was in Henry Ford Hospital and wanted me to speak with the doctor who was attending him. The doctor began with a description of his problems, and was going into the plan of care when I interrupted and said, "Please, Doc, do what you think is best, and do not call me for approval for any care of this person. He is my father, but I have no regard for what goes on with him medically, and I want you to understand that he will make his own decisions. Please do not involve me." I hung up.

How ashamed I am now to have said that then. But we do what we do when we do it, with the tools we have at the time. He did what he did when he left me. I did what I did when I "left" him. The Henry Ford Hospital doctors did an amputation above the knee, and he lived for a few years afterward. Sydney told me when he died, and I came to Detroit because I was his closest living relative.

All his cousins and relatives where excited to see me. His nephew, James, met with me at the funeral home on West Grand Blvd. That was an impressive place, and it was designed to be that way because the funeral home business was a major commercial endeavor in Black Detroit.

Undertaking was one of the few professions that allowed Black Americans to enter—teaching and ministry were very open for us, medicine and law to a lesser extent. These professions were wonderfully supported by the HBCUs (Historically Black Colleges and Universities). Those were places that sprang up in and after Reconstruction, and persist today. Thank goodness.

The undertaker's desk was a huge slab of mahogany, polished and massive in an elegantly restrained, large office. We sat and discussed what to do. James opted for every option offered by the funeral director—flowers in multiple large urns, an organ, a piano, a vocalist, a cortege to the burial site, a silk-lined casket with a lead casing, and a minister to lead the burial service in the chapel and at the grave site. I sat quietly.

At the end of the plan, I said, "I have one thousand dollars to contribute to all of this. I am assuming you, James, will foot the bill for the rest of what you want. If you cannot or will not, then I will elect for a simple cremation with ashes given to me, which I will split with Sydney."

Turning to the undertaker, I said, "I think all the State requires for cremation is to have is a pine box, right?"

James was silent for a while, and then said my plan seemed better than his.

"Yes, all that we'll need is a pine box," the undertaker said.

We went with the Roast and Toast carry out box plan.

After the funeral, the family wanted me to open the package he left for me. They kept talking about the huge insurance fund that he had told them he prepared for me. I feared that what I would find inside would be hugely disappointing, either to me or to them, and so I demurred and did not open the papers there, pleading a need for privacy after the death of my father.

I took the folder of personal papers back to my home in Greenville, Michigan, where I lived at the time, and opened it up. It was a term policy to age 70, life insurance policy, worth $30,000. My goodness! He had paid on that for all the years I was alive; and you have to understand how much money that was in his mind, and how hard it must have been to keep the policy active all those years, even though he never saw me.

I think he took that policy out, and that is when he called me way back, when I was living with Mom on Trowbridge. I like to think that was the purpose of that call, to tell me he had prepared for my life and sustenance with an insurance policy; that he was trying to be a good father in the only way he knew how. I have no way to know if this is true or not; June never said anything about him all the time she was alive. But I am writing this, so my book will say what I want to believe.

It was a term policy to age 70. He died at age 73, outliving the policy, and thus rendering it invalid. Oh well, it was the thought that counts.

Max got cremated. I got a cup of his ashes; Sydney got the rest of them in a large, 20-pound box. I placed his ashes in a commemorative holder, shaped like a proud horse, and have it in my family honor shrine to this day. I never really knew him, but I now know why he was the way he was, and have forgiven him because he did really love me. I can only hope he will forgive me for leaving him alone with those medicos at Henry Ford Hospital.

## DIGRESSION #10: MAKING BIG PHARMA PAY BIG MONEY

Big Pharma . . . Big ideas . . . Big money.

No doubt about it, the American pharmaceutical industry is a health care behemoth. It is wonderful, creative, and profitable. But the excesses it has demonstrated make many of us angry and frustrated.

Is Big Pharma innovative? Yes, if there is money in it. If there is no way to monetize a development, then I think they put it on a shelf and let it molder away in a hole of forgotten failures. Big Pharma is also a copycat business. For example, when propranolol came along, it was the first in its class. It was a beta blocker blood pressure pill. Over the course of 17 years of patent protection, the drug raked in millions of dollars. After the patent protection was ended, dozens of other companies came out with dozens of copycat beta blockers. Each one was better than the previous one, true, but the heavy lifting had been done by the original developer. Not that that mattered, because, as one drug rep told me, "We only need to get one percent of the hypertension market to make a profit from our new beta blocker drug."

See, it is all about the Benjamins.

So, what can we do about Big Pharma and the Big Dollars that go with it? Try this.

A new drug that is not a copy of a previous molecule, gets a five-year protection of its patent. After that, anyone can make a generic. All pharmaceutical companies pay one percent of gross profits to support medical schools, another one percent to the national patient compensation fund, another one percent to the advocates fund, and a final one percent to support substance abuse treatment centers in all states and territories. This just makes so much sense.

They need to support the medical schools that turn out the physicians who will write prescriptions for the medications that Big Pharma creates. They need to support the national patient compensation fund because of the harm done to people who have taken their drugs and been injured or killed. They need to support the advocates who take care of injured people who are unable to manage their own lives, such as the mentally ill, the homeless, and abandoned people in our cities.

They definitely need to support substance abuse centers and programs because it is those drugs made by Big Pharma that cause addiction. They can pay fines as easily as you can blow your nose, but substance abuse support would be a forever proposition that keeps a steady tap open on their bottom line of profit.

There is no need to hate Big Pharma, but there is no need to let them off the hook when it comes to funding a better method of health care in America.

WE'RE BACK . . .

### Popoff Clinic in the Heart of Detroit's Drug Land

As I mentioned earlier, late in 2017, I had an opportunity to revisit the east side of Detroit, where I grew up. I worked at the Popoff clinic located at 10809 Mack Avenue, just north of Indian Village. It was owned by Michigan State University's College of Osteopathic

Medicine, having been donated to the school by Michael Popoff's widow, Linda. Michael was an MSUCOM grad, and opened his clinic when it was mostly a Polish and Russian immigrant community, and he stayed as it changed to a mostly Black community. More power to him for his willingness to care for indigent patients for the entirety of his life.

The neighborhood has changed. When I was young, we walked to Nichols Elementary School, and the gas station on the corner was a place to get a bottle of soda on the way home. Now from East Grand Boulevard to the Popoff clinic on Mack, there are 17 churches all thriving. There are probably 1700 drug- and alcohol-addicted people living in and around that stretch, who are not being served or saved by those churches. How sad.

America woke up to the drug problem when it found that the sons and daughters of the ruling class—white middle class and white lower class—were being sucked into the maelstrom of drug addiction, incarceration, and death, just like countless generations of Black and brown people. How sad. That vision of life along Mack Avenue generated my next digression.

The drug abuse problem, like so many other ills that afflict lower income people of all colors, and especially Black Americans, is caused by the person at the top of our national leadership hierarchy: Mr. President. I have come to believe that, like Isaac Newton had three laws of motion, I have three laws of presidential behavior:

One: No sitting president has ever, nor ever will, independently, willingly, or voluntarily promote, enact, or call for any activity or legislation that supports, improves, protects, or uplifts Black Americans while in office, unless . . .

Two: He is forced into that position by political expediency, wherein he needs the votes of Black Americans in order to get through a primary, or get elected, reelected, and otherwise maintain in power and . . .

Three: That same political expediency pressure is a direct result of the vote being given to Black men and women, and the willingness of those men and women to use their vote to get the rightful benefits, which otherwise would be denied to them.

My message is go vote. That is another WIIIFY moment.

## DIGRESSION #11: WORTHWHILE SUBSTANCE ABUSE TREATMENT

Centers will be funded by the federal government. Not only that, but the prisons will no longer bulge with drug user offenders, and drugs of abuse will be treated as misdemeanors, not felony criminal offenses. We will wake up and follow the direction taken by Portugal in 2000 when they realized you must treat addicts, not jail them.

This is the outgrowth of the Harm Reduction initiative from The Substance Abuse and Mental Health Services Administration (SAMHSA), which is part of the U.S. Department of Health and Human Services (HHS). The primary goal of the Harm Reduction initiative is treatment, not incarceration. Its mission is to "meet them where they are" with, for example, the needle exchange programs and marijuana decriminalization programs that have gained traction across the nation.

How would my future vision of this program work? Try this.

Drug detox centers will be located next to the National Drug Distribution Centers (NDDC). Because addictive drugs are decriminalized, not the same as legalized, they will be sold exclusively by the federal government.

Why not give the DEA (Drug Enforcement Administration) some real and meaningful activity by letting that agency set up and run the DEA NDDCs? Each user has an ID card, or perhaps a designation on the back of his/her driver's license or state ID card. Users come in and purchase what they want, get their needles if necessary, and can go to the injection room which is located near the DEA NDDC. The more important option is that they can come in and seek admission to the detox unit, which is also next door to the NDDC.

Therapists, psychiatrists, and other physicians work in the National Drug Distribution Centers, providing care to addicts who want to quit. There is also an in-patient housing unit, located as close as possible to the NDDC detox center, so that addicts do not have to return immediately to the places that enable them to continue being addicts. They stay until they qualify for halfway house lodging, and each halfway house allows for a year of residential care. These locations are franchised by the federal government and are supported by funds from the pharmaceutical industry, so there are adequate inspections and standards, plus follow-up on outcomes. Without data on the post-treatment lives of addicts, it would be impossible to adjust the programs that are run by the DEA.

The ideal situation would be to have acute detoxification facilities hand off a person to an in-patient residential facility, which then hands them off to an out-patient halfway house. This would include: five days of acute detox; next, one month of in-patient residential post-withdrawal syndrome care; then one to two years of halfway house life; five years of mandatory out-patient therapy; and finally, five years of mandatory self-help support group attendance, which might be adequate treatment and would certainly provide data to adjust programs.

I am so suspicious of drug and alcohol addiction treatment institutions that make great claims about success, but unfortunately have high recidivism rates. What is the definition of success? That needs to be defined, because the lure of relapse is lifelong. Like smokers, how long must a person be abstinent from tobacco before he/she can say, "I am clean?" I do not think the definition of "free of drug addiction" has been determined or agreed upon as of now.

We need a drug detox program that:

1. treats the biological, neuroanatomical deformations that occur as a result of drug use;
2. addresses the underlying emotional traumas that generate the desire for drug abuse; and
3. provides coping skills to address the societal stressors that drive so much of our recidivism rates.

Employers will be allowed to ask to see your ID, to find out if you are a registered addict. If you are, they can hire you or not, and can require you to take drug testing or not. The employer will know your status on the treatment timeline.

Like in Portugal, those who are drug distributors will be prosecuted as the felons they are. But the small-time users will be treated and given the opportunity for detoxification and return to a clean life. In my life as a physician, every addict I have ever seen has always wanted to get off the stuff, but may not have had anything more than the feeble encouragement I could provide. The infrastructure to help them cross over from addiction to cure was lacking at every level of life. Medical care, education, housing, employment, mental health services should be the right of all Americans who are trapped in the world of drug addiction. Instead, we punish them to placate the uninformed community, pacify the police community, and promote some politician's goal of reelection.

In my future vision for a better system, our method for obtaining the drugs is simple: our DEA purchases the drugs from those who produce them. Anyone else who purchases the drugs will be prosecuted by the DEA. The drugs provided by the DEA are certified for purity and controlled for dosing. The federal government will not allow any competition to survive, forcing users to come in get registered, and have a daily option for treatment that actually works.

In addition, we should select the staff at halfway houses from people who are previously addicted, while other staff members can be social workers and counselors. There should be in-house education facilities for those who need to finish high school. People with addiction/substance abuse disorders need to be destigmatized, re-humanized and loved, not incarcerated and hated.

WE'RE BACK . . .

**Warren Carroll Garner and June Belle Malone: Power Couple**

My mother married Warren Carroll Garner in 1960, and he was the best dad ever.

As I've said, he and Mom were both in the real estate business. He was a broker and she was the manager of the classified ad section of the *Michigan Chronicle*. That newspaper, known on the street as the *Green Sheet*, was the voice of Black Detroit from the '50s to the '80s, and it was a place where I learned the value of work and learned the joy of putting words on paper.

My mother headed the classified ad sales department and had two women working with her. Mr. Quinn was the boss, and it was a small enterprise that had big clout. Black-owned businesses advertised there, and real estate sales were listed there. White-owned papers did not court the Black community, and real estate red lining was still present.

Red lining is the process of delineating the population by race and marking the heavily Black neighborhoods with a red line on a map. This, then, was used by insurance companies, real estate agents, grocery chains, and so many more commercial ventures as they decided whether or not to provide services inside the red (Black neighborhood) lined areas.

My mother reached out to every Black real estate company, and then to every white real estate company she could, to get them to advertise in her newspaper. They responded and the ad sales grew exponentially. She met Warren and they fell for each other in a big way. He had been previously married, with one adopted son. And as I shared earlier, he also had a daughter in Germany, as a result of a wartime liaison with a German woman when he was stationed in Stuttgart. He was mostly a family man who craved the good life of home and family. June was alone and craved a stable man who would value her and accept her teenage daughter.

Perfect match, as far as I could tell.

They got married and we moved to a house on the west side, Atkinson Street, just off Woodward. Then we moved to the Dexter-Davison area, and then we moved back to Taylor, just west of Woodward Avenue, near Clairmont. It seemed that every time Warren found a good property, we moved into it first, fixed it up, and then sold and moved again. I was in Cass Tech High School at the time. During the start of every semester, the office would ask me what my new address was this time, because they saw a pattern and knew I would be somewhere else every six months.

Warren gave me the love he would have shown to the daughter he had to leave behind in Germany, and gave me the training he would have given to his adopted son, who had denied him. Not a day went by without a lesson from him, either through direct speech to me or by observation. I learned what it was to be a hardworking person, how to lovingly relate to someone, how to be competitive, and how to enjoy life without destroying yourself.

Warren was a man of great character, and every young man he encountered was changed for the better by associating with him. My cousin Keith Ledbetter, my cousin Wade Kirksey, and my cousin Dennis Archer all developed into healthy, adult, Black manhood because of him. A lot of my male-oriented behavior was also based on his role model—assertiveness, hard work, competition, careful analysis of human character, and a conservative financial posture.

Warren and June became a power couple in the Black Detroit business community. She also branched out at the *Chronicle* by writing one of the first gossip columns, called "Other People's Business." It was a compilation of stories, sent in from readers, and written to shield anonymity of the perpetrator of the various deeds and misdeeds. It was like trolling on the Internet before the Internet was invented.

If you had a piece of dirt on your local minister, you could write it up and send it to June, and she would publish it. No names were ever used, but everyone would know who the bad person was. And if you had a good joke, you could also send it in and she would publish it. Most of them were, when filtered through today's sensibilities, crude, racist, sexist, and totally not politically correct, but the Black community bought the paper just to read her column for the jokes and gossip.

She was so popular that she left the *Chronicle* to write her column for *The Detroit News*. This happened after the riot of 1967 when

*The News* was looking for more contact with the Black community. She eventually landed an afternoon TV show, called "June Brown's Detroit," which interviewed Black Detroiters of interest and/or notoriety. It may have lasted for a season, and was very popular, but she was not able to give it the time and energy it needed while also maintaining a full-time real estate business with Warren.

He eventually worked his way up in the real estate world, to the point that he was appointed to be the realtor for all the VA (The U.S. Department of Veterans Affairs) homes in the city; these were homes provided exclusively for veterans. He was the first person of color to have that appointment, and it gave him a pile of houses that he managed. He had some for sale and some for rent all the time. At one point, he and June had more than 150 VA homes in their control. New ones came into the market all the time, so they were extremely busy. This gave them the chance to open a real estate office, which was located in Southfield. Then they moved to Holly, Michigan to build a home there.

Warren had always liked the area near Holly, and used to go squirrel and rabbit hunting here. He would take me, and as I shared earlier, even bought me a .410 shotgun and tried to teach me how to hunt. I was good enough to shoot a squirrel in the eye, but it disgusted me to do so. I never bothered to keep up with my hunting skills.

He found a place in Holly on a lake and bought the property, and then put an Avion travel trailer there for them to dwell until their home was built. He insisted on having the garage made into a family room, and put in a wood burning stove, which made the place really cozy. Over time, they added barns and storage buildings, got dogs and horses, and obtained more acreage because Warren decided he could feed the horses at a lower cost by growing their food, than buying food for them.

They got interested in horses because they bought a horse for me for my birthday. I lived in Crystal, Michigan, and they lived in Holly—a two-hour drive. I had no place for a horse, no interest in riding a horse, and no time for a horse. I think Mom wanted one, and this was her way to get around Warren's objection. Of course, I wanted to send the animal to their farm to have it boarded there, and Mom was ever so happy to say yes.

The horse was called Flicka. Once they had one, they decided to get a second one so Warren could ride. Then Wade Kirksey came to stay with them, and they needed a third horse. Then it was time to expand the barn, get a tractor, raise some hay, get a truck to haul things around, and so on and so forth, until they had a real ranch.

I think June came up with the idea of developing a business with the horses. As I shared earlier, she combined a horseback riding enterprise with a dating club for Black single people and called it the G2 Ranch. She advertised it, organized it, had Wade serve as the chief wrangler, and the club took off like a rocket. Single males and females came up for the Saturday horse trail ride, followed by the dinner-dance and BBQ. The hook-ups were fast and furious, and everybody really loved it. There was no alcohol, no drugs, no gangs, and no fights—all of which were a common problem in the club dating scene. Their enterprise grew and, for several years, was the focal point for the Black singles dating community.

But it took a lot of energy and a lot of insurance. When the rates went up to cover liability for horseback injuries, Warren and June decided to end the G2 Ranch. Gradually, they found buyers for the horses and got down to just one, an old gray sway-back Percheron named Sam. Wade was growing up and soon left the ranch, so then they had to offload Sam, too. Warren still had his real estate business. How they did all that with the G2 Ranch, I will never know, but they were filled with energy and love for what they did, and for each other.

I think if former President Barack Obama and former First Lady Michelle Obama needed role models, then Warren and June would have shown them how to be a power couple beloved by all.

## DIGRESSION #12: PATIENTS CAN ORDER THEIR OWN TESTS

What a strange thought. How would the medical world function if every patient could ask for and receive labs, X-rays, and other diagnostic tests on their own?

The caveat is that they would have to pay for them out of pocket and not kick the cost back to some third party, like an insurance company. I think many people would love to be able to do this. Lots of information on the Internet about medicine is full of personal, unsupported bullshit, but lots of it is actually very helpful. If a person can follow along with the discussion, and not get caught up or tripped up on the medical terminology, there is a wealth of information about practically everything that bothers you.

There are hundreds of legitimate sources that are doing their best to provide information and education to the lay population. That could be made into a more targeted approach if patients had the option to find the right test and order it, get the results, and take them to an open-minded physician, who would follow-up and go the rest of the distance toward treatment.

In Fort Wayne, Indiana, there was a free-standing radiology office. The place would do every imaging study that would be done in either of the local hospitals, at half the cost or less, with just as much technical quality and an equal amount of professional oversight. The facility was owned by the same group of radiologists who were providing services to one of the hospitals, so there was no question in my mind about quality equivalency.

Patients who had no insurance got their test done at an affordable price. How could that happen? The radiologists performed their work without the crushing burden of administrative overhead imposed by the structure of a large health care system. They did not cut corners or avoid rules and regulations from HIPAA or EPA or NRC; they just did not have to provide a piece of their income toward the paycheck of a CEO, COO, CFO, etc.

There are places now here in Ohio where patients can get an imaging study done that is not in a hospital. Many times, the insurance company will direct the patient to one of these places because it is less expensive than a hospital. Amazing, that an insurance company would even let that happen.

There was a time when a physician, asking for an imaging study, had to speak with another physician employed by the patient's insurance company, and beg permission to let the study be conducted. Without that permission, the company would not pay. I sometimes wondered how those physician gate keepers slept at night, knowing that their purpose was to deny care and deny diagnostic studies to people who had true health conditions. How does repeating a non-diagnostic ultrasound instead of obtaining a non-contrast CT scan speed diagnosis of a pelvic mass? Those tumor cells are dividing at a rate that is dizzying. So, if you see the mass today, then believe that by next month it will be double in size. In six months, it will be pressing on something important, and in a year, it will have metastasized to lymph nodes and other organs.

I recall one fantastic patient who was able to take control of her own health and order a few tests that rapidly moved her from problem symptom to full recovery, in what amounts to lightspeed in the universe of medical diagnosis.

Let's call her Miss M; she came to me for a routine new patient visit, and in the course of talking with her, she told me that she had been diagnosed with ovarian cancer in the past. I asked her to tell me what happened. She said that she began experiencing weight loss that was unintended and fairly rapid. She checked her diet, and could not discover a reason for it. A few weeks later, she noticed some abdominal bloating.

She was very cognizant of her family history, and started asking relatives to fill her in on other medical conditions that were present in her family line. Breast cancer and ovarian cancer were present in a couple of female relatives. She began searching for more information on both conditions online at Mayo Clinic, the American Cancer

Society, and other legitimate resources. She performed an abdominal exam on herself, as well as a breast exam, and discovered a small tender area and mass in her right pelvic area.

She looked for all the differential diagnoses for this, and then scheduled herself for a pelvic ultrasound. A mass was found, and she took the report to her primary care family doctor, who conducted the remainder of the exam, confirmed what was on the scan, and sent her to the oncology department, where she had surgery, which was done in a timely fashion. From the start of her symptoms to the completion of her oncology care was just three months.

Here is one example of a well-informed, intelligent woman, possessed with enough medical agency to figure out what steps to take to get better. She paid for her ultrasound out of pocket at a free-standing facility. She knew her insurance would have given her the run around, much less denied her the right to order a test on her own.

The other piece of good fortune was that she had a family physician who did not scornfully or angrily turn her away because she obtained a test on her own. Instead, that doctor embraced his patient's intelligent approach and joined her in seeking the next right thing to do.

If doctors and patients were allowed time to collaborate in order to find problems, intervene in a timely fashion, and coordinate care, money and lives would be saved.

We must hope for this to occur in some future that is yet to be determined.

WE'RE BACK . . .

**Fourth Street Campus Life and Roommates**

I worked at the *Chronicle* as a young teenager, helping cut ads from the paper, writing ads, editing articles, covering weddings and church socials as a reporter. I recall going to Hamtramck to Unique Press, where the paper was actually set in type and printed. It was fascinating to see the linotype machines, to hear the roar and roll of the printing press, to screen the "hot sheet" for editing just before going to a solid copy, all done at my mother's side. She was one of the first to embark on the "bring your child to work" day, before that was even a thing to do.

At first, I worked with her in the classified ad section, and then I worked as a society reporter. "Society" in the Black community meant anything that anybody did that was celebratory. Weddings, funerals, garden parties, but not church. Church events and news had its own section because the Black church community was hugely important. So, I covered weddings and learned how beautiful they could be. They were all the same; I just had to change the names and locations, and I could write the story from a template in my head.

Because of my experience there, I decided on a career in journalism. My mother was certainly a big influence, and my love of reading made me feel like writing was the thing to do.

I paid no tuition because I was the daughter of a war veteran, George Hutchinson, so that was truly one good thing that came from being his adopted child. I went to Wayne State University, back in the day when they called their football team Tartars instead of Warriors, as they are called today. No one knew what a tartar was, and the team did not win either, so it was pretty much a wash. But I loved campus and had a marvelous time.

Even though my tuition was due to Hutchinson, my life was lived with Warren and June when I started university. My first semester, I lived at home. I could take the bus to school because it was located in the heart of Detroit. But, as I shared earlier, after I came home from a date at 5 AM and found Warren and June waiting up for me, I realized that living at home was not the ideal thing to do for a party animal girl like myself.

My first move was into the Helen DeRoy dormitory. It was literally behind a wall of brick to protect us young women. I found it crushingly restrictive, and asked my folks if I could move out. Warren happened to have a property located on Fourth Street; it was a three-bedroom duplex, and it was ideal.

The location was in a blind cul-de-sac where the Edsel Ford Freeway and the John Lodge Freeway intersected. The majority of people living in the apartments and duplexes were students at WSU. Warren's rental house was a three-bedroom duplex. I was the manager, and rented it from Warren. I found roommates: Linda and Shelley (not their real names), intelligent, exciting, and talented women.

Linda was from downriver, Ecorse, and could sing and play the guitar. She and I got along immediately because we liked BBQ ribs from Tastee Restaurant on Woodward, and Lambrusco red wine.

As I said earlier, we asked our roommate whom we called Patricia the Pig to move out. As manager, it was my duty to evict her. Fortunately, she did not mount any major protest, and the way was open for Shelley to move in. She was reform Jewish, and very much a feminist, going into social work. Shelley had never been around Black people and was very delighted to know that we would accept her as a roommate on full and equal terms.

The other half of the duplex was occupied by three men, all members of a Jewish fraternity. While they were close and neighbors and single, they were just friends, not anyone we wanted to date; that would have been too close for comfort. All three of us girls found boyfriends from various places and groups on campus.

One weekend, we invited Shelley to come with us to a party being held downriver near Linda's home to enjoy authentic soul food. I recall watching her work her way down the buffet line, taking a sample of most everything. She got to the hot cooker and took some of the meat from it, tasted it, and said it was a little salty and greasy, but otherwise flavorful. She turned and asked me what it was.

I said, "Shelley, you just had chitlins."

"What are chitlins?"

"You don't know?" I asked

"No, I don't," Shelley said.

"They come from a pig," I said.

Then it hit me like a ton of bricks, unclean food is pork in the Torah, and she is Jewish.

I stopped her hand before she could lift the fork up any higher and said, "Oh shit, can you eat that if you are Jewish?"

I let go of her hand, and I was concerned about her being in trouble.

"I'm OK with pork because I am a reformed Jewish person. So, what part of the hog has chitterlings on it?"

She pronounced all the syllables, saying chit-ER-lings.

I told her, "You are supposed to say it as 'chitlins,' and it is from the inside of the pig; really way deep inside. It is the large intestine."

There was a long silence here.

She stopped chewing the food on her plate and just looked at me, her fork held halfway to her mouth with a shred of pale chitlins dangling off the tine, a bead of fatty juice dripping down.

"Do *you* eat them?" finally came from her lovely face as she paused in her chew and swallow action.

"You know damn straight I do, Shelley, and it is OK with me if you do or do not. No one here will think badly of you for any decision you make."

She swallowed, I smiled, and we moved on.

Strong, brave, intelligent women are the best friends to have. She finished her bit of chitlins and smiled and went back to the buffet table. She and I remained friends all of our lives. She passed away in 2018, having achieved a life full of accomplishments on behalf of women, and on behalf of herself. She raised a biracial son, making him a strong man proud of his combined heritage, and she did it without benefit of marriage or the encumbrances of a relationship.

**Meeting Arney E. Mustonen**

I met Arney E. Mustonen while I was living on Fourth Street. He saw me at a party, not sure which one, and then found out where I lived and what my name was. He also figured out my school schedule at Wayne State, and was sitting on a bench on a walking path when I first met him. Basically, he stalked me.

He called me by name and said hello. I had no clue who he was, but was curious because he knew my name. I must confess, I was at the height of fashion at the time, with a plaid mini skirt, tight red tank top and white go-go boots; I looked so '60s sharp. I sat with him and we became acquainted. He eventually asked me for a date. We went to the movies and saw *A Fistful of Dollars* with Clint Eastwood. I tumbled for him on the first date. He was so smart, good-looking, and funny, which was everything I needed in a man. He could sing, too—baritone. We hung out together as a regular couple for the rest of our lives on campus, and eventually got married. Yes, I left out the sexy parts, the breakup, and the reunion before we were married. Just use your imagination. You won't be wrong.

He lived with three other roommates in a huge carriage house on Second Avenue in the Wayne State Campus Canfield and Cass area. Pat, Fred, and Jim were his buddies. I would come over and spend time with them, and sometimes stay overnight. He would not stay overnight at my place because it was much smaller.

The carriage house also had a reputation for great parties. The front house was occupied by a popular professor who hosted parties. Arney, Pat, Fred, and Jim also threw parties. The professor knew all the cultural icons and glitterati in Detroit, and folks in the art scene. Arney, Pat, Fred, and Jim knew all the cool people and political activists on campus and around town.

They both threw a party one summer Saturday, and the entire backyard was filled with wall to wall, belly to belly people, smoking, dancing, drinking, talking, singing, laughing, kissing, yelling, and so forth. But at one moment, someone said, "Nureyev!" The word was shouted out by more and more of the crowd in the yard as the incomparable Russian ballet super star Rudolf Nureyev himself showed up at the party. A great cheer came from the crowd when he waved his hands, grabbed a drink, grabbed a girl and a guy, and kissed them both. What a night.

We quickly found out that our immunity from racism only existed on campus. One night, Arney was driving me back to my house when we were stopped by the city police. The officer, a white man, looked into the car, shining his flashlight on the two of us. He stopped Arney for a taillight violation. He looked at Arney, then at me, then at Arney, then at me again. I could see him forming his opinion of what was going on.

He leered at me and asked Arney who I was, Arney said I was his fiancé, and the officer's face went through a multitude of changes, ending up with violent disgust.

He thought I was a prostitute and that Arney was just getting a piece of Black strange. The fact that Arney identified me as a legitimate partner infuriated the cop.

He took Arney and me to the station on Woodward (it is not there anymore), and booked him, fingerprinted him, and gave him a hard time. We were able to leave without encountering anything more than a ticket and lots of hassle. It was good that Arney was a law student who knew his rights and let the officer know he was not going to be pushed around.

We ran into more of this kind of BS episodically in Detroit and, after the riot, it was even worse because then Black people looked at us with hate, too. Racism is so complex and stupid.

**We Got Married in a Riot, Hotter Than a Pepper Sprout**

We were married in St. Andrews chapel on a Friday afternoon on the Wayne State University campus. John and Kathy Klimek were best man and maid of honor. I told my parents about the wedding the weekend before it happened. He told his mom and sisters the day after he graduated, which was three days before the wedding. They were in town for his law school graduation and had to stay for the wedding. Our ceremony was presided over by Hubert Locke, a Black minister who was also the City of Detroit Police Commissioner. My stepdad, Warren Garner, also had a CCW (Carrying a Concealed Weapon) permit. He and Pastor Locke were both packing at my wedding.

Poor Arney was covered front and back, and very nervous at the sight of two armed Black men at the wedding. We had a reception in the Traffic Jam Bar on Cass Avenue, and honeymooned at the Pontchartrain Hotel. We steamed up the shower and made a mess of the room. We ate in the fancy French restaurant. Arney ordered steak tartare, not knowing it was just rare sirloin with an egg on top. We were so naïve, but so very happy together.

Then the riot happened. We were married June 30th and the Detroit riot broke out a week later. I was working at WJBK TV 2 as a news reporter, and he was working for the Interfaith Action Council as an attorney.

On the first day of the riot, we were coming back into town on Sunday with Arney's old roommate, Patrick, and as we were driving back south into town on the Lodge Freeway, I saw a column of smoke on the right side of the freeway behind Henry Ford Hospital. Arney said he could see smoke on the left, and Pat saw smoke straight ahead. We knew there was a major problem and, when I got home, there was a frantic message on the answering machine—no cellular phones back then—from the TV station asking me to come in. I did, and I was put to work going to interview people on the scene as the riot unfolded.

There were cops, firefighters, and rioters everywhere and true chaos in the streets. It quickly got worse, and the State Police and National Guard showed up on the second day. They were largely ineffective as the burning and looting escalated. My color gave me access to locations where Black riot "leaders" were gathered, and my status as a reporter gave me access to white leaders downtown. I was the only reporter in the city who could freely access both venues.

I recall going to a meeting around Dexter Avenue, and as I was going inside, the participants stopped Bud, my camera operator, and Bill, my sound engineer, because they were both white. I looked at the guard and told him that if he wanted his group's voice to be heard, he had to let me AND my crew inside or it was no deal. He was surprised by my assertiveness, but let us inside. Our film that night was the exclusive footage of Kenny Cockrell's speech.

By the third day of the riot, President Lyndon B. Johnson was on the phone with Detroit Mayor Jerome Cavanagh, demanding that something be done PDQ, and the something was going to be the U.S. Army's 101st Airborne Division, which specializes in air assaults. The National Guard rolled into town that night, and Arney and I could hear the treads of the tanks coming up the Ford-Lodge freeway interchange. We still lived on Fourth Street in a cul-de-sac where the west bound Ford merged into the northbound Lodge, and the sound was eerie.

By morning of the fourth day, there was only sporadic gunfire. By day five, most of the city was quiet. By day six, there were no new fires, and by day seven, it was pretty much done. The big event was the shooting and death at the Algiers Motel on Woodward. The city was a wasteland in its heart—the Woodward corridor.

As the riot passed into uncomfortable, immediate history, Arney and I moved to another location. We both were working. I was still on TV and very popular. He worked for the Detroit Interfaith Action Council as their legal advisor.

We left the place on Fourth Street and moved to a carriage house on East Boston Boulevard. Boston and Chicago boulevards were the place in Detroit where, in the '30s, if you had lots of money, you built a house there. The Archbishop of the Catholic Diocese of Detroit had a parish home there across Woodward, from the Cathedral. Father Divine, a Black minister of local fame in the '30s and '40s, also lived in a house on the other side of Woodward. Each home was magnificent, like the homes in Shaker Heights in Cleveland. Each one had a garage with a carriage house, and that is what we lived in.

Our little place was probably 1,000 square feet, but for two people, it was totally enough. Kitchen, bath, living room, sunroom, bedroom, and a view overlooking a landscaped garden.

This is where I lived when I realized my husband was an alcoholic. I knew he drank. I drank; we all drank. We were in college, and so that was what you did on weekends and during gametime. But soon, I saw that he drank a lot more than once in a while or once a week. He was a three to four days a week drinker, with a liking for gin and tonic. I have tasted gin and tonic, and it is bitter and noxious as far as I can tell, but it was his drink of choice.

I got mad at him when he was drunk, because he was so fucking drunk! One night, I decided to fix him. I moved the furniture in the bedroom so that it was opposite of where he knew, and when he came home drunk—I knew it was one of his drinking days—he went to the bed and collapsed upon it, only to discover that it was not there, so he hit the floor and just passed out right there. I put a blanket over him and went to sleep by myself.

His addiction to alcohol was the reason for the disintegration of our marriage. So many people suffer from the effects of it, and physicians are so clueless about what to do for treatment. Like addictive drugs, alcohol destroys the interconnectedness of the brain, as well as damages every other organ in the body. Most times, doctors do not screen people for alcohol problems, and so it goes undetected, untreated, and like any disease, eventually destroys not only the person who uses it, but also the people who are living and working with the addict.

If only we had time to be better for our patients, so much more could be done by every primary care family physician. We need to know more about what is the most current treatment or intervention, but we barely have time in the office to say hello, refill pills, and order lab work before it is time to see the next patient. And in actuality, all you can do is "see" them and move on.

Shame on us/U.S.

## DIGRESSION #13: PHYSICIANS WILL BECOME AUGMENTED CYBORGS

Resistance is futile, and the future is knocking on the edge of this as I write. Elon Musk—think what you will of him—is a visionary genius; he is wealthy and unafraid. He plans to test his device called Neuralink,[2] which implants an AI program into a living brain. It is designed to treat neurologic diseases such as Parkinson's disease by controlling the area of the brain that is damaged so it can prevent the tremors that trouble a Parkinson's patient.

The advent of this type of technology opens infinite possibilities. Besides curing diseases, these brain implants could control many other activities.

Imagine having a brain implant that connected you to an AI supercomputer. The wealth of information that would be available to tap into would make every physician as intellectually equal to the character Dr. House, from the television show *House*. No one doctor can possibly know as much as the character played by Hugh Laurie, but with a brain implant that accesses a centralized supercomputer, a regular physician now becomes as intellectually potent as that TV character.

Once a physician has the information base, why not provide real healing power in the hands of that doctor? Can you envision a scenario where the physician can take samples from a patient using special implants in each of his/her fingertips, such as saliva, blood urine, tissue, all of which can be obtained on the spot and tested without going to a lab?

If diagnostics are possible, why shouldn't therapeutics also be possible from the physician's hands? Imagine being able to inject antispasmodics, pain relievers, sedatives, antipsychotics, antibiotics, antipyretics from your fingers.

There is something that is scary about this, but something else that is mind boggling and so very, very attractive. What kind of people would be selected to go to medical schools? Graduation would involve getting your brain implants, putting on your academic hood, and tossing your cap into the air. And completion of residency would involve the implantation of a final piece of the software for your brain.

But in order for this higher order physician-cyborg to occur, medical school education will have to change. One change I will advocate for is that the process be expanded to a five- or six-year program.

I went through in three years, and it was year-round with no breaks. I think we had 10 days between semesters. Wisely, my college eliminated the soul-crushing, three-year program, realizing that it produced flawed, anxious people, which confused those who might hire us. I had to explain over and over again, every time I applied for privileges or a job, why I only had three years of medical school. But when I went to medical school, there was so much less to know. Seriously, I am not kidding. There were only 100 elements in the periodic table of the elements when I entered practice in 1980; now there are 118 in 2021.

Medical students need more time and training to become better physicians.

Consider a six-year curriculum where each section is six months long, from January to June, and from July to December. Time off will be the last week of June and first week of July, then the last week of December and first week of January.

Here is my proposed schedule:

**Year 0.5, July to December**

Anatomy
History of Medicine
Doctor-Patient Relationship
Palpatory Skills/OMM
History of Osteopathic Medicine, A.T. Still
Doctor-Patient Relationship

**Year 1.0, January to June**

Biochemistry
OMM
Molecular Biology
Simulated Patient
Cultural Competency/Europe
Microbiology

**Year 1.5, July to December**

Nutrition, Sanitation
Cultural Competency/South America
Human Physiology
Genetic/Molecular biology
Pharmacology, Level 1
Endocrinology

**Year 2.0, January to June**

Female Genito Urinary

**Year 2.5, July to December**

Cultural Competency/Middle East

Medical Jurisprudence
Male Genito Urinary
Neurology
Simulated Patient
Cultural Competency/Africa

Gastro-Intestinal System
Musculoskeletal
Pharmacology, Level 2
Simulated Patient
OB/GYN

**Year 3.0, January to June**

Hematology/Lymph
Cardiology
Nephrology
Pulmonary

Special Senses EENT
Primary Clinic
Cultural Competency/BIPOC

**Year 3.5, July to December**

Integumentary
Respiratory
Orthopedics
Population Health, Research Epidemiology
Psychiatry
Primary Clinic
Cultural Competency/Australia

**Year 4.0, January to June**

Cultural Competency/Asia
Pediatrics
Pathology
Dentistry
Toxicology
Hospital
Brain Implants, Basic

**Year 4.5, July to December**

Rheumatology
Geriatrics
Forensics
Podiatry
Brain Implants, Advanced
Hospital
Cultural Competency/India, SE Asia

**Year 5.0, January to June**

Oncology
Anesthesiology
Medical Reimbursement
Pain Management
Implant of Therapeutics
Hospital

**Year 5.5, July to December**

Addictionology
Radiology
Medicine/Government
Surgical Principles
Implant of Diagnostics
Hospital

**Year 6.0, January to December**

Practicum Apprenticeship

As students rotate through each of the sections that deal with the systems of the body, they will return to the anatomy lab for a refresher training specific to that subject matter. This return to anatomy reinforces the didactic knowledge, and this is how it is taught now at Ohio Heritage College of Osteopathic Medicine.

There should be more time for pharmacology because of the explosion of research; it will be vitally important to know as much as possible to help prevent medical errors, to develop genome specific treatments, and to avoid adverse reactions in patients.

Within each of the six-month sections, beginning in Year 1.0, students begin live clinical preceptorships. They must have a six-month-long session in each of the following areas: emergency medical care, pediatrics, family medicine, obstetrics, internal medicine, and in-hospital care.

Topics on how a physician gets paid, as well as the interface between medicine and government, are overlooked and ignored today. Also, the future physician needs to understand the rest of the real world, so a cultural competency class covering the major demographic world regions will be preparatory for practice anywhere in the world. They will need this, because the cyborg physician will be one of the most highly sought-after employees ever. Anyone who has a lot of money will want a personal physician who is augmented, and national leaders will want one or more. Major health systems will want to staff their hospitals with augmented cyborg physicians.

After medical school, with diagnostic and therapeutic implants in place, these new graduates will begin their training. They will not need a residency because the apprenticeship will replace that. That is enough, because at the start of year five, they receive their brain implants and will have access to the entirety of medical knowledge, as well as current, past, and most recent research to guide their decisions. It may turn out that physicians go back to the most basic distinctions—physicians or surgeons. Hand skills will be important, so some people will turn to just surgery while others will be more interactive with patients as physicians only. Those who specialize in OMM will be equivalent to surgeons because of their hand skills.

They will have to spend time learning and gaining experience. Even though they may have all the knowledge that exists of research and practice, they still lack experience. So, they will be rotated to each of those world areas in which they took cultural competency classes. They will learn to interact with people from all nations, all races, all cultures, all religions, and understand they are here to treat all humanity.

Physicians will have their phones, which continue to have all the current smart phone functions, but there will also be the addition of a portable view projector screen. The device will project a screen upon which the brain-implanted physician can show any view, formula, information, photo, drawing, etc., and share with those around him or her. It will be like having the ability to create a PowerPoint slide show with your mind and instantly display it to those in the room.

The fact that these future physicians have implants in their hands and brains will not lessen their ability to be empathetic and caring human beings. They are augmented with new skills, not diminished in their humanity. In fact, it may be possible to select people for medical school who score high on empathy more than they do on scientific knowledge, because society needs physicians who are more altruistic, empathetic, and caring. And with the brain implants, an empathetic physician can also be a highly scientific knowledgeable physician, too.

The wealthy already have access to fast, discreet medical care, thanks to concierge medicine groups, which cater to people who can pay for physicians to make house calls on yachts and private jets, in mansions and board rooms, and at upscale events. During the COVID-19 pandemic, concierge medical groups provided private coronavirus testing by physicians who were transported via planes, helicopters, and chauffeured vehicles. They catered to families who wanted testing before a wedding or holiday gathering, CEOs who needed testing of all parties before a meeting, and high-profile people engaged in all kinds of activities that required secrecy and total discretion. This service is expensive because it includes testing, house/location call charges, special services fees, and even higher prices during holidays and on weekends.

Since this is already occurring with human physicians, imagine the access and level of care if cyborg doctors were able to provide this service.

WE'RE BACK . . .

**Moving to 3455 Sloan Road, Crystal, Michigan**

People were frightened and still very angry on both sides of the color line in Detroit. No one knew what to do, but Arney knew that we should not be living in the city as an interracial couple. He feared what would happen to us and to any children we had in such a charged and angry environment.

He found a place in Stanton, Michigan where an attorney named Ben Franklin (honest to God that was his name) had just been elected to the newly created judicial position of district court judge in Montcalm County, and this attorney wanted to sell his practice. Arney reached him and agreed to take over the practice. This was in 1970, and I left my TV station job and stood by my man as we moved to our first home together in Crystal.

The old farmhouse at 3455 Sloan Road was built in the late 1940s or '50s, and it was owned by one of the two Black families in the county. They sold it to us on a land contract and we were so happy. It had two buildings and a garage, and was located on a three-acre site in the middle of a horseshoe bend of a river called Fish Creek. There were two small islands just off the shore, and a barbeque pit. On the other side of the house was a swamp filled with mosquitoes and scrub, but also filled with promise; it could be a pond.

I had nothing to do—no job there for a TV reporter. There was not even a newspaper in the county worth talking about. I was going to be a homemaker. It was very scary, but Arney had his law practice, and we were going to be just fine.

Our first big adventure involved getting educated about septic tanks. Understand that we were both city-born and bred and knew nothing about drain fields or septic tanks.

Our two-story farmhouse had three small bedrooms upstairs and one bathroom downstairs. There was a gas stove that was very primitive, and a wretched kitchen. The land outside was gorgeous. There was a Concord grape arbor and leafy maple, pine, and arbor vitae trees all along the property. The river was a gently flowing shallow stream that had recently been stocked with brown trout, and was a popular place for fishermen.

The home's interior was covered in wallpaper, the windows were old and leaky, the floors were squeaky, and the upstairs was just barely high enough for us to stand up. But all we saw was an opportunity to make it what we wanted. We wanted to be self-sufficient and live as much off the grid as possible. I invested in a subscription to the *Rodale's Organic Gardening* magazine and learned as much as I could. It was fascinating, and I continued to love organic gardening long past my time living on Sloan Road.

We moved in and set up life together. One day, I heard a lot of dripping noises coming from the basement and told Arney that we needed to find out what was leaking. He went down to the basement, and we saw a pool of water.

You must understand that the "basement" was a Michigan cellar, an area dug out under the first floor of the house into the subsoil. There was a furnace there but no floor or walls, no concrete or dry wall, or any of the stuff that is used in home construction today.

The bathroom—we only had one on the lower level—had a tub and shower. Each evening I would shower, and each morning Arney would shower. The water from the tub actually ran down a hose into the subsoil floor and was absorbed into the ground. This works fine, as long as there is only one person who showers once or twice a month, and that was indeed the case with the previous owner. But two people running showers every day was a stress on the ground's ability to absorb the water, and so I heard the result of accumulated bath drain water as a dripping sound.

What about the toilet, you may ask? Well, that involves the septic tank and drain field. The septic tank is a large concrete holding tank buried in the ground with an overflow valve that leads out into the drain field. The drain field is a terracotta tile-lined pathway of ceramic tiles that carries the wastewater out of the septic tank across several yards of "perkable" soil so that the bacterial waste is deposited into the land and naturally decomposed over time. "Perk" is short for percolating, and the county requires that the drain field pass a perk test before you install a new septic.

Again, here we had a 250-gallon septic tank, which was the minimum for one person under the building codes of the time when the house was built. In 1970, it was not at all up to code. Five thousand dollars later, we had an up-to-code septic tank, holding 1,500 gallons, a new 40-yard drain field, and a bathtub that was hooked up to the septic.

This was the starting point of the multiple upgrades that we made to the home. Over time we: removed five layers of wallpaper; raised the second story from six feet to eight feet; added a bedroom with a Scandinavian fireplace, a bathroom, a sitting porch upstairs, a new bathroom, kitchen downstairs, and then the south side addition.

This was Arney's dream work. In addition to lawyering, he also dabbled in ecologically friendly home remodeling. His dream was to have a 40 by 20 sunroom and woodburning fireplace in our home, with sky lights and insulation. Most of the work was done by Bill Nestle, who was a local contractor. His wife, Norma, was a babysitter for my kids for a while. Arney and I pitched in and did as much of the work as we could.

### Days of Lumber, Woodburning Nights; Not Days of Thunder or Talladega Nights

The sunroom was a beautiful addition when it was done. The floor was black, heat-absorbing concrete flagstones, and the south wall was filled with floor-to-ceiling windows. The roof was sloping with two skylights, illuminating a Vermont soapstone woodburning fireplace. There was a wooden storage chest for the firewood. I filled the room with a large, eight-piece sectional couch. We heated the house with wood, and each year in September, had to find and cut down a tree, chop it into burnable pieces, and stack it into cords before snowfall. There was still a furnace, but we tried not to use it until late January or February, when we were low on wood. In retrospect, it was idyllic.

The children would be asleep upstairs in their cozy bedrooms, the radio was on with Garrison Keillor hosting *A Prairie Home Companion* show on Minnesota Public Radio, and the fireplace was emitting great warmth. I was on the couch, Arney was on his computer. Life was so good. In actuality, we worked hard to get a few days like this.

Finding and cutting the tree for the wood was hard and hazardous. Splitting the wood was even more dangerous. I learned to use a maul and hammer to make kindling and that is probably how I hurt my right shoulder, which bothers me to this day. The wood was stored inside, which took all four of us—Arney, me, and both kids—an afternoon to haul it in.

Arney was forever looking to find the right wood splitter; the market was full of them, and they were all dangerous widow- or amputee-makers. He bought one that was shaped like a pyramidal cone with groves on the side in a spiral pattern. The idea was to attach this device onto the wheel of your car after removing the tire, prop up the car, and have someone feather the gas pedal, making the wheel rotate while another person pushed the cut log onto the pointed end of the rotating spiral of death, and thereby split the wood.

I got to sit and feather the accelerator while Arney pushed the wood onto the rotating device. He and his buddy were working together because they were both going to share what they had cut. I could see that they were getting tired, and I could see that they were unaware of their Mackinaw jacket sleeves getting closer to the spinner as they got more tired and sloppy.

I turned off the ignition, pocketed the keys and told them, "We are done. I am not ready to be a widow today."

They could both see that I was a Seriously Angry Black Woman, and so that stopped the death show of wood splitting.

We kept the pests in the wood under control with the Shell No Pest strip, which was probably one of the most toxic chemicals known to mankind. We had wood ash in the air all year round; even in summer, it was hard to remove from walls and furniture. So, I am sure we were breathing it in 365. The fireplace ashes had to be hauled out each day and dumped onto the compost pile we kept by the edge of the garden.

Winter was a never-ending line of fireplace related chores for all of us. But I remember it fondly. We were so determined to be self-sufficient and off the grid that we even decided to have our own source of renewable protein in the form of fish.

We had a large garden after the pond was dug. You may recall the pond-site swamp that was present when we bought the place. Well, we got it dug out and found there was an artesian well that flowed into the depression, so we had a clear-flowing fresh water source and a large pond. Arney filled it with trout, and I started a compost pile on one corner of the shore. Later, we added a pile of sand to make a play beach for the girls, and put up a swing set, too.

We even bought ducks to swim on the pond. My garden was as long as the pond, about 80 feet long by 30 feet wide. I tried to grow as much as possible. I was an avid Rodale Press organic gardener. Tomatoes, peas, green beans, corn, squash, head and red leaf lettuce, two kinds of Swiss chard, white potatoes, pumpkins, gourds, cucumbers, dill, cilantro, celery, pole beans, summer squash, zucchini beets, carrots, turnip greens, collard greens, were all in there. I learned to can, freeze, and preserve food, and would routinely put up 60 quarts of spaghetti sauce, plus make kosher dills and freeze whatever else I could grow and save. We eventually added a large deck and hot tub to the south side of the house, and lived in a wonderful country paradise.

We were ready to start our family. We had two dogs: George, the black Labrador, and Heidi, the white German Shepard. I am an only child, and Arney is the first of five children. He always said he wanted a large family. I was not at all certain I wanted more than two. I thought no child should grow up alone, but no parent or pair of parents should have more than three.

So, I made a bargain with Arney. I told him I would have the first two children, and then he could have the second two children, and I would have the last two children. We laughed about that and agreed that a couple of kids to match the couple of dogs would be plenty for a couple like us.

Any parents who have more than two children are just plain outnumbered because each kid takes two people to handle, and when you have two kids, you need four people to take care of all their needs. I know this is not good math, but I think most parents will understand the philosophy behind it.

We began our family—no training, no close family support—just the two of us.

## DIGRESSION #14: THE EVE

**The EVE—Extra-Uterine Viability Environment.**

Too many women have problems with fertility, pregnancy, and delivery. There is a huge market for an unoccupied uterus in the world today; just witness the women in India who have had C-sections to deliver babies for foreign couples who have undergone IVF procedures and need a place for the fertilized embryo to develop. Those poor women receive perhaps an amount of money that would equal one year's income. India's surrogate market rose to $400 million in 2012[3] but in 2015, the country banned the practice of foreign couples paying Indian surrogates to have babies for them. Other countries such as Ukraine developed thriving surrogate markets for foreign couples.

I know it is possible to support a 28-week infant outside of the uterus, because it was done in 2017. The first steps for this were accomplished when a premature baby, born at 28-weeks' gestation, was kept alive in an upgraded plastic bag filled with placental fluids, nutrients, and oxygen, that mimicked the uterine environment and brought to maturity.

Now just imagine how that might work if science took the next step. Who would want one? Every Hollywood actress who could not afford (the time and body changes) to have a pregnancy, corporate ladder climbers who could not tolerate the time off from work, wealthy women who fear the physical demands of a pregnancy, and infertile couples who want a child without the danger and litigation of a surrogacy, and, of course, same-sex couples who want to start a family. These would be people at the top of the economic pile because the initial EVE would be costly. But once it became better engineered and more acceptable, the cost would decline.

Imagine a couple who can afford the EVE and who decide not to have the risk of a normal pregnancy interfere with the running of their lives, for any reason. The IVF procedure is completed, and the viable embryo is inserted into a sterile chamber, which is then filled with placental-type nutrients. This chamber is maintained at the home of the couple.

There are a huge number of problems and risks that are eliminated with an EVE. These include: intrauterine infections, STDs in pregnancy, placental problems, fetal alcohol syndrome, fetal narcotic syndrome, mal-presentations that result in C-sections, pregnancy-induced hypertension, pregnancy-induced diabetes, postpartum and intrapartum bleeding disorders, weight gain of pregnancy or lack of adequate weight gain, trauma to the mother that kills her and/or kills or injures the fetus. Sexual activity between the parents can continue undisturbed.

The fetus is not going to be exposed to bacterial, protozoal viral or fungal infections, trauma, alcohol, tobacco, illegal drugs, side effects from legal pharmaceuticals, poor nutrition, a kinked umbilical cord, a difficult birth canal passage, or other birth trauma.

No women who use an EVE will have pre-eclampsia, premature birth, a low-birth-weight child, cerebral palsy children, C-section scars, or birth canal passage trauma. All people using the EVE will maintain their normal lives with regard to employment, physical activity, sexual activity, and lifestyle in general.

Amniocentesis would be a simple procedure of taking a sample from the EVE tank to check for genetic disorders at the second week, or sooner, of gestation. Fetal malformations can be observed and corrected while in the EVE, just as they are now done by intrapartum trans-utero surgery.

I mentioned above that India has had a large number of poor women who earned money by serving as surrogate mothers for infertile couples. Though banned in India, and disrupted in Ukraine due to war, this remains a thriving industry in countries such as Mexico, Greece, and Colombia, according to the website globalsurrogacy.baby. Serving as a surrogate helps many poor women earn far more money than they might otherwise earn.

Here is what happens. A wealthy couple undergoes IVF and the egg is transferred to the uterus of the surrogate woman. The woman is housed for the duration of her pregnancy in a carefully controlled living arrangement, given food and prenatal care, and monitored until the week prior to her due date.

She is then taken to the OR for a planned C-section to deliver the baby. The couple takes possession of their child, the woman is paid, and she's sent home on the third post-op day.

These surrogate women can have as many C-sections as is humanely possible, and as long as their uterus is not in danger of rupture, which would probably be a maximum of four times.

I believe this is a vile practice of using some other woman as a surrogate. With the EVE, this would end. Surrogacy is a boon for some, but as a method of earning a livelihood, seems to be economic oppression. A woman can only have a limited number of C-sections before she becomes such a high risk for uterine rupture during pregnancy, that she is no longer a candidate. Then what becomes of her life? C-sections are not without risk, as they are major surgeries that require long recovery, and leave lasting problems for the woman.

I can hear objections arising now from the legal and religious communities. I cannot answer all their objections, but I do know that once Pandora's box is opened, there will be those who will find a way to use what has been let out. First, it will be done in secret, next just for the wealthy, then overseas, for the famous, then there will be legal battles, and *then* there will be acceptance. More and more women will find a reason to have an EVE. Women will be able to control their fertility and control their reproductive activity. This will be a private, at-home activity, not under control or surveillance of a hospital, where government regulations will be in effect.

What becomes of the OB/GYN community, of physicians and the midwives who work with them, or without them? Great changes will occur because these physicians will now have to do deliveries on women who do not have or want the EVE, or who cannot afford it. They will need to level up their skills and learn how to use forceps again, and manage deliveries and pregnancies in a more humane and gentle fashion.

Women and their families with an EVE can do a home delivery. They only need help when there is a malfunction in the EVE or a developmental or genetic problem with the fetus. Just as you can send in saliva and obtain a genetic study, families can send in a placental fluid sample and obtain genetic information of their child. The decision to have an abortion is now completely private, and always available before any date of any minimal-known viability—as early as two weeks. Cerebral palsy, Down Syndrome, Tay-Sachs, sickle cell disease, muscular dystrophies, and many others are known early, counseling occurs in the privacy of one's home, and decisions are made without outside pressure or threats. Is this utopian or dystopian? I have no crystal ball to say which is possible. I just say that if it can be done, then it will be done, especially if there is a dollar to be made, and the EVE will come to be a fact of life.

I do believe—and you should also believe—that a lot of progress in health care comes about as a result of being able to monetize an idea, and not because it is an idea that is needed, good, or important in the provision health care, but rather because there is money to be made.

Using that premise, I can see a time when there will be an end to surrogacy motherhood, and it will be brought about by the development on an Extra-Uterine Viability Environment—the EVE.

The kind of people who use surrogate mothers are also the kind of people who would use an EVE. So are also women who have uterine anatomical disorders, all couples who have failed IVF implants to achieve a viable pregnancy, gay/same-sex couples, and older couples.

With an EVE available, that list could expand to include women who are entertainers and cannot take the risk of a pregnancy disrupting a career path, women who are professional athletes, women who are in business or other leadership roles, and single women who do not wish to be married, but who want a child. And the final category will be any man or woman who can afford it.

The EVE would consist of a large sterile tank filled with artificial amniotic fluid that is temperature and pH balanced, and accessible only to the OB/GYN who owns it. The tank remains in the home of the person who has contracted with the OB/GYN for this service.

The parent(s) can watch the development of the child together, and bonding can begin prior to birth with music specially developed for the fetus, while both parents can speak to the developing fetus and show love as it grows.

No doubt the EVE will be the province of the truly wealthy, for a while. But as the technology evolves, the cost will decline. No health insurance will cover it, at first, but advocates will make it happen for women who can demonstrate extraordinary need for a child from this methodology. Once that happens, other insurances will develop a way to tap into the market and offer policies that cover and provide for EVE delivered processes.

Abortion will continue to be a difficulty to navigate. Suppose the genetic testing reveals a deadly or less-than-lethal problem, such as cystic fibrosis or sickle cell disease. Does the parent/parents terminate the embryo? Is that a crime if it is done in the second week of gestation or less? Can the EVE be moved to a state that allows for abortion if medically necessary? These and other questions are beyond my pay grade, but someone—physicians, ethicists, legislators—will have to pass on them as the EVE becomes more widespread.

And what about the market for human female womb surrogates? It is hard to tell if the market will decrease, increase, or become more affordable. If the EVE is readily available, will there be any move to limit the number of children a parent/couple can have? Why not have 19 and counting for everyone who wants a large family. Octo-Mom—the woman who underwent IVF and delivered eight babies—will be surpassed by Deca-Mom, Duo-Deca-Mom, and Tri-Deca-Mom.

The EVE will develop because there is a way to make it happen, and a way to make a profit from it. John Varley, the Hugo Award winning science fiction writer, mentions a device like the EVE in his book *Steel Beach*. Perhaps his idea has been percolating in my mind all this time. The EVE does not need to fill a medical or social need; it just needs to find a venture capitalist and willing physician to partner up and a marketer to launch it.

*Brave New World*—as English author Aldous Huxley describes in his 1932 dystopian novel—is not far behind.

## WE'RE BACK . . .

### Ophelia & Veronica, *Mes Belles*, Are Born

In 1970, I got pregnant with Ophelia, our first daughter. She was born in Sheridan Hospital, delivered by Henry Beckmeyer, DO, who was also my mentor for medical school at Michigan State University. People came to see her after she was born—family drove up, friends stopped by, neighbors moseyed into the newborn's nursery, and even folks we did not know came to see the baby. I was confused about her popularity until I realized that these Good White People (GWP) had never seen the product of an interracial marriage and were intensely curious about what color she would be.

In retrospect, it is just funny as all get-out. At the time, it was insulting, but as I have grown and lived and learned, I understand that it was part of the educational aspect of my life—teaching GWP about Black people.

When she and I came home from the hospital, our two dogs were there to greet us—Heidi, the white German Shepherd, and George, the black Labrador. The Steere family—excellent neighbors who had befriended us—had given us a rocking cradle, and I placed her in it and let the dogs in. Both dogs came to the cradle, sniffed the baby, and then each dog took up a place at the head or foot of the cradle, laid down, and guarded their new pack member.

Ophelia was a marvelous child, learning so quickly and being so cheerful.

In 1974, I learned I was pregnant again. Our second daughter was a double footling breech presentation. This means both feet were going to try to come out first, and then her head would rip me open, and I would bleed out and die. The only way I knew about her positioning was because of an X-ray procedure that is no longer done now. Dr. Beckmeyer ordered a pelvis measurement called Snow's pelvimetry to determine if I could deliver her vaginally, and seeing that was not an option, scheduled a C-section.

Veronica was gorgeous and huge, nine pounds of joy. She was the culmination of everything Arney and I wanted. He wanted six kids; I only wanted two. I told him I would have the first two, he could have the second two, and I would have the last two. Somehow, he never came through on his part of that arrangement. He said he would have a vasectomy after Veronica was born, but never made those arrangements prior to the delivery, so I calculated that his commitment to that process was low, and told my doctors to do the tubal.

Like her sister, Veronica was bright, beautiful, and athletic. Both girls were so good together. They played in the woods that surrounded our home, and enjoyed fantastic imaginations as a result of living in a home with two intellectuals and a 3,000-book science fiction library. They built forts in the forest and joined our neighbors for sugar bush maple syrup sap season. They were called the Sap Queens because they could tap and empty syrup buckets the fastest of all those who participated.

Memories of my daughters sustain me. One is a memory video that plays in my head of them going onto the school bus and the dogs watching them get on. And then the dogs barking as the bus returns, and the girls hop off and run up the hill and driveway into the house at the end of the school day.

At school, our daughters excelled in sports. Ophelia starred in track, field, and volleyball, while Veronica was a champion in track, volleyball, and basketball. Both girls hold records in their high school, to this day.

Both daughters attended a top-ranked university and earned master's degrees at other esteemed universities.

## DIGRESSION #15: YOUR HEALTH RECORD IS ON VIDEO

In my vision for the future, the medical record will be a video document.

One of the current drivers of discussion in the medical community is physician burnout and the EMR (Electronic Medical Record). Most physicians will tell you that the EMR they are using is slow, cumbersome, difficult to use for input and output, and interferes with the doctor-patient relationship because of the time that is eaten up with typing, typing, typing. They will state that the emergence of the EMR into clinical care is a big reason for burnout and early retirement from active clinical practice. They are right.

The EMR became a favorite of the business gurus who brought their ideas into health care to transform a system into something that would be data driven, more efficient, and that would help simplify billing, as well as control health care spending. None of that was true then, nor is it true now. That was the ugly intersection of business management with medicine in the late 1970s.

They made physicians talk about total quality management and continuous quality improvement. They, like Jon Snow in *Game of Thrones*, know nothing, but because they run hospitals, they made the EMR happen.

The EMR is nothing more than a device to generate a bill to the insurers. If there is any meaningful clinical information in a chart, it is buried, or otherwise hidden in layers of administrative garbage, required "macro" paragraphs, redundant phraseology that is designed to protect against legal attack, and mind-numbing graphs that do not tell you what actually happened when a patient saw a doctor.

Obamacare, the Affordable Care Act (ACA), embraced the EMRs and required physicians to use the damn things. First, they offered a Medicare payment bonus for each year of use in the three-year run up to the start of ACA, but the bonus declined as you approached the "go live" deadline. Then they used a penalty for each year a physician failed to implement an EMR, with the penalty increasing over time after the roll-out of the ACA. The EMR is the child of the insurance companies and federal government, and is the tool of the medical software developers and computer hardware companies.

It is a most ugly child holding a most unwieldy tool.

The EMR required selection to be sure it was able to perform the convoluted tricks of documentation required by the ACA, then it required purchase, installation, and then training of staff before "go live" dates in the office. Physicians quickly found that within six weeks, there were bugs, incompatibilities, and the inability to transfer information from paper charts to the EMR, or to move information from one company's EMR to another company's EMR. Therefore, if you bought one from GE Centricity, you had probably better stick with them through each upgrade and change. You would have major problems moving the Centricity generated documentation to the Athena system.

Plus, each corporate health care entity was required to have HIPPA firewalls so that information from one system could not be stolen, which meant that it cannot be shared with information from another system. The result is that patients cannot go to health systems outside of the one they are in because their records are not readily available to doctors in a different system. We—doctors and patients—are all stuck on the island of EMR insanity. Hospitals capture patients with the EMR while insurance companies capture covered lives.

I used a half-dozen different EMRs; all of them were cumbersome and prevented me from having meaningful interaction with patients. Plus, every other clinical person was allowed to add stuff to the chart, so that if my nurse wrote one thing and I wrote something different, there was a conflict in the documentation, which might not be discovered until next-to-forever, or when the chart is given to the plaintiff's attorney who is just looking for conflicting shit like that.

The other problem with EMR documentation is the "he said/she said" problem of what actually happened in the exam room. Patients do not remember and, actually, physicians do not either. Plus, there is no time to get all of it into the record.

Additionally, physicians who are problems—sex offenders, substance abusers—can say whatever they want and no one can disclaim what they said happened.

When I served on the State of Michigan Board of Osteopathic Medicine and Surgery, we had reports every month in which a patient charged a doctor with inappropriate touch, but how are we to know? The outrage in the Osteopathic medical community over the Larry Nassar case is that his touch was medically correct, but he applied it in absolutely the wrong way, because he could hide his hands from view of the young women who were his patients and their families who were sometimes in the treatment area with him. Nassar, the former team doctor of the United States women's national gymnastics team, is now serving a 60-year prison term for sexually abusing hundreds of girls and women.

A video record of the doctor-patient encounter will put a rest to many of these problems.

Documentation would no longer require typing till a clinician's fingers fall off.

Doctor-patient encounters would be meaningful because the interaction would be between the two, and not between the doctor and the EMR.

Accuracy of statements made to the patient and made by the patient would be preserved.

Avoidance of inappropriate touch activities would be easier to achieve.

Patients would be able to leave the encounter with a thumb drive or CD of their visit. Their visit would reside on their Cloud chart and be available to all legitimate users. Billers could look at the video and decide how to code it—assuming we are still using billing systems as are currently being employed—so that no doctor would have to count elements and figure out what level of work was done.

Malpractice suits for office-based activities would drastically drop in frequency.

The office is not the only place where direct visualization of activities would produce a major change in behavior. Imagine if you could watch the surgery or procedure being done on your family member?

If you wanted to, would you like to see what goes in the OR or procedure room? For those who elect to do this, why not set aside a TV monitor showing the activity and have a private viewing area for the family to watch. The people watching should be able to hear and see what transpires. The people working would certainly be more professional in their speech and actions.

To draw a harsh parallel, think about executions, which are witnessed by members of the law enforcement community, the family of the victim, and the members of the penal institution. When people are watched, people tend to behave better.

I have seen a lot of horsing around, bad language, angry behavior, sexist taunting, racial slurs, and vicious, dangerous throwing of instruments in my years. Then there are the lawsuits involving sexual activity performed on anesthetized patients by surgeons in the privacy of the OR.

No one knows, except maybe a nurse, but how likely is a nurse to accuse the surgeon or anesthesiologist of something like that? Unlikely, but it has happened. Most of the time, the nurse is not believed and is then punished by the administration. But occasionally, the nurse is believed, and then investigations must be carried out to find the truth. A video camera seen by family members, or a recording that starts when the patient is placed in the procedure room will put an end to 99 percent of the problem.

The big barrier is physicians. We/they do not want the general public to watch what goes on in their private domains of surgery and clinical office settings. I understand that, but at some point, the desire for transparency will become so pervasive, not only in medicine, but in all other professional endeavors. Citizens abused by bad and/or racist police clamber for body cameras on police officers. How much longer before patients demand the same for physicians?

Maybe we should put body cams on our politicians too, because CSPAN is not enough.

WE'RE BACK . . .

**Arney Emerges as an Alcoholic**

Arney was drinking heavily. I was unhappy with my entrapment in the backwoods with rednecks, saddened to know that my husband was killing himself with alcohol, and suspicious that he was with someone else.

Arney excelled at drinking and carrying on an affair with a married woman until we moved to Wisconsin in 2000. They were together every chance they had, she thereby making her husband a cuckold, and he making me unhappy beyond belief. I turned a blind eye to it for as long as I could.

One day, I decided that Arney was going to leave me, either by vehicular suicide or divorce, and then what would I do? First, I decided to go to Al-Anon, and second, I decided to go to medical school. Dr. Beckmeyer encouraged me, as did Dr. Robert Ricketts, the surgeon who did my C-section and later my gall bladder surgery.

I realized that I needed to make up credits in science that I had avoided in undergraduate school at Wayne State University, so I went to Montcalm Community College and Central Michigan University to get classes in biology, physics, and chemistry before applying to

MSU and other schools. I then applied to MSUCOM, Cornell Medical School, and the University of Michigan. I was accepted at Cornell, U of M, and MSU. I chose MSU because it was in-state tuition and close to home. I have never regretted that pathway.

I got to Al-Anon after finishing medical school. I wish it had been sooner, but what the hey, I found it, and that is all that really matters. The Alcoholics Anonymous support group for drinkers in recovery is called AA. The support program for those who live with or work with alcoholics is called Al-Anon. Please visit both of their websites for all the information you may need on each of these groups. I joined Al-Anon in April of 1985.

By all rights, I should have been just fine. I was married with a thriving medical practice, lots of respect, most of my medical school debt paid off, two wonderful children, and a husband who was a district court judge. That is what the outside world saw. I saw an entirely different life. Arney had become wretched and twisted due to the guilt he felt at being my husband while being in love with another man's wife. He kept up his façade as best he could, but he tried to soak away the pain with alcohol. He spent most nights in Brownie's Tavern, which was on the way home, and would roll in drunk, clamber into bed, and fall asleep.

I seethed and raged internally. I suspected he was with his mistress, but could prove nothing, and really did not want to find out. The rage and anger solidified into resentment and despair and hopelessness, and it burrowed internally and made me hate myself. There must have been something wrong with me that resulted in my husband being unfaithful, right? So that was my mind set.

I needed to die.

Both children were at school and Arney had gone to work. I was home alone, not yet dressed, sitting with my cold cup of coffee in my fuzzy brown housecoat in the living room of our house on Sloan Road. I was sitting in the large recliner, the bookcase behind me filled with books and our 33-record album collection. The blue carpet was filled with scraps of pet hair and trash from the previous night of arguing and fighting with Arney, who had come home drunk, again.

Since I was still a smoker, I had a cigarette with my coffee and was looking at my day to come. I saw oblivion, loss, disappointment, abandonment in my future, and no way to remove myself from the onrushing juggernaut barreling down a path to defeat me in marriage. I was unloved, unloving, unlovable, and thought I did not need to live anymore.

I cried and smoked and cried and smoked. Then I took the butane lighter and touched it to the area of the housecoat just above my right thigh. The flame slowly caught and made a char, and then some smoke. I kept applying the lighter to the robe, willing it to catch flame and consume me. It seemed as if there was a hood of darkness around me, and the living room was shrinking and compressing around me. Finally, a small flame caught and remained, weakly burning in the fabric of the robe. I just looked at it and never heard the door open.

For some reason—Al-Anon would say there definitely was a reason beyond our understanding—Arney had to return to the house, and he saw what I was doing to myself, rushed in, and put out the flame. He was horrified, and angry with me, at first, then apologetic, and then honestly ashamed that I was this distraught because of his drinking.

I honestly do not recall what we said to each other, but the end result was that he called his lawyer friend in St. Louis, Michigan, who was also a recovering alcoholic, and said, "Henry, we need help."

Henry K. and his wife, Shirley, both came to the house that afternoon.

They split us up and took us to the Alano House in Grand Rapids on April 13th, 1985. I went to the Al-Anon meeting with Shirley, and Arney went to the AA meeting with Henry. I was so frightened, and I am not sure what was making me feel that way. I had just tried to kill myself and was rescued by the person who was the cause of my abject pain, and I felt afraid because I was being rescued?

That is how twisted the thinking becomes when a person is subjected to being the codependent partner on the merry-go-round of alcoholism.

Up is down, down is good, help is pain, life is wrong, nothing makes any sense, and each day slogs along thicker and slower in the mire of so many negative thoughts, arguments, anger, repressed feelings, and despondency, and it is all so incoherent and no one cares. That is where I was mentally when I went to my first Al-Anon meeting.

I came home a new woman.

I heard that people did not live like that, that there was a way to live fully, gratefully, happily, and free of mental anguish. Even if your partner was a practicing alcoholic, that help was available, that I was a loveable, loving, loved human being and I was not alone with this problem. Most importantly, I learned that I was not responsible for causing Arney to take up drinking, nor could I cure him, nor was it my responsibility to even try to cure him.

I kept going back to those meetings. I found a way to put that meeting into my regular routine, and every Saturday morning I was there. I bought books, got pamphlets, listened to speakers, and made connections with other Al-Anon members. I changed my way of thinking. Arney decided he was OK now that I was in Al-Anon and did not immediately return to AA meetings. I got a book, *One Day at a Time in Al-Anon,* known as the ODAAT, and read it every morning. I still do that daily reading.

I swear that from April 13th, 1985 to April 12th, 1986, each day in that book was written specifically to address the problem, situation, or feeling that was consuming me at the time. No lie. No matter how I felt or what was facing me or what had transpired in the previous 24 hours, the words of the day in the ODAAT seemed to be a spot-on target for my needs for an entire year. I think back on that year, and it seems eerie, but it was true, and remains true even to this day for me.

On June 23rd, 1985, Arney left the house. He told me that I was just too different and he could not live with me anymore. I was not angry, saddened, frightened, unhappy, or even distressed in any fashion by his announcement. I was ready for it. I did not even know I was ready for it, but when I called Shirley, she said he was right because I was different, and he had to figure out what he needed to do.

But what was I supposed to do? She told me to do the dishes, take a walk, read some Al-Anon literature, and go to a meeting as soon as possible, because all I needed to do was take care of me, my needs, and the needs of my children, and not worry about whatever Arney was going to do. She told me it was my first test of the principle of detachment. Letting go with love so that the person he was could move down his path, and the person I was could move down my path, but love each other and learn to love ourselves.

I never called him; he never called me. Our daughters asked where Daddy was, and I told them he was visiting friends, because as far as I knew, that was probably what he was doing. I was so free and happy while he was gone, that it was a shock to see him return on June 28th.

Not only did he come back, he also decided to go into treatment for his alcoholism. That was when, if you had good insurance, you could be placed into a recognized, professionally-competent substance abuse treatment center for 28 days. He found a place, and we spent some time gathering what he needed for his stay, making plans to get court coverage from a visiting judge, and taking care of all those minutiae that comprise a person's day to day life.

He came home from the detox center a new man. He was happy, clean, and sober, and he and I both attended meetings on a regular basis. He stopped hanging out with his old buddies at the bar and spent more time with his children and me. It was truly a blissful three months. Then, one day, he played golf with some friends and had a beer after golfing.

They say that lapses happen for both partners in recovery, and the best course of action is to remember how you found recovery, and strive to find it again without devolving into arguments and recriminations and blame, blame, blame about why it happened and whose fault it was.

He fell off the wagon and, sometime later, went back to a recovery program. But the second time was harder on him, and he fell off again and back into alcoholic behavior. The people around him did not think drinking was bad, or that being an alcoholic was bad. His best friend was a serious alcoholic, and gravitated to Arney whenever Arney was wavering between sobriety and alcoholism. That was just enough of a push to take Arney over the edge and back into active drinking. It was just too hard for him to go to AA meetings on a regular basis. I stuck with Al-Anon and continued meetings for 36 years and more, even to this day.

There were some times when it was really hard to find a meeting, some times when it was really hard to go to a meeting, and some times when it was really hard to speak at a meeting, but I kept up the program. His drinking was making our marriage difficult, and I found a meeting where the members were combined AA and Al-Anon people. Many of them were couples in the program, and many of them were divorced people in the program.

They gave me what I needed to make my decision to seek divorce in 1990. I needed a support group that would not judge me for my choice to leave, and it was the best thing I did for myself. I could not see how I would live with him and remain in recovery myself. It is said that two sober people, or two alcoholics, can live together in perfect harmony, but if one is sober and the other is not, then the partnership is doomed. That was true for Arney and me. Either I had to become an alcoholic, or he had to remain sober for us to remain together; that was my viewpoint.

And so, I decided to get divorced, and did in January, 1990.

**Vignettes de Arney**

How do I possibly sum up the experiences of 47 years spent with one person? Arney and I met in 1965, married in 1976, divorced in 1991, lived apart until we returned to living with each other in 2000, and more or less remained together until his death in 2012.

I was with him longer than with my parents, and we shared so much, loved so passionately, fought so frequently, argued so eloquently, and shared the best life together I could hope for.

Perhaps a few vignettes showing his personality and characteristics would be one way to share his memory within my memory.

To my grandchildren: You two only saw him when he was at the end of life, in a wheelchair with continuous oxygen, singing a Finnish baby song in front of your fireplace on Willow Wood Lane. Here are other glimpses of Grandpa Arney.

*Arney and Me Hang Out on a Weekend on Campus*

After we had met, we knew that we would be dating on a steady basis. One weekend, we had to go run some errands. All we had between us was five dollars. I insisted on getting my birth control pills first because, you know, first things first. He understood and then said we need gas, too. I paid 50 cents for the pills, hopped back into his old Chevy beater, and we stopped at the gas station. He got two packs of Kool Mild's/Menthol, one for me and one for him, and paid a dollar for them, then pumped in 50 cents worth of gasoline, maybe two gallons. With our remaining $3.50, we went to the Traffic Jam Bar on Cass Avenue, had a couple of burgers and a pitcher of beer, and spent the rest of the afternoon enjoying each other, and all our campus friends' intellectual conversations. This is how we learned to manage money and share resources.

*I Meet His Grandmother, Mrs. H*

Arney told me he was Finnish. I looked up where the country was and said, "So, you are Scandinavian?"

He said, "NO, I'm Finnish."

I could not fathom the difference, because to me, they were all from up there in Nordic/Viking Land. Later he told me that the Finns were disparaged in Nordic Land because so many of them had intermarried with the indigenous people, Laplanders, and were not considered "pure." In fact, he said that when the Finn people came to America, there were classified at Ellis Island as non-white.

He was getting serious about us and wanted to trot me out to see a relative, his grandmother, Mrs. H Piilo. She was his mother's mother, and lived in the Rosedale Park section of Detroit. I got dressed to go. I put on a blue scoop neck, long-sleeved mini-dress that reached just to my upper thighs.

He took a look and said, "No way are we going there with you in that dress."

Hey, I looked good: long shapely legs, slender waist, ponytailed hair, just so fine—for campus. Definitely not for meeting my BF's gramma. I changed to something longer and covered up a lot more, and we drove out there.

She was sitting in her living room and opened the door to greet us. She paused for a long time before she moved to let us in. Then she said something to him in Finnish, and he replied in a mix of broken Finnish and English. This went on for a while, and then she shrugged and said something in Finnish that must have meant, "We'll see how she is."

She made homemade Finnish sweet bread, called pulla. I don't think I've ever had such good food as that cardamom-flavored buttery bread, hot from the oven, sprinkled with sugar. We all had that with strong coffee. Afterwards, I cleaned up the kitchen and asked for the recipe. She was impressed with my willingness to do that and actually smiled when we left. Arney told me that I had passed the house guest test. He was unafraid to show his family that he could transcend racism, and they should, too.

*The Party at My Place on Fourth Street*

One weekend, on campus, not during exam time, my roommates and I decided to have a party. We each had a boyfriend, so that made for six of us. The three guys who lived on the other side of the duplex each had girlfriends, so now we were up to 12 people. I said we had to invite Arney's roommates, Pat, Fred, and Jim, who each had a girlfriends, so that was 18 people. I said it would be wrong to leave out the people who lived on either side of our house and across the street from us. What the heck, we invited the whole street.

Everybody brought something to eat. I remember we made lasagna, and the house was full of food and drinks, and the smell of marijuana was redolent inside and outside. I'm sure I do not know how that got there. People flooded out to the porch and steps, front and backyard, and up and down the street. Enough alcohol had been poured down enough throats, that eventually somebody wanted to have a car race, like you may have seen in the *Fast and Furious* movies. Linda was the starter, standing between Fred and Arney's cars, who were going to race their respective cars. Both cars were beat up—Arney had a Chevy and Fred had a Ford—needing repairs of all kinds—interiors, body, frame, engine, chassis, you name it.

They started at one end of the street and roared down to the other end, which was blocked off with the freeway barrier fence, slammed on their faulty brakes and came to a halt. Except that Fred's brakes quit and he slammed into the fence. He was unhurt, but the car was mushed in, smoking and leaking. Fred was so angry, he jumped on top of the hood and started smashing it, saying, "This fucking piece of shit car lost!"

The whole crowd took up Fred's cry and began chanting it. Then every other guy decided that was a good idea, and soon enough, there were a dozen drunken guys and a half-dozen drunken girls also doing a demolition dance on Fred's car.

Dear grandchildren, your grandpa was capable of being outlandish and had wild a side that he kept quiet when he was on the bench or in public.

*Our First Night in Crystal, Michigan*

After the riot in Detroit of 1967, we moved to Crystal, Michigan, and bought a ramshackle place in the backwoods. Our house was literally in the woods, with no lights of any kind, on a dirt road with only a landline/party line telephone for communication. We had moved in planning to unload the U-Haul the next morning.

Sometime around the time that bars close, we were awakened by the sound of shouting and shooting. Some people who did not like the idea of a white man and a Black woman being together had come into our driveway, which was circular, and started shooting their guns. We hunkered down together, and Arney told me not to worry, they would never do that again. I am not sure what he did but, please recall, he was the lawyer in town, and I am sure he made his wishes known to the local sheriff. We never had another incident like the Montcalm County Welcome Wagon again. He was very protective of me and all his family.

*Snowmobile Adventures*

In mid-Michigan, in the '70s, every man who was a Man had a snowmobile. Arney got a pair of Arctic Cats and we rode them as much as we could. He would frequently go with a group of his buddies on night rides. They would gas up and oil up their machines, and Schnapps up themselves. They had flasks and flashlights, and were feeling good, roaring across the snow. One night they decided to race to the local bar on Crystal Lake (not the uptown bar because it did not have lake access). They took off, planning to race around the shoreline to the bar, but Arney decided he wanted to win, and so he cut across, going closer to the center of the lake.

Everyone started waving and shouting at him, and he thought it was because he was ahead, but he realized they were telling him to go faster. He looked behind his snowmobile only to see that the lake ice was breaking underneath the vibration and weight of his snowmobile, and if he did not veer toward the shore or speed up, he was going to drop into the lake and drown, freeze, or die. He made the right choice and got closer to the shore before a huge hole in the ice broke open behind and ahead of him. He learned to not ride across a frozen lake in March, because he knew life was precious.

*Harriett the Goat*

Arney was the world's best dad and would deny nothing for his daughters. One day, he brought home a goat. We already had two dogs, a cat, and a pond filled with trout, but he thought a goat would be just the ticket. He told me the goat would eat the grass out back of the house, so he would not have to mow it. The girls loved that animal and named her Harriett. I was doubtful about a goat for a pet, but decided to go along with the plan.

He put Harriett in a fenced-in area, which had a small outbuilding to serve as her "shed." She opened the gate, pranced to my garden, and began eating everything there. I put a lock on the gate. She jumped the fence and began eating everything in my garden. Arney put up a layer of concertina wire on top of the fencing. She jumped the fence like an Olympic high jumper, with inches to spare, and finished eating everything in my garden. We staked her out on a rope, tied down in the ground. She pulled it up and continued eating what was in the garden. The dogs harried her, and she butted them into submission, pulled up the stake, and began to eat my Concord grape arbor. Arney thought all of this was so cute, and the girls were totally forgiving of the goat's behavior. I was furious.

One night, we lay abed with the window open to enjoy the summer night air, when we heard a noise, waking us up: *TAP-tap, TAP-tap, TAP-tap, TAP-tap*. Arney sprang out of bed and went to look outside. We heard a bleat, and he saw Harriett perched on the roof of his Chevy soft top SUV, putting hoof shaped dings and dents into the vehicle. Suddenly, the goat lost her charm, and Arney took a shot at her with the Daisy BB rifle. She bolted off the car and he began to plan her demise. He knew he could not outright slaughter the animal because Ophelia and Veronica would be heartbroken.

He was saved by Uncle Danny. Danny was his first cousin, and one of the only people who could out-drink Arney. Danny called and said he wanted to come visit with his girlfriend. Arney said yes, and Danny showed up in an RV on Friday afternoon with his latest female acquisition. We had a marvelous weekend.

NO, let me be honest. They had a drunken weekend. Arney, Danny, and his girlfriend soaked up as much beer and booze as we could buy, and I was fit to be tied, but what could I do? Sunday morning, Arney and Danny got up extra early, and I watched as Arney loaded a fifty-pound sack of Purina Goat Chow into the RV with Danny and Female Friend, and they drove off—with Harriett the goat in their RV!

"What are you going to tell the girls?" I asked. "How did you get Danny to do this? Where is he taking the girls' goat?"

"Don't sweat the small stuff," Arney said. "I gave him the goat, the goat food, a six-pack of beer, and $20 for gas, and he took the goat. We will tell the kids that Uncle Danny wanted to take Harriett to the petting zoo so she can meet her future goat 'husband' and have a family and babies there."

They story worked. I never did find out what really happened to Harriett, but I like to think Danny really did get her to a zoo. Arney always had a way to solve a problem and soothe people's feelings.

*We Both Encountered My Worst Patient*

When he was District Judge and I was on staff at Sheridan Community Hospital, we frequently encountered the same couples. I would see the wife for a medical reason, and he would see the husband for a legal mishap. One night, we both met a man whom I call my worst best patient.

I was on ER call and was summoned to the ER because the sheriff deputies had a man there who needed stitches before being transferred to the jail. It was Thursday night and the man, let's call him Mr. B, had been tossed out of a bar in Stanton. He was picked up for drunk and disorderly conduct, resisting arrest, and public drunkenness. He resisted just enough that the officers had to "touch him up" with the night stick, and so he was in the ER awaiting stitches.

I got up, dressed, drove to the ER, and walked in. You know it is bad when there are three sheriff deputies present. Cherie, the night ER RN, knew what I would need and had the suture tray ready to go. I walked up to the patient and introduced myself: "Hello, Mr. B, I am Doctor Mustonen, and I am here to help you tonight."

He was lying on the gurney, drunk as the proverbial skunk, with blood congealing on his forehead where the nightstick had been applied, and one eye closed from the blood and swelling. He rolled his head to the sound of my voice, opened his good eye, and greeted me with, "I don't need no nigger doctor bitch working on me."

The whole ER went into silent stasis. I was the doctor. My husband was the judge. The deputies and the RN just looked at me, mouths open, waiting.

I said, "Mr. B, I understand your desires, but tonight you only have one choice and it is me, and I am going to do my best for you. After that, you may pick whom you want."

Cherie gave him a tetanus booster after I put in the stitches, pulling them nice and tight for sure, applied the dressing, and then I gave my business card to the deputy. I told him that Mr. B would need to have the stitches out in seven days, and I would make an appointment for him in that time to come in to be taken care of. My bill would go to the county for the care, and would the deputy be sure that Mr. B got my card with the appointment time and day? The deputy assured me he would take care of it.

I went home, back to bed, and told Arney, "You might be seeing him."

Arney told me the rest of the story. Mr. B went to court the next day, and he got to stand before Arney because the morning was arraignments for all the people picked up overnight and tossed in the county jail. Friday afternoon would be small claims court.

He said Mr. B was in line behind several others, looking hungover and unhappy to be there. The Deputy gave Mr. B my business card as the line moved along and said, "Good luck."

Mr. B shuffled along as the line moved up, one defendant arrestee at a time, holding my business card, which said S. G. Mustonen, DOPC, with his appointment day and time on the back. In between shuffles, he was looking up at the bench where Arney was seated behind a sign that read "Honorable A. E. Mustonen 64 B District Judge."

Looking up at the sign on the bench and down at the card in his hand, the connection between the names suddenly slapping into his consciousness like a sledgehammer, the enormity of his racial faux-pas the previous night and his impending judicial doom descended darkly like a pool of squid ink to smother him and his shitty future.

He showed up one week later to have his stitches removed. I saw his name on the chart before I entered and steeled myself for more racist silence. I entered with a professional face plastered on, but was shocked when he jumped off the exam table, stood up, and began to cry.

"I am so sorry, I am so sorry, please forgive me, I never meant to say any of those things. I did not mean it. I was so drunk, that is not how I am. Please, Doctor Mustonen," and so forth.

Not what I had expected at all! I told him to sit down, relax, no hard feelings, and that if he needed a family doctor, I would be happy to take him, and could I please take out his stitches, and tell me if he thought drinking was a problem for him?

We hit it off just perfectly. He became one of my favorite patients. He sobered up, got a job, met a nice lady and got married, and moved on to a much better life. He only got a fine and an admonition from Arney of, "Get your life in order, quit drinking, and don't let me see you here again for this."

I think he saved Mr. B's life by setting him on a path away from alcohol, which is so ironic a statement, considering the way that Arney's life went.

I loved that man. Good, bad, ugly, alcoholic-driven character defects and all, I loved Arney.

## DIGRESSION #16: WE ARE SUCH CHARLATANS

As a physician, I get a lot of respect. I really am not sure how that came to be, because I was such a blunt and plain-spoken interactor with people in my clinics. I always enjoyed talking to people and hearing them tell me their stories. My training and career in journalism and TV news reporting gave me a leg up on other physicians who find it hard to speak to strangers. For me, getting to know a person was the goal of each day. I realized everyone who was my patient had a very unique story to tell, and I would benefit if I just listened.

Maybe that is why I got a lot of respect. Most physicians deserve whatever respect they do get because it is a really hard job. But there is a group—small, thank goodness—that are such a bunch of charlatans, that I am sometimes ashamed of the profession. They include:

- The skanks, who grope and molest patients under the guise of doing an exam.
- The greedy bastards, who sell their names and signatures for money to buy things they do not need.
- The pompous assholes, who proclaim by word and deed that they know everything.
- The arrogant jerks, who tell a patient that the problem is psychosomatic, which is a fancy word that means the doctor has no clue about what is wrong with you and is not willing to try harder to find out what your problem really is.
- The morally corrupt, who join forces with the administrations of hospitals to squash physicians who speak up on behalf of patients, or on their own behalf, for better care or better conditions.
- The addicted, who hide their problem until it cannot be hidden and someone dies in their care because they were high or twisted on some illegal or legal mind-altering substance.
- The ignorant fools, who never bother to keep up on the latest treatments and let patients suffer.
- The careless, who fail to understand when they don't know what to do, that the right thing to do is to refer the patient to someone who does know what to do.
- The chronically insensitive pricks, who think that they do not have to listen to what a person is saying, or watch the patient receive a piece of devastating bad news.
- And the ones who are sexist or racist and think it is OK to be that way.

Every patient should be willing and able to ask as many questions as he/she wants, and to get answers that are honest and accurate.

# WE'RE BACK . . .

**Arney's Drinking Leads to Divorce**

Arney and I were moving more apart with each year. His drinking and his extramarital affair inflicted a painful emotional trauma. I buried myself in work and ignored him. He drowned himself in alcohol and ignored me.

He eventually had to run for reelection to Montcalm County District 64 B judgeship. The first campaign was great. We were like Bill and Hilary Clinton, pulling rich and poor, Black and white people into support for him. The second campaign was fairly automatic because the opponent was not well-known, and because Arney was not yet a complete disgrace due to his drinking.

He drank at least four times a week, and got sloppy, deadly drunk each time. You cannot hide a habit like that, but because he was a District Court Judge (and white), he got a pass on most of his transgressions.

But the third election was the end of it because his opponent was the son of a local preacher, and a sober man. All his opponent had to say was, "I am a sober Christian," and that was enough of a campaign speech to which Arney had no rejoinder, not being sober, and not setting foot in any church in the county. Neither of us was very religious, but I insisted that both girls get baptized. Like Elvis Presley said, "It would be a shame to miss out on going to Heaven on a technicality."

Before the vote, I made a grid to try and decide if I would stay with him or not. My decision was, if he won and was still drinking, I would leave. If he lost and was drinking, I would leave. If he won and stopped drinking, I would stay. If he lost and stopped drinking, I would stay. The operative word was drinking, and so I realized that winning or losing was not important.

He lost, and I filed for divorce. I did not care what people thought of me. Some may have said that I left because he lost, others may have said I left because he was with another woman. I know why I left, and so did he, so to hell with what other people said.

He moved out of the house, took his cat, and rented a place on Baldwin Lake. It was a strange 16 months. I hired a lady attorney, and he represented himself. My attorney had to remind me that, as participants in a divorce, we were opponents and adversaries, and could not be nice to each other. That was really hard to hang on to in small towns like Crystal, Sheridan, and Greenville, Michigan.

No judge in Montcalm County would hear the case, so the divorce took place in a county to the north. It was over so quickly, I hardly knew what happened, but it was just like the attorney said. We had previously hashed out all the details in the prior agreements, so all I had to do was tell the judge that, "I am not pregnant and I do want to proceed with the divorce." Done and done.

Every year for 14 years after the divorce, I had a divorce party, inviting my best female friends for dinner, drinks, and hot tub time at my house to celebrate my freedom from alcoholic life. Those were great parties and great women. I tried to hold them around a theme, so we would have reason to dress up and drink lots of wine—Roman togas, cowgirls, James Bond, Medieval Queens, Betty Crocker celebration, and many more occurred over the years with fond memories.

**Life Transitions**

Veronica and her husband moved to the Midwest, found jobs and a home, and had two children—first Ezekiel, then Magdalana.

Over the course of time, Arney's health declined, and he moved into a retirement community in Ohio, where he spent his last days able to see his youngest daughter and two grandchildren. He died in 2012, and our daughter made his life so wonderful in those last years.

In 2014, I decided that I, too, should just hang it up from the active practice of medicine, and so I left Indiana and came to Ohio, and landed a deal on a condo, not far from my daughter and her family.

**Dogs and Cats**

Dagmar, George, Heidi, Rom, Tyrian, Blitz, Jessie, Alia, Conan, Jane, Daweed, Drucilla, Seal, Shadow Icon, Trump, and more dogs and cats all have shared my life and pathway. I know that they are on the other side of the rainbow bridge, waiting for me to come and play with them and love them again. These are the dogs and cats we had over the years.

The best animal was Heidi, the white German Shepard. She probably had some kind of seizure disorder because whenever a two-cycle engine started, she began to chase herself into a circle trying to bite her tail. When Arney used the chainsaw, she turned into a whirling dervish and would collapse, exhausted, on the ground when he was done. Her partner was George, the black lab. Arney named her before we looked to see what she really was. Her best attribute was chasing skunks. One night, we woke up to a horrible smell coming into the bedroom on a summer night. Then we heard George barking and we went to see what was happening. She had cornered a skunk and the skunk had discharged a load of skunkum onto the dog's face and then ran away.

We washed George in everything—water, soap and water, tomato juice, milk, baking soda, vinegar—trying to remove the skunk smell. The dog did not mind; her sense of smell was gone for a couple of weeks as the skunk had hit her right in the nose.

One year, we had a massive outdoor party. Gus, a fellow we both knew and admired, set up his much-admired BBQ roaster and put on a quarter of beef to cook. We had 50 to 70 people roaming the place on Sloan Road, and everybody was drinking. This was in 1974 when Veronica was only six or eight months old, and we had a large pond fed by an artesian well on the property. Somehow or other, Veronica got put down on the sand by the edge of the pond and left alone. She crawled to the water and tipped in, face down.

The only one who saw her distress was Heidi the Shepard. Heidi dragged Veronica out of the water by the diaper and began to bark like a crazy banshee. Everybody saw what had happened and ran toward the dog and child. Heidi went ballistic and barred her teeth, ruffled up her fur, and started barking, keeping everyone away except Arney and me. We pulled Veronica out of the sand and saw that she was crying and breathing and OK. Rest assured that that dog never wanted for anything in the world after that. And when she died, we buried her on the property and planted a memorial pine tree over her grave.

Your pets will become fond memories for you, too, as you grow and develop. Remember, they are here to be your pets and serve as trainers for other relationships. If you can care for both a young pet and keep a plant alive for a year or more, then you may be ready to have a relationship with a human being. I learned that from the Sandra Bullock movie, *28 Days*, and I think it is a good lesson to hold on to.

**WJBK TV and My Journalism Career**

I was a television news reporter and local star on Detroit television in the mid-1960s. Betcha didn't know that.

Somewhere in the basement of my Ohio home is a container that holds old 16mm film rolls of me on TV, and there is a photo, hanging in my master bathroom, of me when I was starting as a reporter.

My mother worked for the *Michigan Chronicle,* had a great reputation in the Black community, and she was known in the white journalistic community as a person of influence. She got me my first real job in journalism by letting me work at the *Michigan Chronicle* as a reporter. As I said earlier, they assigned me to the wedding news. It was easy, weddings were frequent, and the writing was in a pro forma style. The photos were also nice to look at, and there was nothing controversial about the story. It was so boring, but it was steady.

The racial unrest, marching, civil rights activities, and problems of the '60s put a lot of pressure on the journalism/news communities across the nation. At some point, they decided it would be good to have a Black face on their news shows and Black reporters on their radio and newspaper staffs. WJBK was a CBS affiliate, owned by Storer Broadcasting and operating in Detroit. This was the time before cable, before the Internet, before cell phones. Television in Detroit had only one UVH TV channel and three VHF stations: channel two, CBS; channel four, the NBC outlet; and channel seven, the ABC outlet. There was a Fox station on the horizon, along with a Canadian station that most Detroiters could pick up easily. So, competition for viewers was between the three major outlet affiliates, and it was fierce.

The TV news shows went on at 6 PM, then the national news show followed. Having a lot of people looking at the local stuff was important to the national management, and the national management must have leaned on the locals to get a Black talking head in there to pull in viewers.

Initially, WBJK approached my mom because they had heard of her and knew she was known in the Black community. Bob McBride, the station manager, however, from what I understood, decided that she lacked photogenic acceptance—meaning, she was too old. He did not ask her to be on TV when he met her, rather, he asked if she knew anyone who might fit the bill. She gave him my name and I showed up for the job interview.

There was a Black woman already at the station, Trudy Haynes, but she lacked the charisma they were looking for, she was older than I was, and she was not pulling in the numbers they wanted. Plus, they did not feature her in any large or positive airings. She only got small stories and was not an announcer, just a feature reporter. I was lucky to get the spot. Trudy would have been great if they had trusted her to do the work. They did not, and she moved to another state and did very well on the air elsewhere.

Bob McBride seemed to have made his decision when I showed up, and so the interview was just to be sure I did not have horns and a tail, so to speak. I got hired.

The first thing he did was change my name. It seemed like all white owners wanted to do that to the Black people around them. Kunta Kinte became Toby. I became Sylvia Wayne.

I was still going to Wayne State University, finishing up my degree in journalism in 1966, so he told me that I should plan to either go to night school or drop out. I elected to go to night school and work for him. Then he said my name was too difficult. It was Hutchinson, because I was not yet married to Arney Mustonen. Either name would have been a problem, because both had three syllables, and were not easy to spell, either.

McBride then pronounced me Sylvia Wayne, because I was at Wayne State University, and it was similar to Haynes, the other Black woman who was on the way out. I'm sure he figured, because WE all looked alike, it would be just fine to give me a name that also sounded alike.

I started work in 1965, late in the year, and got assigned to a camera man whom I perceived as a resurrected hillbilly with an IBEW (International Brotherhood of Electrical Workers) membership, along with a sound engineer who was silent beyond belief.

In those days, TV news was filed on 16mm film and required a lot of heavy equipment to make things happen. The film had to be rushed back to the studio, developed, edited, spliced, and placed in the broadcast camera in a certain sequence for the announcers to follow. Time was of the essence, and there was a huge team of people making it all happen by 6 PM each night. This was back in the day when there was no Internet, no cell phones, no YouTube, TikTok, Snapchat, Twitter, Facebook, or even digital video cameras. Old school, all the way from story to TV camera.

My cameraman called me "Kid." He sneered a lot. My sound engineer drove the Chevy Suburban that we used as transportation from place to place. I was just a reporter. I went to various places and interviewed people that my editor, Carl Cederberg, lined up for me. At first, Carl told me what questions to ask, but later I figured out how to do it my own way.

My favorite question was "Why?" This was absolutely unheard of in TV news reporting at the time. The people I was interviewing were mostly in soft news stories, like the opening of food banks and charity events, but later I was given the city government reporting, and moved up to county government stories, as well.

The big news—which was any crime, political happenings, and union items—were the provenance of a white male reporter.

Not only would I ask WHY, I would also smile and be sexy while I was interviewing people. I would look them in the eye and cock my head to one side. It was distracting, but it went over with the viewers like gangbusters. Also, because I was usually the only woman and always the only Black person in the crowd of reporters, I got noticed by whomever was on the stage. My questions were always first or second in line to be answered.

I got to interview famous people who came to Detroit. Gene McCarthy, Democratic candidate for President Richard Nixon, the U.S. President himself, and Muhammed Ali, "The Greatest," were some that I actually spoke to. McCarthy had the sexiest green eyes. Nixon was as shifty and cold-natured in person as he appeared on TV. The Champ, Ali, was the most gorgeous physical body I had ever seen. They all had charisma, and if you ever get to see it, you, too, will realize how powerful it is.

My presence on local television was pretty powerful stuff, and viewership went up remarkably fast. I got noticed around town quickly. I loved the work. Who wouldn't? The job let me wear nice clothes and lots of makeup, get driven around town, be on TV, and smile for a living. I made $25,000 a year in 1967. In 2022 value, that would be $222,162, just to give you some perspective. But I was not the highest paid person on the news team; that was Jac LeGoff, the evening news anchor who got $100,000, which calculates to $888,647 in 2022 money.

I bought a Ford Mustang hatchback in a brown sugar-glaze color and loved my life. Arney and I were planning to get married, and things were going just great. He was in law school and was in the background of my life as an on-air personality. I enjoyed having a boyfriend to boast about at work.

No one at work really tried to bond with me. They were all white and older than me, and they were suspicious of my professional longevity. I believed that some were even jealous of my rapid rise.

Marilyn was the weather girl, John Kelly was the co-anchor, Jac LeGoff was the main anchor, Jerry Hodak was the other weather guy, and Joe Weaver was the big reporter. Jack McCarthy was the other white guy reporter. Carl was the managing editor.

Jac LeGoff was almost lured away from the station with an offer of $100,000 a year by the Canadian station, but according to the newsroom grapevine, Bob McBride heard about it, matched the offer, and sweetened it just to keep him. His name and reputation were golden in Detroit, and he was without a doubt the best-known local evening news anchor. All of them were fairly nice to me and friendly in a professional way, and as soon as they realized that the pecking order was not challenged, I was accepted. I even struck up a long-term friendship with reporter Erik Smith.

Unfortunately, one high-ranking person—who shall remain unnamed—made my life a living hell at the station. Not a day passed that he did not do something to harass me or shame me. He would walk through the newsroom, down the row of desks, and as he passed by me, reach into the crack of his pants to pull them out from between his butt cheeks, knowing that I alone would see this gesture.

At the end of the day, as I would go to my car, he would find a way to pull up in the parking lot in his car, roll down the window and make sexual advances to me, and then smile and drive off. He and one of his cohorts once cornered me in the basement near the film editing room and turned on a fire extinguisher aimed at my feet to make me dance. They were careful to do it when no one else was looking and quickly walked away when someone came around the corner. These and other indignities went on every week.

Who would I tell? My word against a powerful white man? Accusing him of any of this would be pushed aside. I told Arney, but he was not my husband yet and in no position to do or say anything either. There were no equal rights laws, whistleblower, or sexual harassment statutes, or #MeToo activities going on. I was on my own.

One white male colleague thought the whole situation was funny, but in a grudging fashion admitted that maybe "they should lay off a little because it wasn't nice." He thought it was funny, just not nice.

One day, long after I had left TV 2 and was well into my career in medicine, I got a call from some friends who told me that my harasser was interested in speaking to me and connecting. They said he had been terribly distressed by a family member's substance abuse problem and wanted to share his experience with me because he, too, was in Al-Anon.

I was tempted to speak to him, but decided that was not what I needed to do. I told my friends to let him know never to reach out to me again until he had found a way to apologize for all his secret, shameful behavior and cruelty that he had heaped upon me. In the Al-Anon recovery program, the act of recognizing all those whom you have harmed and then making amends to them is one of the 12 steps they encourage us all to practice.

I am still waiting for that Al-Anon Step 9 letter to come from that man.

All this harassment changed on Sunday, July 23rd, 1967.

## DIGRESSION #17: WHY REPARATIONS ARE A MISTAKE, BUT I WILL TAKE THE MONEY IF IT IS GIVEN

In 2020, the first year of COVID-19, there also arose a great resurgence of the movement for social and racial justice, and it was called Black Lives Matter. It started after a Black man named George Floyd was killed on May 25th, 2020 in Minneapolis, Minnesota.

A white police officer arrested him for supposedly passing a counterfeit $20 bill, handcuffed him, and put him in the police cruiser, then pulled him out of the back of the patrol cruiser, tossed him, handcuffed to the pavement, and kneeled on his neck for eight minutes and 46 seconds. Mr. Floyd died crying for breath, for Jesus, for his momma, in front of regular people on the street, in front of three other police officers, in front of the world. The world was able to watch because people pulled out their phone cameras, recorded it, and posted this gruesome video on YouTube.

The nation, and then the world, erupted into cries for social justice, an end to killing Black people, and the call for monetary reparations for 400 years of slavery here in the USA. Riots, marches, and demonstrations, as well as counter demonstrations, rocked the nation and the world. Figures in Black Lives Matter, as well as all the sports world, spoke out. Laws were changed, and confederate statues were pulled down, like the way the Iraqis toppled statues of Saddam Hussein. There were similar calls for justice for Native American people and LGBTQ+ people, as well. There was a call for reparations for Black Americans. We were supposed to get money for the horror that started in North America in 1619, and in South America in 1509, and continued into 2020.

I think that is a flawed idea.

If white people are given a chance to pay Black people for some crime against Black humanity that was committed by people who were not at all related to today's white people, then I think today's white people will take the opportunity to do it and slink back to a position that lets them feel that they no longer are part of the problem. White people can say, "We paid you Black people, now shut up and quit bothering us, quit asking for anything more. You got your money." They are let off the hook by the salve of the green poultice.

If you look at how Europeans in America "negotiated" with native populations, betrayed contracts and treaties, passed laws to create ethnic cleansing of entire regions (the Indian Removal Act, which allowed the Morrill Land-Grant Acts to function effectively, created Michigan State University, for example) so that white populations can claim land, you will see that giving money is not difficult for racist white leaders. The racist leaders and policy makers spoke with a forked tongue, then, to the Incas and Aztecs, to the Arawaks and Potawatomi, and Apache and the Sioux, and they will speak with a forked tongue to Black people in America, too. Giving money is not hurtful to the white racist leaders. They will be willing to pay a lump sum any day because that does not hurt them.

Making money in amounts equal to their racist leaders is what is hurtful. Keeping the money we rightfully create and/or earn is what is hurtful to them. Not paying money into their racist institutions is what hurts them.

Here is my suggestion.

My current property tax is $4,442.50 a year. In 30 years, if I did not have to pay that tax, that would come to $133,275 of income in my pocket. That sum does not include what I would save in sales tax. If I rounded up the figure to $10,000 to include all the sales and other taxes I pay, the amount over 30 years would be $300,000. Imagine if my grandchildren had $300,000 in savings, or in some kind of investment fund, by age 48. How much wealth would they have if they were able to work and earn, and keep all that they earn to use for positive purposes? A dollar would be a true and real dollar, not a portion of a dollar with the rest sent to the government that promotes their destruction.

I know Ta-Nehisi Coates made a marvelous argument in favor of reparations. I read his article in *The Atlantic* magazine, and was appalled at how horrifically Black people in America had been treated. Our history of suffering was worse than I could imagine, and it persisted longer than I even thought. He is right to quote the person who said that we, Black people, are poor now because of what happened to us back then. We are not poor because of how we are now at all. We have been subject to theft for centuries.

I would argue that instead of giving every Black American a lump sum and letting white people get off the hook, why not give every Black American a lifetime exemption from paying any taxes of any kind?

Taxes are a form of wealth accumulation for government. War and money, money and war, are intricately intertwined. Think of taxes this way. They are what we pay to a government that uses those funds to oppress Black people and people of color. So we are, in effect, paying to promote our own oppression. That needs to stop.

No more property taxes, income taxes, estate taxes, sale taxes, inheritance taxes, transfer taxes, FICA, FUTA, Medicare and Social Security taxes, or capital gains taxes, hotel taxes, or gasoline taxes for Black people.

Huey P. Newton, the co-founder of the Black Panther Party, wrote a book, *Revolutionary Suicide*, which made me think that, as Black Americans, we are subjected to taxation without representation, and that was one of the reasons white colonialists demanded independence. So, Black Americans should have independence from taxation, and maybe military service, too, because we are paying for no representation in our government, and are also forced to fight the government's wars of aggression against a world of POC and Black people.

I can only imagine how many people would decide to quit passing as white and claim to be Black for the money.

My dear grandchildren, you would come to this largess at age 18, and for the rest of your lives have no tax burden. White people might not feel that money is being taken from them and given to Black people, but rather look at it as money Black people are not paying, not what whites are losing. This method does not allow white people to shirk their duty of growing up into being socially just and accepting of racial equality. That struggle can and should continue.

Remember also that cash in hand is cash in hand. How you decide how much to give each Black person could be a problem. Does a person have to prove he/she is Black? Does a person have to prove he/she is descended from people in slavery?

Former President Barak Obama, as I understand it, would get nothing (his father was Kenyan and his mother was white American), but former First Lady Michelle Obama (her parents are African American) would get something. Is that fair?

Do you give the money to the people who are incarcerated? If not, then what happens to their share, and why are they not being included in the count? What if you are a person with Black blood and very light skin who has passed for white? Do you now declare that you are Black? What if you are just a person who was raised with Black people, and now you claim you identify as a Black person because of how you were raised? Does that count? Do poor Black people get more than well-to-do and wealthy Black people, or is the distribution completely equal? There is no adequate sum that you can calculate for all Black Americans.

Tax exemption is the only truly equal method.

I asked Siri on my iPhone to calculate the total dollars if every Black American got $1,000, assuming there are 30 million Black people, as of this writing. The poor thing, she said, 3e10, which looks like this: $30,000,000,000.

No way will white people give up cash like that to Black folks. Nor should they. First of all, they cannot. Even billionaires such as Warren Buffet, the Koch brothers, Jeff Bezos, Elon Musk, and the U.S. government do not have, in aggregate, enough money to do that and still run the country.

Secondly, once you let a criminal perpetrate a crime against you and then agree to settle for cash instead of true justice, you give the perp permission to harm another, and you create yourself as a paid victim sell out.

In addition to not ever paying taxes, I think reparations should be tangible and should directly address the areas where Black people have been systematically oppressed, repressed, excluded, and punished since 1619.

Consider this system as my alternative to reparations:

1. Black people are allowed but not required to serve in any branch of the military.
2. Every county sheriff's department and every state police department should have numbers of Black officers proportionate to the numbers of Black people in the county and the state served.
3. Every tertiary educational institution should have free tuition for any qualified Black student who pursues a Doctorate level or Master's level degree. Law, medicine, architecture, engineering,

business, education, nursing, theology, philosophy, arts, literature, and more will blossom.

4. Every county will have polling places located in every public building. Schools, libraries, police stations, fire houses, township offices, city halls, and county halls, should be available for this.
5. No Black person will pay any interest on any home mortgage or business loan. No Black person will pay any tax on any property, personal, or commercial activity.
6. All banks will have more than one Black officer on the board of directors and in C-level positions.
7. All Black people who are renting space of any kind, will pay one-half of the current rent.
8. All Black prisoners who were convicted of a drug-related charge, and have served at least one year, will be released out of jail and given parole. They will also be entered into drug rehab, job training, and education programs.
9. No Black person will pay for any kind of health care. All doctors, hospitals, clinics, dentists, and other health professionals will treat us for free.
10. All food purchases made by Black people will be at half price in any store.

These 10 points will continue for 400 years.

Reparations need to directly touch the people who have benefited from the oppression of slavery and the uneven legacy of wealth that accrued to them.

I would take the money and I would be happy to get anything. But I would not want white people to be able to say that they are now off the hook and no longer need to worry about being racist or participating in racist activities anymore. Money is good, but it may not be the way to end the horrible inequity that has made America so racially cracked apart.

It is just a thought.

WE'RE BACK . . .

**Married in Detroit During the 1967 Riot**

The tensions across the country fueled by racism came to a head when the city of Detroit erupted in a race riot one hot July night. The police busted a blind pig—which is an after-hours illegal bar—on the near east side of town, and people exploded in violence during the arrest. Legal drinking establishments had to close at 2 AM, but Black people, who were not allowed into those places, set up their own illegal drinking locations with no closing hour except sunrise.

Word spread and pockets of violent outbursts quickly developed. First, fights and fires began on the east side and spread across Woodward to the west side.

It was on the first Sunday of riot week, early afternoon, when Arney and I and his old college roommate, Patrick, were coming back from the Milford, Michigan shooting range. We were driving back home along the Lodge Freeway when I saw smoke coming from behind Henry Ford Hospital. Patrick called out that he saw smoke coming from the other side of the freeway, and Arney saw smoke coming from points in front of us in the downtown area. We went to our home. I called the TV station.

"Come in quick," Carl said. "We need you. There's a riot in the city!"

Arney and I had recently gotten married, on June 30th, 1967, and the riot broke out shortly afterward. He and I had both graduated in June of 1967—him from law school, me from journalism studies. He was working for the Detroit Interfaith Action Council as their attorney, and I was working at the TV station, but we were still living on the house on Fourth Street—the dead-end where the westbound Ford Freeway exit ramp took traffic to the northbound Lodge Freeway. Our house was across the street from the rental unit that Warren owned, which I had lived in with my roommates, Linda and Shelley.

I went to work, and the newsroom was buzzing like an overturned wasp's nest (sorry about the pun). Everybody was there, and assignments were being given out. I went with Ken and Bill somewhere up Woodward for "action shots." Other reporters were sent to city hall and police headquarters.

It did not take too long for all news organizations to realize that the rioters would not have anything to do with any white face coming in for an interview. Also, no white face was safe in any of the areas where rioting was still happening. I was the only Black TV personality in the city, so I got to go everywhere.

Because he was old and probably frightened, my cameraman was reassigned to another reporter. I got the new guy, Bud. He was full-on Irish, and proud of it, too. And he was the most helpful, caring, generous coworker I ever had at the station.

Early in the riot, I was informed of a meeting that was going to be held by the "Black coalition of peacemakers" at a church near the Dexter-Davison area on the city's west side. It was closed to white people. All the leaders of Black Detroit would be there, and many of them were college friends I knew from Wayne State. Carl asked me if I would go and try to get a statement, or at least make some B-roll action footage to be used for a voice-over report. I said yes, taking Bud and my silent sound engineer with me.

We threaded our way along West Grand Boulevard, past Motown's headquarters, then passed looters running along Dexter Avenue before arriving at the church where the meeting was being held.

I walked to the door, leaving my cameraman and sound engineer at the car, getting equipment set up outside. I recognized one of the leaders of the meeting and asked if I could get an interview when it was over. He and I knew each other, peripherally from Wayne State University campus days. He said I could come in, so I motioned to Bud and my sound guy, and as they walked up to the entry, they were accosted by the group behind my friend.

They were decidedly not nice to my crew. They began with:

"Ain't no white mutherfuckers coming in here."

"Get whitey the fuck out of here."

"Take your weak shit white asses and get the fuck out."

"She's OK, but we don't want none of y'all crackers."

More statements like this began to boil up. I looked at my friend. I pinned him in place with my most professional stare and I said:

"I know you have a message, and you know you have a message, and I know you know you have a message. But if you want that message heard, you will say it to me. There is no other reporter here, local, state, or national. And, rest assured, everything you say to me will be televised local, state, and fucking national. If you are going to say it to me, you are going to let my crew come in with me, or the deal is off and no one will hear you."

We had a brief stare-down, but I smiled and then he smiled, and signaled to let all three of us in the room. He made me keep the cameras turned off during the open meeting, but afterward, I interviewed him and gave him plenty of time to make his point. I even told him how to structure it so that his point would not get edited out back in the film room. People crowded around behind him as he spoke, doing the equivalent of "photo bombing," as he answered my questions.

We drove back to the studio with the hottest story of the day. In fact, it ran on the 11 PM news, and the noon and 6 PM news the next day. The leader who gave that interview later went on to become a member of the Detroit City Council a few years after the riots and racial tension calmed down.

That riot lasted from the 23rd till the 28th of July, and left 43 people dead, 342 injured, and 1,400 buildings burned. It took 7,000 National Guard and U.S. Army troops to quell the event. The city changed a lot, mostly for the better, as a result of that riot. That year, there were riots in Newark, New Jersey and Gary, Indiana, and the entire nation was filled with violence, anger, and fear.

I was hot stuff on the air during this time. The national CBS network sent its top reporters into town because the city was under martial law for a week, and the U.S. Army 82nd Airborne unit was in town, too. The night they came into the city, Arney and I could hear them moving up along the westbound Ford Freeway. The noise was very strange to my ears, but Arney said it was the sound of metal treads on pavement: "Those are tanks." He knew that sound because he had served in the U.S. Army.

President Lyndon B. Johnson was not taking any more shit from the rioters—the troops were in town. President Johnson was livid because of the disorder, and was turning up the heat on all levels of government. It was BIG news.

I was everywhere. There was no door closed to me for interviews during, as well as after, the riot. The top white male reporter lost a lot of traction in the newsroom power ranking. The CBS reporter gave my name to the people at CBS headquarters and told them to approach me for a national job.

I was told by CBS national reporter Jon Hart that I would get a phone call from THEM to come in and have an interview. Bob McBride heard about it, of course, and he called me to his office for "a serious talk." This was about a month after the riot was officially over. He told me that I was going to get a $5,000 raise immediately, as well as a bonus, and all I had to do was sign a new contract. The phone call had not come, and I was not sure it really would. I signed the contract.

Later CBS hired another Black woman, Michelle Clark. She rose to fame and did a fabulous job. She later perished in an airplane flight on assignment. I would have been in her spot had I not signed the contract that prevented me from accepting work with CBS. Fate is powerful, baffling, and cunning. What I wanted—a job at CBS—would have been the end of my marriage and my death. And for my dear grandchildren, it would have meant no birth of your mom or Aunt Ophelia, and more importantly, no YOU.

I think on that and wonder what would have been my life path if I had said no to McBride and yes to CBS. Would I have perished on that flight or not? Fate is wonderfully weird and unpredictably twisty.

Bud and my sound engineer remained as my primary work crew,

but I also worked with Mike and Sid. Sid taught me a lot about camera presence and editing, and served as a mentor and director when we worked together.

I was at WJBK from December 1966 to June 1969. Great times, and lots of fame and recognition. That one prominent white man at the station stopped harassing me because I was a star in the pecking order.

Arney got a job in Detroit, being "of counsel" with a law firm in the Penobscot Building downtown, but was never happy with the work. He later saw an ad in the legal news about a small country practice for sale in Montcalm County. He inquired about it, visited it, and liked it and accepted the offer. He told me we were moving to mid-Michigan, and I had to let the job at WJBK go.

He was my husband and I did not want to lose him. I made the decision to leave my life at WJBK and move to Crystal with Arney. We talked a long time about making this move. The occurrence of the riot made us fearful of being an interracial couple in the city, and fearful of how we would raise any children in such an atmosphere of racial hatred. It turned out to be the best decision I could have made.

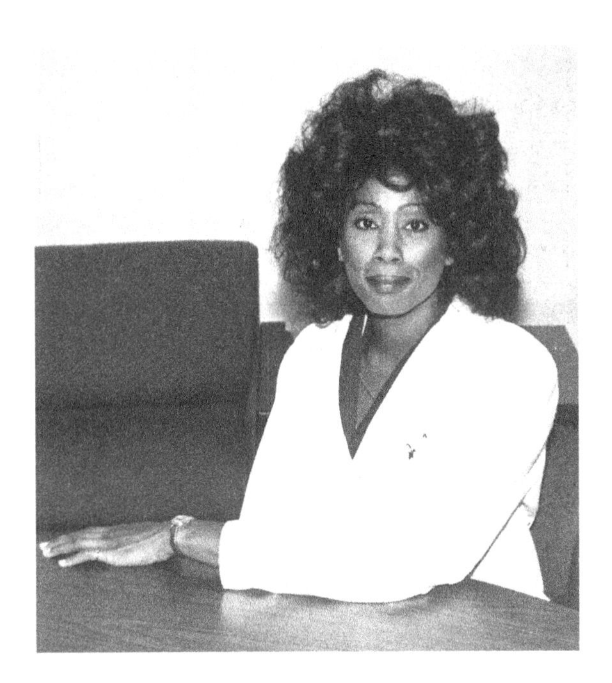

# SECTION THREE
# MY LIFE IN ACTIVE PRACTICE, STEP BY STEP, PLACE BY PLACE

**Crystal, Michigan**

So, we left Detroit and moved to Crystal, Michigan in the summer of 1970.

Living in Crystal was an idyllic sojourn from city life and would have been perfect except for the boredom and Arney's drinking. One day, he got drunk, stayed late at the bar, and drove his car off the road into a small tree trunk. He lived and was not seriously injured, and did not even get a ticket because he was the lawyer.

That gave me a jolt. I had two children, no job, and a husband who was unintentionally suicidal when drunk, and he was drunk a lot. What would happen when and if he died like that? Unpaid home, not enough insurance money, no chance for college for my kids, and no work opportunity for me! All this was on the horizon down that path. I had to do something.

I decided to go to medical school.

Back when I was a sophomore at Cass Tech High School, my guidance counselor told me that my grades in math were not so good, and because of that, I should think about learning to type, get a job as a secretary, and meet someone I could marry. Of course, you listened to your elders back then, and he was a Black man of impressive bearing and intelligence. So, I learned to type in a summer class at the local community center. I got up to 67 words a minute with no errors, 90 with errors, and later, after graduation and during my last year of undergraduate life at Wayne State, I found a job at the free legal aid clinic, which was also where Arney worked as a law student.

I told Arney I wanted to apply to med school, and he reluctantly said OK. I knew that I had a lot to make up because I had avoided science and math classes in my undergraduate life, so I had to take those prerequisites before I could even apply. Thank goodness there was Montcalm Community College and Central Michigan University close to where we lived. The biology and science classes at MCC were a breeze. The chemistry at CMU was a challenge, but the physics classes were simple. I got done with all of those in two years and applied.

**Michigan State University College of Osteopathic Medicine**

Michigan State had just opened the College of Osteopathic Medicine, and because it was in-state, I applied. I really did not know much about Osteopathic medicine, even though both my family doctor and my surgeon were DOs. I also applied to Cornell and the University of Michigan. I was accepted into all three. Because I got letters of recommendation from my physicians, and because it was close, I picked MSUCOM.

One other factor that made me pick MSU was my personal interview with John Upledger, DO, famous or infamous in the profession (it depends on who you ask), and he was motivational and inspirational to me. He also became my mentor in COM, and we remained close friends all my professional life up till he died.

I had to live on campus at MSU for five days a week, and I drove home on weekends to see my family. Arney was in charge of child raising, and like a good father and confirmed alcoholic, he found someone else to shoulder the load. We hired a lady named Mrs. Z, a person who was, to put it politely, a sick controller trash collector. Nowadays, they are called hoarders, and I am sure there is a psychological diagnosis that also fits.

She occupied the rental unit on the back of our property on Sloan Road, and when her family moved her in, they grinned and laughed on the way out, saying, "She's all yours now." She collected and kept EVERYTHING. Bottles, *National Geographic* magazines, newspapers, potholders, cups, bows, ribbons, bottles, photos, plastic gallon milk jugs, plates, Christmas decor, stuffed kewpie dolls, cooking paraphernalia, and 50 years of collected bullshit filled up her living quarters.

The place was easily 1,200 square feet in size, but she had just a narrow pathway from the door to her bed because all the rest was filled with boxes of her collectibles. My children suffered under her harsh care and their father's benign neglect. He was working and never saw what went on; I was at school and never saw what went on. I am so sad now thinking about how much neglect was going on in their lives as I pursued a lifelong dream, and their father pursued a doomed relationship. It is amazing that my children came out as good as they did, given their circumstances.

The first year was all academics. We attended class by day and studied notes by night. Some of us formed study-buddy groups; some did not. I served as a scribe and sold notes to classmates so that they could focus on listening to the lecture. This was before lectures were on video format in the school library, or on YouTube, or live on-demand learning formats now, which meant students actually had to show up to learn.

I was trained in journalism, so it was natural for me to work as a scribe. Remember, this is before the Internet and everything being on video, so you had to take notes as the lecture proceeded. I took notes for three or four people, and they paid me to do so. I think I got the most out of the class, because taking notes, reviewing, and rewriting them really pushed the information into my brain. I was a scribe and I researched the textbooks, too, to back up the notes.

**Intersection of Sexism and Medical Education at MSUCOM**

How sad that I even have to mention this, but sexism is part of life in America. One of our first-year classes was biochemistry, which for me was a real ass kicker. I studied hard but the professor was even harder. I do recall one of his lectures was on the formation of sex hormones from cholesterol. At last, a real good reason to have cholesterol. I heard him say that estrogen, which is the end of the pathway of sex hormone formation, was just the by-product of testosterone. One could argue that this is entirely correct if you look at the pathway from a structural viewpoint only, a cleavage of one carbon group creates estrogen C18 from testosterone C19. But there is never any mention of hierarchy of either hormone in the chemical discussions I read then or now.

His opinion was that testosterone was the product of importance. I did not see him smile as he said this, or indicate that he was just joking. We were sitting so quietly and taking it all down on our note papers because he was a PhD in a major Midwestern Big 10 university, and we were first year, first semester medical students. Who would challenge him? None of us ever did, but it was a statement that rankled me a lot then as it does now. That sexist shit was a pervasive poison then, and seems to remain one now.

**My Clinical Office Rotations**

The second year, we were placed in clinical rotations at various family medicine offices in the state. I was at Harry DeVore's office in a small town just north of Lansing, Michigan, and he was absolutely the nicest doctor I had ever met. He and his wife took me under their wings and helped me learn so much about practical office skills. Suturing, casting, script writing, and much more came to me as a result of his kind oversight. I made it a point to get rotations in the area served by doctors on staff at Carson City Hospital. I knew I wanted to do my internship there and I naturally planned to practice in that same area.

The worst family physician I saw (who shall remain nameless out of respect for his legacy), claimed that he saw 80 patients a day and was proud of it. He literally just saw them and did not even go in the exam room.

He employed two PAs (Physician Assistants) in his office who did the grunt work and heavy lifting, and had an RN (Registered Nurse) who told the PAs what they were supposed to do. This is the same way he made hospital rounds.

He would look at the chart, look in the room, say something to the patient about what was going to happen next, and move on. He dictated orders to the RN at his side and she wrote them down. Then the intern came back and performed whatever it was he had ordered. He was the biggest admitting physician to the hospital, so the administration loved him. His list of patients was never less than 20 each week, and they all had some high impact imaging, multiple labs, and a consult with everybody for every body part that had any kind of problem.

He was a money machine back in the days of fee for service with high reimbursements. No patient complained of his care because no one thought it was wrong. He kept people in the hospital for a week minimum, and longer if he could. He never showed up on time for any delivery, which was fine because we interns would always get lots of OB experience if it were one of his patients who was in labor. He usually came in two or three hours post-delivery, well-dressed and rested, and congratulated the new mom on her birth. His patients loved him.

If he had a patient who was really critical, he would always transfer care and management to either the internist or the surgeon, and step out of the line of fire. The specialists loved him because they always got a nice challenging case to work up, and lots of consults that were bread and butter in the money train for them. As long as insurances and Medicaid and Medicare were paying, this was how he rolled.

**Dr. Musta Mustonen**

The best rotation I did was with my brother-in-law, Mike Mustonen, and it was in Michigan's Upper Peninsula, in Ewen (pronounced YOU-win).

Arney had two younger brothers who both went to medical school in Kirksville, Missouri. Mike went into family medicine; Jon went into ER medicine. Mike had loans to repay to the Federal Health Services and they placed him in this part of the country because it was underserved. It also had a goodly number of people who were Finnish, and since Mike was also Finnish, it was a good fit. He and his wife, Sara, located there and enjoyed the rough woodsy beauty of the place.

I came up there for a six-week stint and really looked forward to it. I would be staying with family and working in a truly rural clinic. Looking at the map, it is easy to see there is difficulty getting to the western part of the state, but I did it. It was a 10-hour drive and I made it. The hardest part was driving across the Mackinac Bridge, a five-mile-long suspension bridge spanning the connecting point of Lake Michigan and Lake Huron, where winds can be strong enough to flip a car over the edge and plunge it into the water far below. So my mantra while driving over the bridge was, "Don't look down!" Then, the boring part was the six-hour drive across the UP, with the world's dullest highway from Seney to Shingleton before I got to Ewen.

How dull was the drive you ask? It was so dull that there was only one bar/tavern on the whole stretch, and it had gone out of business in the UP, which is almost impossible to do.

Mike's clinic was a double wide trailer. There were two exam rooms. Three days of the week, I worked with him, and the other two days of the week, I drove to Ontonagon to work with another MD family physician, who also served as the region's surgeon. Say "AUNT nah gun" and move all the air out through your nose and you will be speaking it UP style. Ontonagon was at the base of the Keweenaw Peninsula, and the entry to Michigan's famous old Copper Country. I got to see Lake Superior in all its fall glory from August to September.

The surgeon was remarkable. He did tonsils and adenoids, hernias, appendectomies, C-sections, hysterectomies, GSW (Gun Shot Wound) extractions, circumcisions, skin and breast biopsies, and PE (Pressure Equalizer) tubes for the ears. He was a family physician, and his patients loved him. He was a good teacher and inspired me to try to add as many of those hand skills as possible into my clinical repertoire.

Mike was equally loved by his patients, not just because he was a Finn, but because he was a musician and a loving, caring doctor who practiced the tenets of Osteopathy with all his heart and soul.

I recall one Monday when we opened for the day, a man came in with a terrible fish hook injury, which occurred on Saturday night. The hook was still in the hypothenar area, the side of the palm just below the baby finger. He had put a dressing over it and covered it in some kind of salve, and waited till Monday to be seen.

When I asked why he waited so long he said, "I didn't want to wake Doctor up. He works so hard; he needs his rest."

We extracted the hook, repaired the damage, applied a dressing, and gave him a shot of hope-we're-not-too-late-with-this-cillin and a tetanus booster. He got better and did just fine. What wonderful people they were.

The entire region was devoid of cultural diversity. There were a few people who were Native Americans, but they mostly stayed away. The rest were descendants of Finnish and Cornish settlers who came over for the logging work, mining iron, and copper industries in the late 1800s. They were rugged, hardworking, honest, friendly, quiet people who drank when they did not work, and worked when they did not drink, and hunted in-between. Amazingly, there were no people of color. (I paste a snide look here.)

I think the last Black person I saw was probably 200 miles south of the Mackinac Bridge.

I got looked at a lot, but when they were told that I was Dr. Mustonen's sister-in-law, studying medicine and learning from him, I got immediate acceptance.

I did not speak Finnish, but fortunately I did not have to. Mike knew some and his nurse knew the rest. But I found that the language of medicine, and always showing compassionate awareness and caring, is fairly easy. It is the way you greet a person, touch them, smile, or listen that mattered. Over the six-week time, I got to meet and treat a lot of his regular patients and establish rapport with them as well as develop diagnostic skills. It was truly hands-on and rewarding to be there. I am always, even now, grateful for the time my brother-in-law took with me, and for what he taught me.

On my last week of rotation, a patient came to the clinic asking to see Dr. Mustonen. The receptionist asked him, "Which one?" in Finnish:

"Valkoinen henkilo or musta ihminen."

He said, "Laakari Musta Mustonen," which means Doctor Black Mustonen. I was Black and he was white, but I was his doctor and he was my patient, and he was happy to have it that way.

In Finnish, the name Mustonen, loosely translated, means gypsy or dark person, so I was finally accepted and recognized as part of the treating team in the Ewen clinic. I was so happy to have that moniker bestowed on me.

Once we finished our second year, we had to do our third year, which was spent in hospital rotations. I picked Grand Rapids Osteopathic Hospital, which was known then as GROH, but now has changed its name to Metropolitan Hospital—dropping the city and the professional identification completely.

Shame on them, to stop wanting to be identified as Osteopathic. In my stretch of professional life, I have seen most of the Osteopathic hospitals do the same thing. They quit using "Osteopathic" and merge with some larger allopathic institution, giving up all the things that made them distinct.

## DIGRESSION #18: MD AND DO PROFESSIONS WILL MERGE

There will come a time when the DO and the MD professions are the same. For the past 150 or so years, that trajectory has been gaining momentum. The final culmination is not far off.

Andrew Taylor Still, MD, DO, was the founder of the Osteopathic profession in 1874 in America, and in 1892, established the first school of Osteopathic Medicine. In 1899, Daniel David Palmer—who was the founder of the Chiropractic profession in America—wrote that he was one of Still's students. Still also employed John Martin Littlejohn, who was the founder of the British School of Osteopathy Medicine in Great Britain in 1913. A.T. Still was a son of a Methodist preacher, a military physician for the Union in the Civil War, and was convinced that medicine as he saw it was deeply flawed.

Over the course of decades, he developed his theory and put it into practice with astonishing results. He was excommunicated from his church, which said that laying hands on people to cure them was work that only Jesus/God could do. He started the first College of Osteopathic Medicine in 1892, and admitted men and women. He treated all who needed his skill and care.

The Osteopathic profession avoided all medications, surgeries, and vaccinations at its inception, and used only the skill of the practitioner's hands to restore blood flow to diseased organs, which then resumed normal function.

The MD profession ignored Osteopathy, vilified it, then finally, grudgingly accepted it after WWII. That acceptance occurred because no DO was allowed in the ranks of service, so they became the physicians for their communities while the MDs were overseas. Can you believe that the US government would let Black men go overseas, give them guns and pensions, but would not let a DO physician go? Stupid racism is the worst kind.

After the war, there was no way to disallow the gains DOs had made and the acceptance by the public, and no way to deny them the right to set up clinics, open hospitals and colleges. They did. They thrived.

The American Osteopathic Association (AOA) preached that DOs were distinctive and different in how they treated patients, but the same as MDs in their training and skillset. That does not make sense philosophically or epistemologically. The professions can be equal, similar, or related. I do not think they can be the same. The terminology was as stupid as the phrase "separate but equal." You cannot be the same but different; either you are the same or you are different.

The AOA was making us the same. The AOA sought the same payment structure as the MDs in the halls of Congress, and the AOA supported the American Medical Association (AMA) whenever there was a need to keep reimbursements equally flowing to both practitioners. The AOA supported the same quality reporting bullshit that the AMA wanted under the ACA/Obamacare era. The AOA supported and copied the same recertification bullshit that the

AMA imposed on its membership. The AOA lost membership of its family physicians, just as the AMA did. In fact, the AMA at one time encouraged DOs to join its ranks, but as non-voting members. Yeah, that old separate but equal bullshit came into play there, too.

ACGME, COMLEX, FLEX, AOCGME, and all other MD-DO designations are going to merge into one large conglomerate. We DOs will become subsumed by the MDs because there are more of them than there are of us. Our only hope to remain professionally alive is to be sure that the MD-DO degree designation evolves to recognize both sets of professions.

Patients loved DOs for the honest communication and hands-on healing. But the profession changed as science marched on. The Flexner Report in 1910 exposed the problems of medical education, and DOs had to step up or be left out. Vaccinations were accepted, some became surgeons, and all began to use pharmaceutical medications. Over time, there was an erosion in the number of DOs who used manual skills alone, so those practitioners became a specialty—the Academy of American Osteopathy—to preserve those skills in the profession.

MD hospitals routinely refused privileges to DOs, the same as they did to Black physicians in the first half of the twentieth century. Both DOs and Black MD physicians set up their own hospitals in response to this shutout.

Both kinds of hospitals were eventually absorbed by the MD institutions, for different reasons ostensibly, but actually because of money and bed counts. Hospitals got funded by Medicare for training new doctors and for caring for patients. Much of that funding was based on bed count. The more beds a hospital had, the higher its funding from Medicare would be.

MD hospitals receiving Medicare funds to train physicians accepted DO students (for the money) and found their training was equal or better than the MD students. Competition for students developed between MD and DO hospitals. Because there were more MD hospital spots open for graduates, more and more DO graduates went to MD hospitals for post-doctoral training. DO hospitals began to lose students, and then lose patients, and then, worst of all, lose income. They were usually situated in the older, poorer part of town, and reliant on Medicaid and low-reimbursement insurances. Their income dropped, and mergers became the way to stay alive as an institution.

Even though the number of DO colleges increased, the number of training program spots in DO hospitals was hard pressed to keep up with the number of slots needed for both MD and DO graduates. There were not enough DO hospitals with specialty and sub-specialty training programs to service the demands DO students were making. Those students were defecting to MD hospitals that offered the sub-specialty training they wanted.

So, in 2017, the change occurred where there was a merger of post graduate training programs between the MD and DO entities. This means that any DO can go train in any MD hospital, and alternatively, any MD can train in any DO hospital. It also allows the MD board exams to be open to DO students. State licensing boards by this time have already accepted DOs to practice in all 50 states—Louisiana was the last one to open up and recognize the DO degree.

So, it is a natural progression that the DO and MD degrees will also merge. When? Who knows, but it is on the horizon.

One day, a student who graduates from my alma mater, MSUCOM, will have the initials DO, MD, and a student who graduates from University of Michigan Medical School will have the initials MD, DO, behind his or her name. MD students and practitioners routinely seek out Osteopathic post-doctoral training in all the myriad varieties of skilled hands-on healing that has been developed and researched by DOs over the 150 plus years of the profession's founding.

Holistic healing, the keystone of Osteopathy, is now a catchphrase in allopathic medicine. Patients appreciate the demeanor of the DO physician because we are taught to be patient-centered, and

MDs see how attractive this is and strive to copy it.

Maybe we DOs will become incorporated into the MD structures of education and training and work our magic from within and convert them to our philosophy by stealth.

WE'RE BACK . . .

**Externship at Grand Rapids Osteopathic Hospital**

My time at GROH was great.

I had to find a place to live while I was there, and rented a room in a complex owned by the hospital. It was on the hospital grounds so I could be ready for rounds by 7 AM, or ready for surgery by 6 AM, without difficulty. That meant that I was living away from home again, only able to come back on a Saturday to see my husband and kids.

This is where physicians are made. The clinical skills I learned in offices gave me the heart of a physician, and the clinical skills I learned in hospitals gave me the hands of a physician. Nurse Practitioners (NPs) do not have this, nor do Physicians Assistants (PAs), and one must not forget that training does matter. No amount of book learning will replace actual experience.

Look at it this way. If you read about impressionist art, travel around the world to look at, write papers about, give speeches and lead discussion groups about impressionist art, or even hold Zoom meetings for discussing impressionist art, but never pick up a paint brush and *create* it, are you, therefore, an impressionist artist? I think not. NP does not equal doctor.

The first day of orientation, Neil Natkow, DO, announced that he was our DME, Director of Medical Education, and he wanted us all to know that he was our friend, possibly our only friend, for the next year of externship. God, was he right!

Externship—which means shadowing a medical professional to observe and learn—is the title you receive for the last year of medical school. The next step up the ladder is internship, which is your first year of hospital training after you have graduated from medical school. Then, if it is called for, your next training level is resident, in which you spend the final years of training in your specialty.

Fellowship is the final level of training and is optional, but is done by those who are going into a sub-specialty or an affiliated specialty. For example, you can become a family physician who has completed his residency in Family Medicine, then completed a fellowship in Sports Medicine by completing a CAQ (Certificate of Additional Qualification). Or, you complete a residency in gastroenterology, and then do a fellowship in hepatology for two more years, to specialize in disorders of the liver.

But as an extern, we were the bottom feeders in the pool of medical education. We ranked just above slime, mold, and water bears in the hospital system of respect and responsibility.

That system goes like this for physicians in hospitals: VP of Medical Affairs, Chief of Staff, Department Head, section chief, committee chair, chief resident, resident, chief intern, intern, and finally, extern, who is also known as the POS scut monkey.

For nursing staff: VP of Nursing, Director of Nursing, Charge Nurse, Department Charge Nurse, RN, Licensed Practical Nurse (LPN), medical assistant, nurse's aide, patient care worker, then volunteer.

The similarity is that both externs and volunteers were unpaid and bossed around by everybody else in the hospital.

The hospital was exciting and full of merry medical adventures. Because I was married and not a fool, I kept to myself. I showed up, did my work, attended rounds, read, and went back to my apartment at the end of the day. Getting involved in hospital hanky-panky is the path to social death. I saw it happen and avoided it.

There were good days and there were bad days, and there were days that my momma never told me about while I was at GROH.

My first attendance at a death was horrible. A young woman came in for delivery, and I am not sure what degree of prenatal care she had, but she was complete and ready to push and at term. It was her first child and I was going to be allowed to do the delivery with my resident supervisor, Dr. William Nowak. He was so good at teaching because he was patient and explained everything. The lady was on the table, and Nowak was at my side. The baby came out pale, gray, and limp, and not breathing or crying, but had a slow heartbeat. Bill took the baby after I had completed the delivery and began to resuscitate it.

If you have never had a baby or seen one delivered, the kid looks horrible coming out: bloody, gooey, a creamy-gray color or ashy mauve, and sometimes there is baby poop called meconium in the fluid. Then it starts to wriggle, and you suck the amniotic fluid out of its mouth and nose with the syringe or bulb before it cries. And then it cries and wriggles, and everything gets better, pinker, and louder.

This baby did not do any of that.

Bill told me, "Deliver the placenta. Just wait and massage her uterus, it will come out. I'm busy over here."

The stress in his voice was obvious. I could see the infant was limp in his arms as he rushed over to the far side of the room to begin working on the child.

He called a code and for the pediatricians to come into L and D, and both showed up. They then got the newborn crash cart, and more nurses and respiratory techs showed up. There were three doctors and four nurses and techs around that newborn over in the far corner from me and the mom on the delivery table. Neither she nor I could see what was going on, but I knew that it was not good because I never heard a cry from the infant. She looked at me and asked me, "Is my baby OK?"

There is a long moment, in my memory, of time struggling to pass between her question and my answer. *Oh my gosh, she is asking me, and this is my first time helping a woman with a delivery.* I had seen my own children born, but they were OK. This one was not. These words whirled inside my head as I waited for the placenta to fall out.

WTF could I say? My first delivery and her first child, and the situation was critical. I told her they were taking care of her child. I don't even recall the sex of the baby. Eventually her placenta came out. I counted the cotyledons (these are 15 to 20 structures on the placenta that nourish the fetus with oxygen and nutrients from the mother's blood) and massaged the uterus to expel the rest of the blood and fluid, and made sure the uterus contracted down. I inspected the perineum for tears and rips. None seen, so I cleaned her up and stood by her. I held her hand while her baby was given 30 to 60 minutes of CPR in futility.

One of the pediatricians came over and gave her the bad news. We all stood around as he told her what had happened, why the baby died, and what the plan was for now, for her and the baby. I had faded into the background of white coats and green scrubs surrounding her labor and delivery bed. That poor young woman lost a child. Could any of the loss have been prevented? I cried myself to sleep that night, and I am sure that young mom did, too. I knew I wanted to do obstetrics, and this was actually inspirational for me because I never wanted to have a woman lose a child that way ever again. I vowed to be the best family physician doing OB that I could.

That was my first experience with death as an extern; next up was addiction.

Drug addiction is a fact of American life, and those who are in the medical delivery system are not immune to it. In fact, I feel we health providers are more susceptible because of the exposure and access and lack of oversight.

One resident in the ENT (Ear, Nose, Throat) service at GROH was a cocaine addict, but no one knew. He had free access to the tincture of cocaine that was kept under lock and key in the ER opioid cabinet and no one questioned him when he asked for it. His habit caught up with him because he actually passed out on the OR table and was found to have had a huge hit of cocaine and heroin just before coming to do the procedure. His trainer, Stan Kunkle, finished the procedure, and then everyone had to figure out what to do with this young man whose career was flushing away like a large turd. He was moved out of the system in a fashion I do not know at this point in my life. I hope he was placed into the State of Michigan rehabilitation program for addicted physicians, but I do not know for sure.

Besides death and drug addiction, I got to experience racism up close and personal in my training at GROH.

Each month, externs were placed on a service and worked with all the residents and attendings in that service. The externs were required to attend all the meetings, as well as do the scut work in exchange for the great learning experience we were receiving.

**Racism and Sexism at GROH**

On my general surgery rotation, I got to sit in on the department meetings. One meeting involved selecting people for next year's incoming class of residents. In those days, applicants would submit a photo along with the paperwork.

The session started with a hospital administrator, a smiling white man in an expensive suit, passing around each application. He made a statement about each applicant as he sent the forms and photos down and around the circle of attendings. The surgeons all looked and listened and made notes on a piece of paper.

Then the administrator held up one set of papers and said, "Here is applicant Rodriguez (not the real name). As you can see, we don't need to consider this one for very long, do we?"

He laughed and the circle of men also laughed. The administrator tossed the application into the reject pile and never sent it around the table.

I was sitting in the back behind this administrator, and I could see the photo of a man who looked darkly handsome and very Hispanic on the application papers. He never had a chance. Did they not realize I was there (large and Black and female), listening and watching and absorbing? I never wanted to be part of that hospital staff because their happy acquiescence into the realm of racism was sickening. That is one reason I turned down the offer of a residency in Ophthalmology when it was offered to me. Be part of that staff? No way, baby!

I think the cap on the deal next was sexism in medical life and sure enough, that showed up, too. There was an excellent resident in Orthopedics, Cheryl Sales, MD, who became my mentor when I was on Orthopedics service. None of the attendings wanted to bother with me. They dumped my orthopedic education on her.

I had trouble tying sutures. The surgeon on service was left-handed, and as I stood across the table from him, everything I saw him do, all the motions he made with his hands and instruments, seemed to be upside down and backwards. Cheryl saw me in the surgical lounge struggling with a teaching book about sutures and asked if I needed help. I said yes, and she taught me how to hand tie, instrument tie, do subcuticular, mattress, and so many other stitching and suturing techniques. It was how I spent my orthopedic time when I was not doing exams or rounds with the guys.

She was skilled, kind, and intelligent. She was white and the trainers still treated her like shit. I was absolutely amazed to see how sexism trumped racism at that place. Her greatest sin was that she was a woman, and a woman who wanted to be an orthopedist. She was almost sidelined out of the residency, but she agreed to do a track into the hand surgery program because her trainers felt she was not strong enough to hold up a leg or hip in the OR, and her hands were good enough. I do know things have changed since then, and I am so glad. I thanked that woman for all she showed me, which not only included how to suture, but also how to persevere.

Death, sexism, racism, drug addiction—I think that just about covers most of what I learned about the underbelly of medicine while I was an extern at GROH.

The part about patient care came pretty easily. People liked me: patients, staff, other interns and externs, residents, too, as well as all the low-level staff. I loved to talk to people and listen to what they had to say. I spent a lot of time with people who needed admission exams, and I did a very complete note. Usually, I was the only one who knew all the minutiae about a case, and occasionally it came in handy. Most of the time, it was ignored. Unfortunately, that ignorance of the minutiae in a patient's life is still ignored today, as far as I can tell.

When will we ever learn?

## DIGRESSION #19: BEHAVIORAL HEALTH CARE IS JUST CATCH AND RELEASE

It makes no sense to pick people up off the streets because they are a danger to themselves or others, or because they are—can I say this?—crazy, and place them on a psychiatric hold for 72 hours, only to then let them go out to the street against all professional medical advice because they say they do not want to stay there.

Gee whiz, they were nuts when they got picked up! And 72 hours is not at all long enough to figure out what kind of specific mental health disturbance they have. It could be genetic, toxic, metabolic, drug-induced, a combination of all the above, or something else.

"Catch and release" is a popular phrase in the world of hunters because it preserves the animal for other sportsmen to catch, and it assures that the game will not go extinct. That way, everyone, except the animal, benefits. The state gets to sell licenses, the hunters and fishermen get to enjoy the thrill of the sport, and the commercial ventures get to sell equipment and bait. The game animal is tortured repeatedly until it dies. In and out of the water; in and out of the forest; in and out of the mental health system. It is all the same.

How is that any different than how we treat people in the behavioral health system? If there is drug or other substance abuse, please treat this until it is gone, cleared, and cured. If there is also a mental health issue, please treat this until it is gone, cleared, and controlled or cured.

Do not let the person go home just because the person tells you he thinks he is now well. If he is nuts, how and when does he know he is not nuts? How do you know he is well until you have spoken with all who know him, and until you have tested him for all causes of his abnormal behavior?

It is a form of Medicaid churning of the worst kind.

Treatment centers get paid to hold and house a person.

Psychologists get paid to do an evaluation.

Psychiatrists get paid to prescribe some pills.

Social workers get paid and get to feel like they have helped someone.

Drug court judges get paid and get to feel like they are effectively battling drug use.

Police get paid and get to think they have done their duty by picking these patients up and taking them to the ER.

Physicians get paid and get to feel like they have made a good ER diagnosis. A diagnosis which is not a treatment, and it is a long way from a cure.

But nothing changes in the life of the patient who is shunted from one place to another, on and off the street, in and out of treatment facilities, in and out the door of the local ER department again and again.

The person's family is abandoned, ignored, frustrated, and angered by the over-weaning governmental institutional indifference and incompetence, too.

Eventually the patient will die—still sick, unhappy, and untreated because we all have failed.

We must do better. I hope someone will figure out how to make better happen.

## WE'RE BACK . . .

### Internship at Carson City Hospital

Eventually I graduated. I was in the three-year accelerated program, which meant that I did not have any summers off or long breaks between semesters.

I struggled with lots of classes; biochemistry, orthopedics, and neuroanatomy gave me the shits. Thank goodness for the help I got from Bob Swor in biochemistry, and Rick Bratton and Alice Raynesford for their help with all the other hard classes.

It was a cutthroat life trying to stay ahead of flunking out. I recall the day of the biochemistry midterm—there were only two tests. I was prepping with Bob Swor, my hired tutor, when Leon (not his real name) came up to our table and asked to sit in and participate. Leon was one of the Black males in our class. He had worked for a major insurance company before coming to MSU, and fancied himself a ladies man, too.

He had not bothered to study, and had not obtained a tutor. I told him that he would not be able to join me because I needed 100 percent of the help from my tutor. Leon, indignant at being denied a seat with us, accused me of letting him down, a Black man asking for help from a Black woman.

He was entitled to his opinion, but as far as I was concerned, he had let himself down by failing to take the steps necessary to succeed, and Blackness had nothing to do with his success or failure. Eventually, he did drop out of school because his grades were so terrible. I think he went back to work at the insurance company.

But honestly speaking, our attrition rate was high. Our entering class of 100 had a 25 percent dropout by the time of graduation. Some went into the four-year program, some quit, some could not afford the cost, some got ill, and some just flunked. I was never the smartest one, but at the end of it all, we all got a diploma that said "DO" with no mention of individual cumulative grade point average.

The fact that someone had a high GPA coming out of medical school was not then, and is not now, a guarantee of success in medical practice.

One of the most intelligent people in my class was an electrical engineer with a PhD and lots more professional initials. One day in class, this student decided to argue with the cardiologist who was lecturing about Einthoven's Triangle and how it relates to EKG interpretation. They carried on back and forth for five minutes or so and closed awkwardly. This student graduated high on the GPA scale, never flunked a test, but later, according to what I understood, dropped out during internship.

Another brilliant young man in my class was always the first one to finish a test, and prided himself on being able to prove that. He always knew all the right answers. We called him Brainiac, and he went into neurology because he was a smart fellow. His brains failed him, I believe, because he got greedy. Unfortunately, it was my understanding that he got into trouble with the DEA for selling blank signed scripts. He was not smart enough to avoid that pitfall.

Another student who was previously an EMS (Emergency Medical Specialist) was boisterous and eager to raise his hand to answer a question. I perceived him as a show-off, but he was so jovial, my peers and I agreed that no one really thought it was a bad thing.

So, there, put that "smartest in the class" title in your bong and whoof it, because it takes more than brains to succeed in clinical life.

On July 1st, 1979, I started my internship at Carson City Hospital. I was joined by four men from other schools. The five of us bonded one night listening to Pink Floyd's album, *The Wall,* over the idea that I perceived as a sort of the them—patients, trainers, nurses, cooks, housekeeping, administrators, attending physicians, all of them—against us, and we tried our best to help each other.

I remember our guidebook and best source of mental health recovery was the book called *House of God* written by Samuel Shem, and I still have the text today. It was a true life exposé/satire on the life of a medical student extern/intern in a major hospital.

### Intersection of Racism and Sexism in Medical Education and Practice

Prior to starting at the hospital, each student in MSUCOM had to pick a hospital for internship and hope the hospital also picked them as a "match" for each other. This is a strenuous and stressful time for all students, and many of us pick several places hoping that we'll get matched. I only wanted one, and it was Carson City Hospital, because it was just down the road from where we lived. My second choice would have been Grand Rapids Osteopathic, but then I would have had to live away from home for several more years.

Like everybody else in the match process, I was eager enough to schedule a personal interview at the hospital of my choice before graduation. I met a doctor who was a large smiling white man with a goatee that I believe he thought made him look smart and sexy. In my opinion, he was very loud, and the embodiment of the sexist male chauvinist pig. I witnessed many times when he frequently made statements that would rankle and embarrass any woman around him, and he never apologized for his statements, such as, "Women should never wear pants."

I met him in the lobby at the old building, and I treated the meeting as if it were a job interview, and, in a sense, it certainly was. I even wore a dress, nylons, and high heels.

He looked over whatever papers I had given him, probably some written one-page of why I wanted to train at CCH. Then, I vividly recall him asking me, "What are you going to say to the patient who calls you nigger?"

This was his opening comment. No working up to it, no easing into it, no warning discussion leading into it. In one sense, he was being very honest because he knew the population of the area. But he also knew that I lived in the county, and I also knew what the population was like regarding race relations and cultural sensitivity.

His question was a shocker, and I was very much taken aback by it. I said that I would probably ignore it and move on with whatever it was that I was doing because that would be the professional thing to do.

I was dumbfounded and insulted, but I kept my true answer to myself. My true answer is that I would call the person a dumbass peckerwood and remind the patient that his life is in my hands.

In his own way, I would like to believe, this doctor was trying to prepare me for the realities of life at CCH. The patients were rural, evangelical, poorly educated, blue collar white people. I was none of that, therefore I was going to meet the worst, as well as the best, and I had better be prepared.

But you could also argue, I believe, that he was thinking from his elitist point of view as a wealthy, employed, educated man of standing, and was not giving people of color the benefit of the doubt. Maybe these patients he referenced were not all the racist know-nothings he painted them to be, and this was just his pompous, classist, high-caste belief system coming through.

He seemed to accept my answer and we progressed through the rest of the interview. The interview was successful, and I matched with Carson City.

But this doctor was not done with me yet. From my perspective, he was truly cruel, but very clever, too, and had a sly sick sense of humor that manifested as doing his utmost to bring embarrassment into the interaction. For example, once when we were rounding on his service, he and I entered a patient's room. Before I could present the case, he turned to the patient and soberly and bluntly said, "Dr. Mustonen is from Africa, but she speaks very good English, so I think you will have no problem understanding her."

Then he turned to me and said for me to present the case. I was fuming. But I also understood where I stood on the Mountain of Medical Training.

That MOMT has a steep slope, a distant peak, filled with many obstacles and shit. That shit is deeply layered and always runs downhill. You have to know where you are on that mountain slope and behave accordingly. If you are patient and smart, you will move up that mountain—unless you are Black, female, older, handicapped, foreign, or gay. I had three out of those six deficits. Misbehavior on that mountain will result in hotter, heavier, larger streams of shit being directed toward you for the duration of your position. I did not want more shit coming my way, so I went along with the "joke." This doctor, from my perspective, realized he had an easy mark and made my life unhappy any chance he got.

I could see that my internship was going to be somewhat of a struggle. I had yet to meet the adventure that is called the ICU.

My first week was Medicine rotation starting in the ICU. A lady coded on my first day, and she died. She was going to die. Everyone expected her to die. No one thought she would live. She knew she was going to die. Her family figured her death was going to be a release, so they were prepared for her to die. I was the only one who thought she should have lived, and I was devastated when she died, in spite of my best efforts, ladled on heavily with CPR, rescue drugs, oxygen, epinephrine, intubation, and all of that. She died. I was the ICU intern, and she died on my watch. This was just as bad as the dead baby born when I was an extern in GROH.

I recall leaving the ICU after the failed code and hiding in a janitor's closet, crying. Bless the nurse who provided emotional comfort to me at that time. It was Lynn, a man who was actually the Director of Nursing.

After that, I learned that, eventually, all patients die, and my job is to make their time, while alive, the best I can for them. Not to take it personally if they screw up my plan for them, and not to destroy myself.

The nurses in the ICU were all female, all white, all RNs, and all bored and angry with the fact that they knew more than any intern, and yet had to give all us interns the respect we deserved because we were physicians and they were not. I ran into the Angry White Woman in the ICU. After being disrespected for a few days, I finally spoke to the main leader of the pack, and had a heart to heart with her about what my plans were (staying in Montcalm County), what I hoped to achieve (being on staff at this place), where the fuck I was going to practice (Stanton), and that one day I would be an Attending Physician in this hospital, and could she just understand that I am here to learn and I will be back in a higher position on the MOMT?

It seemed to break down some kind of barrier, and after that, we just tried to connect on a woman-to-woman basis. It became better for me once those RNs realized that I was not a threat, that I did respect them for their knowledge, and appreciated all that they taught me.

We went through rotations as interns, serving time in family medicine, internal medicine, surgery, and obstetrics. We got to study with all the attending physicians at the hospital.

Carson City's physician staff was all white and all male. The nurses were all white, and only the Director of Nursing was male. The administrator was a white male.

One of the surgeons proved to be a great teacher, a good friend, and based on his behavior toward me, a sexually frustrated asshole. Every chance he got to grope me, he would try to do so. Making contact over the operating table by trying to hold my hand was one of the more egregious activities I recall. I believe he was just looking for sex with a Black woman.

So, it was especially satisfying to get my social revenge when I became a member of the hospital staff and in my own practice. I recall a patient who needed an emergency procedure of some kind, and I rushed to the hospital with the patient and helped set up for the surgery. That one particular surgeon was on call, so we scrubbed in and did the surgery together. The patient tolerated the procedure very well and went to the post-op room for recovery, while the surgeon and I went to the surgery post-op station just outside of the doctor's lounge to take care of charting.

I remember that he casually tossed the chart to me and told me to write some post-op orders, being sure to add a morphine pain pump with a 15-minute lock out and IV antibiotics.

I casually tossed the chart back at him and told him that I was no longer his intern, but I was one of his "referring men," and he could write his own post-op orders. I left and enjoyed the sight of his mouth hanging open in major surprise at my words.

We had a much better relationship after that.

The internship was not fun, but at least it was only for one year. At that time, in 1980, the AOA did not require a residency program for graduates who wanted to do family medicine. An intern year was enough. Arney did not want me to do a residency, saying he was tired of being alone and it was time for me to "come home." I listened to him, and that was a mistake that has followed me all my professional career.

The AOA fell into line with the AMA in 1986 and made a rule that all DO students who graduated in that year were required to do a residency no matter what specialty they planned to enter. This meant that every time an organization asked me about my training, I had to say "no residency" on that question. And organizations increasingly began to ask for candidates who were "residency-trained." Since I was not, that resulted in an automatic disqualification for several positions in my professional life.

But I am board certified, just like every resident in family medicine, and I was able to do that by completing six years of active practice, 600 hours of CME (Continuing Medical Education), and by taking the same exam taken by those who are residency-trained. Still, the lack of a residency training program in my life was a professional mistake that I hope is not repeated by those who come after me.

**My Stanton Clinic**

I decided to open up my office in Stanton, the town where Arney had his office and where he was serving as Judge of District Court. I went to the bank, borrowed $30,000 on my signature and my degree, rented a building, found two ladies to work for me, bought some office equipment, and opened up for business on the first Monday in August, 1980. I cannot believe how gutsy that was, for me to walk into a bank and walk out with more money than I had ever had in one lump sum in my life. But my husband was well-known and white, and I was well-known and a DOCTOR, so those two factors probably secured the loan approval.

The town had one DO and one MD. The MD welcomed me. The DO ignored me. Neither one of them was on staff at Carson City Hospital. I did not care because I was doing what I loved and was ready for any challenge.

The first week, I saw one person on Monday, one on Tuesday, one on Wednesday, one on Thursday, and one on Friday. The Monday person just wanted a refill because the MD was on vacation. The one on Tuesday was plain fucking nuts and promised not to come back (lucky me). She had actually been sent to me by the MD in town because he was sick and tired of dealing with her nonexistent problems, which were all mental health related. The ones on Wednesday and Thursday had questions, but did not want to become patients.

Friday was the day I met Mrs. H. She came in with her daughter, Miss S (not their real names), and told me her problem.

Mrs. H started with every doctor's most feared chief complaint:

"I am so tired, Doctor."

Most physicians do not know where to begin with this problem. The list of medical conditions that can cause fatigue fills several pages, and that is before you start looking at those which are psychological. We run and hide when we hear "I'm tired." Most patients get an unnecessary workup and are brushed off with a script for unnecessary thyroid pills, which will cause problems that can later be treated. This way the doctor and the patient both feel vindicated, medicated, and remunerated.

Mrs. H said, "All I do is eat, sleep, pee, eat, sleep, pee, day after day, and I am so tired."

I let her continue, thank goodness, and she went on and on and on. In the greatest of detail, she recounted the onset of her problem, the increasing severity of it, the gradual weight loss, the continuing hunger, the nighttime urination, the daytime urinary frequency, and the increasing thirst. Polydipsia, polyuria, polyphagia in medical terms describes her symptomology, and it is absolutely textbook classic for new onset of diabetes mellitus type two.

My mind was totally blank.

No thoughts were sparkling across my mind, and it was good that I never interrupted her because she kept adding details that nailed down the diagnosis. Even a first-year medical student would know the answer. Here was a true patient with true problems who truly wanted me to do the right thing for her. I had managed patients on ventilators, delivered breech babies, taken out tonsils, attended successful codes, but now my mind had shriveled up into a ball of I DO NOT KNOW WHAT TO DO. I did not know because this was the first time I was truly in charge of another person with NO back up. No senior resident, no trainer, no one to tell me what to order or what to do, no book to turn to. I was on my own. I was an Attending Physician. No shit.

My only course of action was to get more history, do a physical, and keep calm. That is exactly what I did. I let her talk, which is something seldom done, then or now. Mrs. H and I were together for three hours. At the end of her exam, I had blood work done in the office, and scheduled her for a follow up visit to go over the blood work early the next week. She and her daughter left.

About 30 minutes after she left, my brain came on and it shouted, "Hey, bozo, she is a diabetic. Dumbo, you ignorant B*^%$. Get her some freaking pills."

Then I got a call from the lab with urgent results on her lab; sugar was elevated at 375.

I sprang into action and told Shirley, my receptionist, to call the patient and tell her I would be coming by with some test results and some medication. I told Nancy, my nurse, to get samples of a diabetic pill ready to take to Mrs. H's house. At 4:55 PM, I left the office, headed for Mrs. H's home with pills, patient education charts, and a diet sheet. I got to her home, which was actually on the way to my own house, and went in. Mrs. H, her daughter, and I sat and talked about her test results, her medication, and how to use it, her condition and what it meant, and how she can control her problem with diet and exercise. I left her house at 6:30 PM and got home feeling like a Boss.

I did not realize how the Mrs. H Influence was about to impact my professional life.

Monday when I arrived at work, Shirley told me that I was in for a very busy week. Shirley was positively beaming and smiling for joy as she told me how she had been inundated with phone calls and had been booking people for new patient visits, spread out all during the week and into the next week. We had five people, each with a one-hour visit on Monday.

Not sure how or why, but very happy that it was happening, I waded into my real practice.

Mrs. H showed up on Thursday and said she was feeling so much better. Her blood sugar numbers were much improved and all of her symptoms were abating. I was so very happy to have made a positive impact.

Later that day, Shirley explained what had happened. Shirley lived in the same town as Mrs. H and knew all the local family connections. She told me this about my first patient.

Mrs. H was the Godmother of the township. She was either related to or in a group with everyone in three contiguous townships, and furthermore, she had a party line telephone. After I left her house that previous Friday, she got on the phone and told everyone on her party line about the new doctor who took time to listen to her, did a thorough exam, answered her questions, gave her a test that revealed the problem, came over to her home with samples of medication, and spent time explaining what she should do to get well.

Never in her life had any doctor ever done that for her. She spread the word to her five children, her eight siblings, their children and friends, her husband's six siblings and their children and friends, her church group, her women's group, and so on. That woman single handedly launched my career in Stanton/Crystal/Sheridan as a family physician. All I did was the right thing: listen, think, listen some more, and explain. Isn't that what every physician should do?

As the only woman physician at CCH in family medicine, I had a large population of obstetrics. The other woman physician was employed by the state correctional system as the prison doctor. There was an internist at another hospital across the county, but she was no competition for me. It was several years before another woman came into the area to practice, and she became a good friend when I was on staff at Greenville Hospital. None of these women physicians practiced obstetrics.

My life as an OB was busy, rewarding, and full of surprises. I hate surprises.

One day, a lady came in and announced she was pregnant, and would I please be her doctor for the delivery? She had already had seven children, all vaginally and all easy deliveries with no complications. She was a recent transfer from somewhere in the deep South, had moved here after divorcing her first husband, had recently met and married her second husband, and they were excited to be starting a new family together.

She was so nice and sweet, and she was an experienced gravida (a woman who has experienced multiple pregnancies), meaning the baby would probably just fall out and all I would have to do is be there to catch. I said yes, and we got along just fine. She was polite, showed up on time for all of her prenatal visits, and was interested in actually breastfeeding this child because she had never done so with any of the others.

When she went into labor, I thought (silly me) that it would be an hour or two from first contractions to delivery, but when we hit 18 hours into labor, I was beginning to have some serious doubts. She struggled and strained, and finally, she dilated to full, dilated 100 effacement, and began pushing in earnest. The baby was a tough delivery with some mild shoulder dystocia (which means the baby's shoulders get stuck inside the mother's pelvis), but I managed to get the arm out, followed the head, and then the rest of the 10-pound giant baby boy slid out of the skinny little country momma. I was so glad that I did an episiotomy because it saved her from having a vaginal tear.

Later, I asked her how much each of her children weighed at birth, and she told me none of them was over five-and-a-half pounds. I was perplexed until I realized that, when she was with her first husband, they were poorer than dirt, with truly no healthy prenatal diet, and that she was lucky to get 1,000 calories a day while pregnant.

When she married her second husband, who had a real job with real money, she was eating 3,000 calories a day and gaining weight just as she was supposed to, and the baby was growing like an avalanche coming down a ski mountain in Utah. She had never had a child this large, so of course all the previous babies just fell out. Let's hear it for maternal nutrition. And I learned to obtain a better prenatal history on all women I subsequently delivered.

Dr. LVS, the anesthesiologist, was the best OB teacher I ever had, and probably every intern at CCH would say the same thing. He did all the epidurals and was a repository of OB knowledge beyond imagination.

Thank God he was there for my first and only aftercoming head breech delivery. As you may know, babies are supposed to come out head first, face down, with their arms neatly by the sides, and mouths closed until you clean out their noses and get them to take a breath.

The nurses called me because the lady in labor was not progressing as she should. They said they checked, but it was hard to tell what the baby's station was. Station is the word used to describe how high up in the pelvis a baby's head was. Station at minus one, two, or three was above the middle, and station plus one, two or three was below the midline. The lady was 100 percent effaced (cervix is thin) and dilated (cervix is wide open) to 10, but the station was still too high.

I came and checked. Then I asked the charge nurse, Jan, to also check. We looked at each other and agreed that what we had felt was not the head. It was a butt. That is why the membranes had not yet ruptured; there was not enough pressure from a head to break the bag of waters, so this was a breech delivery.

"Oh, shit!" hardly describes what I felt. There was not time to do a C-section because, just as we realized what the situation truly was, the bag of waters did break. Now we are committed to a delivery vaginally because the infant suddenly descended to plus two station.

Dr. LVS came to help with the anesthesia, and while he stood at the head of the table, I sat at the end doing the delivery. He asked me if I had ever used Piper aftercoming head forceps. I said no. He said,

"Well, today is your lucky day because you will."

Edmund Piper, in 1924, developed and designed these instruments. There are lots of complications from forceps, even the ones used for a head-first delivery. Injuries such as bleeding from a rip in the mother's tissues, or from inside a baby's skull, damage to the facial nerves of the baby, and trauma to the eyes are just some of the problems. But when you need forceps, they are wonderful. I was trained to use forceps on a head-first delivery, but a breech delivery is special. Nowadays, there is a YouTube video on how to use Piper forceps, but then, it was just me and Dr. LVS. The description, by the US Army Medical Corps, is horribly done, confusing, and dull. It uses a plastic female pelvic model and a cloth-stuffed doll for the baby. No one does these kinds of deliveries anymore because it is automatically an emergency C-section.

Bless his heart, Dr. LVS told me how to put on each blade of the forceps, how to elevate the handle, how to rotate the body, putting a towel around the baby's arms, raising and lowering the baby's body, and how to remove the blade as the head came out. I think no one in the room but him and me knew that he was providing what they call a teachable moment; that is how smooth he was.

The baby and the momma came out fine. I decided that maybe I should help with the search for an OB/GYN to be on staff.

One of my more fun OB patients was the prima gravida who reluctantly married her boyfriend at the start of the pregnancy so that she would not embarrass herself and her family. When she went into labor, she was naturally apprehensive, but even more so because she had decided to skip prenatal classes. She knew nothing about the process, and active labor was not the best time for measured learning. At least her husband showed up to lend support.

She labored badly for several hours, and after a while, it became obvious that she was not going to make it to a vaginal delivery. She started screaming that she wanted a C-section. She made herself heard throughout the hospital, I am sure. The nurses called me and I came to the labor room to examine her. Her cervix was thin as a piece of paper and seemed to be dilated 100 percent, but the baby's head was still too far up for an easy vaginal birth.

She continued to scream. I told her we would have to do a C-section, and at first, she seemed relieved, then suddenly angry. She sat up in bed, in between contractions, turned to her husband and shouted, "YOU DID THIS TO ME, YOU STINKING FUCK," and then she decked him with a right hook to the jaw that would have made Mike Tyson proud. He went down like a ton of bricks, and miraculously, she relaxed somewhere in her pelvis because right then she said, "OH MY GOD, I FEEL THE BABY COMING."

Sure enough, she was now crowning, and I rushed her to the delivery table. Thirty seconds after she was up on it, her baby came out.

Good Times in OB—how I miss them.

My practice in Stanton was a good one, by and large. I gathered patients, grew my practice, supported my hospitals. I was on staff at both Carson City Osteopathic and Sheridan Community Hospital.

**Intersection of Racism and Sexism in the Practice of Medicine**

Sheridan was the place where my personal physician, the man who delivered my first child, and my general surgeon, the man who delivered my second child by C-section—both of whom wrote letters of recommendation for me to get into MSUCOM—were on staff.

The doctors there—we were only five—had a rolling system of advancement at Sheridan to determine who would be Chief of Staff. The term was for one year, and the vice chief became chief, the treasurer became vice chief, the secretary became treasurer, the former chief became a regular member, and the regular member became secretary. I started as regular member, moved up to secretary, moved up to treasurer, and moved up to vice chief. When it was my turn to be Chief of Staff, they got together in a private meeting and made a decision to select the next person by secret ballot, which had never been the process, and the new Chief of Staff, somehow or other, was NOT ME.

I was disappointed. I was insulted. After the election, each one came to me, privately, at later moments through the week, and assured me that I was the person he really wanted, but that he had to go along with what the others wanted, and that it would not be too long before I was actually ready for chief of staff, and he would be wholeheartedly able to support and vote for me, next time. That experience and the workload made me want to change something.

Change happened sooner rather than later because the workload was crushing me. One day, I had a man at Sheridan with crushing chest pain, impending myocardial infarction (MI), and a lady at Carson City fully dilated, effaced, and ready to push. How can I be at two places at once? I was able to send the man via ambulance to Grand Rapids (where he lived), and drive directly to the OB unit at Carson City to deliver the baby.

My brain started talking to me again, and this time it said, "Yo, dumbo, it's Time To Make A Change."

It made sense to drop down to one hospital. I could see that I was never going to rise up the ranks at Sheridan because it was the epitome of the good ole boys' network. That, plus the double trouble of having critical patients at both places, brought sharply home the need to change, and I cast my vote in favor of being fully active at CCH while being courtesy staff at Sheridan.

CCH kept me busy. I was again hit in the face by the good ole boys' network and male chauvinism when the Chief of Staff asked me to be the interim OB department head. Our OB doctor had left, and I was one of four family doctors doing OB. He picked me because I was the one person with the highest volume of OB patients. I said yes. Then, one day, another FP (Family Practitioner) told me that there was an unwritten rule about who could serve as OB department head.

I told him that if it was unwritten, then it was not a rule, and furthermore, the Chief of Staff personally selected me, and so to discuss it with the Chief of Staff and leave me the fuck alone.

I worked ER, did my own minor surgeries, assisted at my major surgeries, made rounds, sat on committees, attended meetings, trained interns and externs, and handled call and OB for six years at that place. It was wonderful. It was a workaholic escape from the crushing pain of my husband's infidelity and alcoholism that was going on in the background of my life.

One day, Arney said that we should make plans to return to Detroit. He wanted to go back to the city, and it would be best for me to get established there in a practice, and have the girls enrolled in a school, so he could move back after stepping down from the bench. He was in his first term as District Court Judge at that time. He also said that the girls would get a better education at a big city private school than they would at a rural system where books were burned or banned because the wolf crawled into bed with grandmother in *Little Red Riding Hood.*

I agreed. But then I agreed with whatever he wanted because I was such a good and obedient enabler.

## DIGRESSION #20: THE FUTURE OF NPs AND PAs

Understanding why there are advanced practice nurses is not hard. There was a need for them. Someone thought it was a good idea to have nurses who could function at a higher level of practice, above what an RN could do, working in the office or hospital, and perhaps be more independent, but still an important part of the health care provision team.

To which I say, that's just bullshit talking.

What was really going on was that someone saw a way to add more money to a clinic, and to keep women subservient to men in health care. The care provided for by a Nurse Practitioner (NP) is billed as an offshoot of what a physician would bill. The patient's insurance is charged the same fee as if a physician provided the care. But the pay the NP receives is much less than that of the physician. The nurse is cheaper to employ than another doctor, and her effort in a clinic pulls in lots of money. Hospitals love NPs, and will even hire them to do hospital work, especially if they have obtained PhD status training somewhere.

Physician Assistants (PAs) were specifically created to be assistants to physicians. NPs were originally nurses, who stepped up their training. Their origins are important distinctions. Many PAs are men, while most NPs are women. True, there are women who are PAs and many men who are NPs, but the gender divide is real. Women, coming up in the ranks of nursing, have had to follow a historically long, hard road, seeking relevance and appreciation in the ranks of health care. They fought for every step they gained. The system balked at allowing them in the field of medicine and yielded only to the extent to allow these "uppity women" the position of helper to the men who dominated the role of MD-land physicians.

In a not-too-distant past time, physicians frequently picked the nurse they wanted to assist them, and then, if she was compliant, would marry her, too. The NP was a step towards independence that flourished, following the gains made by the Suffragettes, the women nurses in both World Wars, and after the push for civil rights and women's liberation in the 1960s. Needless to say, the men in medicine hated that independence. Therefore, NPs were forced away from complete independence, and required to have a working agreement with a supervising physician in order to practice. The physicians lobby keeps the medical licensing boards and legislatures on a leash, and works hard to prevent them from allowing full and complete independence to any NP. The trend is, however, turning away from that because, as of 2021, 28 states now allow NPs to practice fully, independent of physician oversight.

If you think about it, it is one of the remaining vestiges of rampant sexism in America today. No other non-physician health care provider is required to have a working contract of supervision with a physician.

That constraint to have a collaborative agreement with a supervising physician does not apply to chiropractors, physical and occupational therapists, dentists, audiologists, optometrists, psychologists, family therapists, and so many others in ancillary health care professions.

Physicians will argue that because NPs and PAs are trained to a lesser degree, they are not equal in the provision of care that a physician can provide. I agree. They argue that, therefore, NPs and PAs should not be independent. I disagree. Chiropractors are trained to a lesser degree and are independent. Audiologists are trained to a lesser degree and are independent. Dentists are trained to a lesser degree and are independent. I am sure you see where I am going with my point.

Let the NP and PA group become independent, and let the market determine where the patient will go. Equally important is the need to free the physician from the burden of oversight of a person he/she did not hire, cannot fire, did not train, and who will not be physically nearby. Remember that if an NP or PA makes a medical error, the physician gets sued as well.

My particular disagreement with women who become NPs and PAs is that I feel they have betrayed the hard work done by those of us who marched and protested for women's rights in the decades of the '60s and '70s. I have heard many NPs say that they did not think they could be accepted to medical school because they did not feel they were smart enough. That weak shit argument gives tremendous firepower to the sexist jerks who would limit women's admission to medical school on the grounds of intellectual difference. For years, one of my male trainers complained about women residents and interns, and accused them of having "estrogen brain syndrome." There is no such thing.

I have heard NPs say they have problems finding money to go to medical school, and being an NP is good enough and close enough to being a doctor. I say they again have betrayed those women who struggled to get admitted to medical school, piled on the debt of school, and powered through to a full and successful practice. And I argue that if you are an NP, you are not a physician. You are not practicing medicine, you are practicing nursing; that is why your credential says N (nurse), and not D (doctor). The disciplines are different.

I take issue with those NPs who say they could not find the time to put aside family obligations to commit to the years of training required to be a physician. Again, this is a betrayal of those of us who did find the time for home and career. This is another bullet in the gun for those sexists who would limit women's careers in medicine and relegate us to the function of our wombs. It serves to bolster resistance to the full ratification of the ERA—Equal Rights Amendment. These women fully admit they could not become physicians because of their intellectual weakness or femaleness.

PAs are different because they are created to be handmaidens (handmen?) for physicians, and of course, the majority of them are men, so it is a career that has been designed to last a lifetime. Nurses are relegated by the Patriarchy to being just a bunch of women who are here to help the doctor, and who will probably not work for the entirety of their lives, but will quit to have children. Anyone who has nurse in their title must have the working contractual supervision agreement. Certified Registered Nurse Anesthetists (CRNAs) and nurse midwives must have this. Something is dreadfully wrong with this arrangement.

Some states, as I said previously, have already moved to grant full practice authority to NPs, and as of 2021, there are 28 states in that column. I think that physicians should let them go, like Pharaoh Ramses let the Israelites go. The relationship is similar to the physician being in the role of pimp, and the NP in the role of prostitute. She works and pays him. He "protects" her. From what?

Actually, the physician is exposing himself to harm by agreeing to be her "supervisor." When the NP fouls up in a clinical error, the doctor and the NP are both liable to get sued. Therefore, the wise physician will support full practice autonomy for NPs. Let them go where they can, practice as they will, charge what they wish, and attract whomever wishes to see them. Let the marketplace determine who will succeed. Let them be sued like the doctors they claim to emulate.

We could look at clinical outcomes now and see that NPs do not do better than doctors in measurable clinical outcomes, as shown in many valid studies. We can see that NPs get better patient satisfaction scores because they spend more time with patients. What the fuck! Of course they do. They can spend the time with moderately ill and reasonably well patients because they send the sickest and most complicated patients to their supervising physician, and thus, are able to sit and chat with the easy-to-diagnose and the easy-to-care-for patients.

I would caution NPs to be aware that, as they gain full practice autonomy, they also expose themselves to full malpractice lawsuits. The National Practitioner Data Bank reported in 2011 a steady increase of malpractice claims pertaining to NPs. The NPDB said that mistakes relating to diagnosis and/or treatment usually triggered those claims. In addition, the NPDB said that when a location for the claim could be determined, it was usually in an outpatient setting.[4] Another report in 2017 showed the trend continuing.[5]

There you have it. The NPs are not medically trained; they are nursing trained. They do not diagnose; they follow algorithms. Patients who do not fit into the algorithmic tree are triaged to a physician for care.

They will also work for less and be more willing to accept less. Hospitals and large health care organizations have figured out that they can hire a $65,000 a year NP and fire a $165,000 physician from any clinic, and pocket the difference. They hire one $265,000 a year supervising physician to oversee the charting of a dozen NPs, fire a half-dozen $300,000 physicians, and life is good in the corner C-suites of the organization. The physician who stays in that organization is in a race to the bottom with the NPs. That physician, if they are wise, will decamp to Direct Patient Care and leave the NPs to themselves and the health care/hospital organizations that hire them.

Patients will find out that their simple needs are taken care of by an automated process, an Internet search, or a video conference with a physician, and when those thoughts gain traction, that is when NPs will be facing increasing marginalization. Patients will realize that they get what they pay for, and a lower price frequently leads to lower quality care.

Women going into the NP field need to quit promoting the concept of the weak woman, the intellectually inferior female who is not ready for a real career cop out, don't have money for med school bullshit, and powerless female mythology that their mothers and grandmothers pushed aside in the 1960s. We will never get the ERA passed if women behave this way.

Physicians need to give up their role as medical pimp for NPs. They need to give up their role as slave owner of NPs. They need to give up the malpractice risk associated with supervising NPs who are not able to function at the required level of care. They need to give up the desire to work for organizations that are not physician-owned and physician-led. Let the other patients go where they wish.

In the future, when physicians become fully augmented, they will no longer need any kind of assistant, neither NPs nor PAs, and when medical schools have open enrollment and a six- or seven-year training schedule, the people who drop out will flow into the ancillary function of non-augmented health providers. Maybe we will call them NPs or PAs, or something else, but they will be the main providers for the health care needs of the middle class. They will be completely independent, and have their own offices and practice locations.

WE'RE BACK . . .

## DOH, Botsford, and Return to Detroit

We began the search for work for me, and a school for the girls. School was easy. We found Detroit Country Day School, ritzy and pricey, but really good. We also found a nice condo apartment tucked away in a Detroit suburb, just off Lahser Road. We hired a search company—this was before the Internet—to help me find a job. The place was with three doctors in Taylor, Michigan (little Appalachia, or Taylor-Tucky, as they called it) who ran a resident training clinic at an inner-city hospital just off West Chicago Road. Northwest General Hospital could have been the model for the 1980s NBC television drama, *St. Elsewhere*—run down, mostly Medicaid population of patients, with all Black staff and all white doctors. The residents were all white, and I was going to be the resident trainer. I told those three doctors that I wanted to try as hard as I could, and that if I performed to their standards, I would like to become one of their partners.

See, there is the proof that I have always been an honest, hardworking fool. In my opinion, there was no way on God's green Earth that three white guys who graduated, trained, and worked together would ever let a Black girl into their tightly controlled professional practice. I would never call them racists, just practical and close-knit from medical school forward. They did not say no, nor did they say yes. I was too stupid to realize that is how the good ole boys' network operates. Talk is cheap, and they treat you that way, too.

I busted my buns for them. The clinic was busy every day, with all kinds of medical adventures, and with three residents, one intern, and one extern on the floor, it kept me jumping as I moved from direct patient care to teaching, over and over, each day, plus running the drug detox unit upstairs.

One day in the midst of this, my dear Grandchildren, your Auntie Ophelia had a very serious medical condition that required immediate hospitalization. I left work and took her to the hospital, where she was admitted and treated. Afterwards, my mind was churning in the aftermath of this emergency, wondering what would have happened if I had not been able to take her in for care. I still had to go to work.

My bosses had also requested that I keep the clinic open with extended night hours. None of the residents would be working nights, just me. I would have to come in and work from 11 AM till 9 PM each night. I would still teach residents, run the detox unit, make in-patient rounds, and see patients in clinic.

### Intersection of Racism and Sexism in Practice at Botsford

I contemplated this as I sat in the office at my desk. On some strange impulse, I opened the desk and saw a letter from my bosses, discussing how they would use the money given to them by the hospital for hiring the clinic resident trainer (me). They had received $100,000 from the hospital for my fee, but gave me $60,000 and split the remaining $40,000 among the three of them.

Thank goodness I was married to a white person, because the revelations in that letter would have made me become a Black nationalist, except for the fact that I understand how hurtful stereotypes rooted in racism can be, and how powerful the pull of more money is.

But that letter did reaffirm my decision to not let myself be used and abused any more. I chalked their behavior up to simple male chauvinism and greed, which transcend many other labels in life. I decided to make changes that were more protective of myself and my daughters. I told them, flat out, I would not work anymore nights.

They heard me and saw my resolve, and I know they did, so I made my plans to escape before they could make their plan to hurt me. Harriet Tubman would be proud of me. I contacted my friend Bill Anderson, DO, a Black surgeon at Detroit Osteopathic Hospital, and landed a spot over there in a few weeks, gave my notice, and left Botsford, Northwest General Hospital, and my three bosses.

DOH placed me in rotation at several clinics they owned around town. I worked with Dr. Art Bouier, DO. He was arguably the smartest internist on the staff at DOH, and at Junction Clinic over in the Michigan and Trumbull area, as well as a third location on West Grand Boulevard, with Drs. Cooper and Dash.

The West Grand Boulevard clinic was where Steve Swetech, DO, and I got to work together. He was one of the funniest, most enjoyable people in medicine I ever met. Full of ideas, full of fun, and a hardworking person. We energized the clinic, and had one of the best working groups I ever joined. I also worked in Dr. Rose's clinic and met Hal Friedman, another DO who graduated a few years behind me, and was the other most delightful person to work with. Fun, hardworking, full of great ideas, Hal went on to achieve a leadership position in the Michigan Association of Osteopathic Family Physicians. I remained good friends with both those men over the course of my professional life. Who says I can't get along with white people?

My stint with Botsford/Northwest General Hospital was one year, and my stint with DOH was also one year, and then I realized that Arney was not going to move back to Detroit. I had had it with the city.

My blood pressure took a spike while I was living there, and I actually found myself in the ER. I had been placed on Catapres, which is an alpha blocker, and it slowed my heart rate way, way down. The ER physician, Gust Bills, was a former extern who had followed me in a family medicine school rotation in my Stanton office years ago. He came to see me and was stunned to see that it was one of his former teachers. Dr. Bills was thoroughly put off his game and just stammered.

I interrupted him and said, "Gust, do what you know you are trained to do. I was one of your trainers, so I know you will do the right thing."

That broke the logjam, and then he smiled and got busy. I got better. I was taken off that med, and my pressure remained just fine.

But I needed to leave Detroit. I was alone and lonely. Our daughters had returned to Greenville High School, and I needed to return as well. I got in touch with United Memorial Hospital in Greenville, and they were excited to have a family physician interested in joining their staff.

Detroit was an adventure that was good and bad. Among the good things was that I made a lot of new friends and developed more clinical skills. Among the bad things was that I met some truly bad people, got a lawsuit while supervising a resident, and I got sexually molested because I was lonely and vulnerable. The spike in my blood pressure was the final warning sign of things to come if I stayed in the Motor City.

But what was I returning to by coming back to Montcalm County? Just as I had no idea of what to expect in Detroit when I moved there, I was unprepared for what Arney had for me on my return to Montcalm County. He had accumulated a ton of debt. The dear man never had any sense of how to save money or how to spend it wisely. As much as he earned, he spent or wasted. His drinking habit accelerated, and it took a village of friends, buddies, and employees to keep him from going off the rails in his work as District Court Judge.

I was much less trusting when I moved back to Greenville, of everyone. Arney tried to get the hospital to lend me money so that he could get rid of the debt he had accumulated. They refused. At first, I was upset with their decision, but in retrospect, it was the kindest, wisest thing they could have done. They saved me from leveraging his debt on the back of my second start-up clinical practice, and thereby, prevented me from building up more bitterness as the future of our declining marital relationship became clear.

You see, Grandchildren, sometimes we—mindful of our own desires—are unaware of what is best for us, and it is only the will of the Greater Providence of the Universe that prevents us from coming to dreadful grief.

I moved back and started my second clinic, this time in Greenville, in 1989.

## DIGRESSION #21: PATCHWORK HEALTH CARE

Our American health care system is a patchwork of competing insurance methods and applications.

Various groups of people are favored, many groups are underserved, and all groups are overcharged. No one in any group has any say in how the providers will be paid, and that is a major disconnect that makes it possible for hospitals to be profit-driven when patients never have to pay their bills because a third party pays. If you are a patient, why not ask for the most and the best all the time because the government will pay for it. And if you are a hospital being paid by a third party, why not charge the most you can?

Let us imagine how a person could cycle through all our forms of health care.

Imagine a person who was a Native American raised on the reservation and treated all his life by his tribe's national health care system, as long as he's lived there.

If that person, call him John, left the reservation and went to college, he would be able to participate in the school's health care system.

After college, when John got a job, he would sign up for Blue Cross Blue Shield medical benefits offered by his large corporation.

If he lost his job, he could apply for COBRA, which would allow him to privately pay for the same kind of insurance his former employer previously paid for him, but only for 18 months.

If John did not return to his employment but joined the armed forces, he would be covered by U.S. military medical care. After military service was completed, John would be eligible for VA benefits, but only at a VA hospital.

If he had an automobile accident, he would be covered by automotive insurance benefits, provided he had enough money to purchase auto insurance.

If John found another job after his recovery, but it offered no insurance or other benefits because it was part-time, he might sign up for Medicaid, which is a state-run program and varies from state to state.

If he were injured on that job, he would be covered, however, by worker's compensation insurance for a while. He might also apply for permanent disability status, which is a federal benefit program, as a result of that injury. His application would take years for that status to be granted, and frequently requires the help of an attorney.

After recovery, John would drift down the economic slope and find a way into minor crime, get arrested and convicted, and placed into the care of the local municipality's jail health care.

After release, John continued his spiral, got arrested again, convicted of a major crime, and placed in a state-run institution with state-run prison health care, which is privatized.

If, upon release, he were able to obtain Medicaid again and still use his VA benefits, that would be a bonus.

By now, John would be old enough to apply for Medicare because he has Social Security Disability and has health insurance via that pathway.

The sad fact is that none of these systems coordinate care between each other, and obtaining records from one to transfer to another is tedious and difficult, to say the least. Much information is lost, no EMR is shared between any of them, and poor John may not recall all the details of his various diagnoses, treatments, and physicians, much less recall all the medications he may have been given. Each one of these health systems are hugely bureaucratic, as well as interested in its own self-aggrandizement and self-preservation. Patients slip through multiple cracks and suffer and die due to bureaucratic neglect.

The war cry of "Medicare for All," or M4A, by Democratic presidential candidate Bernie Sanders of Vermont in 2016 and 2020, rang a bell, and it resonated with a lot of people. The opponents who said it would take away people's right to keep their own employer's health insurance failed to realize one important fact: the employer will seek the cheapest option. I will always admonish you to Follow the Dollar in health care when you are looking for any reason why a thing is the way it is.

If I am an employer and I know that my workers can have either M4A or I can pay to give them something else, I will quickly run the numbers and drop any private health insurance plan I may have offered if it will save me even one dollar per employee per month. Pretty soon, the entire nation will be on M4A because it will be cheaper. Whether or not it will be better or the same as some high-quality, high-cost, private, commercial plan is another topic that has to do with quality health care.

I am not sure anyone has a real definition for quality health care.

WE'RE BACK . . .

**My Greenville Clinic**

Arney and I sold the house on Sloan Road to a doctor on staff at Carson City Hospital. We bought a place at 1024 Arloa Drive on Burgess Lake. I got hired by UMH and opened a clinic just across the street from the hospital in Greenville.

Solo practice was always my choice, and this was a fresh start.

The building was so sweet: a reception area, manager's office, private office for me, a backroom lab, and four small exam rooms, each one with its own toilet and lavatory. No one builds an office like that anymore; the plumbing cost would be atrociously high.

I hired Linda Huckleberry as my manager, as well as two other ladies to work as LPN (Licensed Practical Nurse) and receptionist. Linda stayed with me, but the other two positions rotated over the years among various people. One person I hired was an LPN (I will not say her name because I do not want to hurt her feelings or memory) and she was chronically late.

I do not know why, but she could never show up on time. I changed her start time to 11 AM, and she still came in late. I asked her what were the barriers at home that prevented her from coming in on time, what, if anything, was the problem here at work that prevented her from coming, were there personal problems, transportation problems, health problems, what the fuck, anything problems. No matter what I did to help, she failed to show up in a timely fashion. I had to let her go. Sometime later, she asked me for a letter of reference for her next job application. I think I wrote something, but I may not have made any statement about her punctuality. It was, after all, a small town.

Another lady was the mother of a person who sold me my first insurance policy. In fact, that policy changed companies about five times and I still have it today as a paid-up, whole life policy. As long as I die before age 107, you grandchildren will get a large sum of money, and at the current rate of inflation and such, it will probably be enough to get a campus bus ticket and a taco salad to split between the two of you. Enjoy!

Hazel, that lady, was spectacular. She was calm, efficient and absolutely wonderful at drawing blood. I asked her if she could draw blood and she said no, she had no medical training at all. I asked her if she would like to learn and her eyes, so luminous, lit up like Times Square on New Year's Eve, and she said yes. I taught her and she excelled. She could poke and get blood from squirming little kids, concrete veins from COPD'ers, ropey wiggle worm veins from old anemic ladies, hidden like Lazarus veins from morbidly obese patients, you name it, she could find it and get a sample. And she was happy in her work, and kind with everyone she phlebotomized.

Sue was another lady who worked for me—funny, happy, and just the best at the front desk. She had the best ideas for parties during the holidays.

We used to dress up for Halloween as an office to celebrate the holiday. One year, Sue came up with an idea we liked. We decided to be Elvis and his motorcycle biker club as a theme. Sue dressed in a complete leather fetish outfit, with mask, high heeled boots, and a whip. Linda was Elvis, and Hazel and I were the remaining bikers. I found a fake nose ring and wore it as I was seeing patients that day.

One gentleman, one of the other Black people in the county, came to see me about his shoulder problem. As I was examining him, I noticed how he kept looking at my nose ring, then down at his shoes, and then back to the nose ring, and down to his shoes, and he would shake his head and make a grimace kind of smile. When we were done with the exam, he paused to ask, "Is that gon' be there on your face permanently?"

I told him it was just a piece of temporary jewelry and he didn't have to worry. He said thank goodness because if "it was gon' be there, I'm not gon' come back, because I can't be sure what you don' turned into." Bless his heart, he thought I had really gotten a piercing to my nose.

When the day ended, we decided to go out and we stopped at a local candy store across the street. I had some play money with a picture of President Bill Clinton on it, so I purchased some candy and placed the phony dollars on the counter for payment as a joke. After all, we were all in costume. The clerk looked at it and then started to ring up the sale and give me some change. I had to stop him and point out that the money was fake. OMG, this is why America will fall into destruction; no one pays attention to the details.

Each year, I would take my staff out for a holiday Christmas dinner and presents. We would rent a limo, bring our husbands, go to a good restaurant in Grand Rapids, and drink and eat till we were stuffed. One year, I gave each lady a nice piece of costume jewelry and a check for a hundred dollars as a gift.

A few weeks later, my accountant called me to say that I couldn't do that.

I exploded with a huff and said, "Why not? We earned it. It is my money and I wanted to reward them."

He asked if I had taken out the taxes from the money.

"Taxes? Taxes? What taxes?" I asked.

He proceeded to explain, so patiently in the short version, the U.S. tax laws that govern employers and the contributions they are required to make on behalf of all their employees. My head was swimming by the time he was done, but I learned that I really did not know much about running a business. He corrected the problem and made all the proper distributions so I would not be afoul of the IRS. My staff kept their bonus. I corrected my ignorance and made sure I spent time going over the Profit and Loss statements, and learning all about FICA, FUTA, and SS and Medicare tax requirement. That was the first time I realized why so many physicians are willing to go to work for a large hospital or health system instead of trying to set up their own practice. A better medical curriculum would strive to cover how a doctor actually gets paid.

In Greenville, I became the competent physician who did what needed to be done, not only for patients, but also for the hospital.

United Memorial Hospital was struggling under poor leadership and poor management. Finally, the Board decided to hire a better CEO and try to turn the place around. I volunteered to be the physician representative on the board of trustees. Every month, I would listen to the crap and drivel from the administration. But I would tell the good burghers of Greenville what they did not know about what their doctors and nurses were undergoing.

I was listened to. When they hired Mike M. to be CEO, he approached me and asked if I would be part of his team and serve as VP of Medical Affairs. I said yes, and we really hit it off. He was energetic and foresighted, and understood what it took to make a business run. He had a great CFO, a sharp HR director, and a clever PR leader, and the five of us were a close knit, productive, cohesive team. We hired doctors, organized departments, energized nursing staff, got the chronic non-signers of charts to sign their charts. I worked with the medical records manager and the risk manager, and together we rewrote the hospital bylaws. We started a high school scholarship program and passed our JCAHCO inspection with flying colors.

Signing charts is important to hospitals because of money.

Hospitals get paid only after the doctor has signed all the necessary pages in the chart. That is still true even with an Electronic Medical Record. Back in my day, charts were all paper. We had one room in the hospital devoted to charts that needed to be signed. They were stacked in bookshelves with the name of each doctor on the edge of the shelf. The orthopedic surgeon and one of the family doctors were neck and neck for the award of most unsigned charts in a month.

The hospital threatened them with removal of admission privileges, except for emergencies. That was not a barrier at all, so it did not work because the doctor only had to state the patient was an emergent admit and bypass the penalty.

I decided to tell these rule-breakers that after a chart passed a certain number of days incomplete and unsigned, they would be kicked off staff. They would then be required to resubmit every piece of paper, application form and filing fee, references, and background checks as any new physician applying for privileges. First time applicants generally get through the admission process in about two to six months, depending on how long it takes to get all the paperwork back from the various sources, to which the hospital must make inquiry. This was a major challenge to them.

They did not believe I would do that. We were playing a game of "chicken" to see who would give up first. I stood my ground. I told them that we would find another traveling orthopedist or recruit another family physician. They caved and came in to sign charts. It took the orthopedist a whole day to complete his. It took the family physician a weekend to complete his. No one on that staff ever played "chicken" with me again.

Then the CEO got into a personal disagreement with the big shot on the board, who also happened to be a big shot in town, and the CEO left. We were devastated, but we were hopeful the next one they hired would be as dynamic as Mike. They hired a man who had a military background.

To call him a rigid personality type would be a kind description. Unyielding and short-sighted would be a more accurate way to speak about him (also nameless to protect his name and memory). He hired Jeff Askenazy, MD, whose ultimate conviction and prison sentence, along with the hospital being indicted and paying fines,[6] played a role, I believe, in the downfall of UMH.

Jeff was from New York and unabashedly Jewish, which was as much of a culture shock to Danish-derived Greenvillians as my being African American had been to them earlier. I took it upon myself to introduce Jeff to the community in my role as VP of Medical Affairs, and my job was orientation of new medical staff members.

I picked him up from the Bed & Breakfast on Main Street, and we went to the one of the local taverns for dinner to talk. He was well-spoken, well-read, and an anesthesiologist by training, who had two pages of published studies in his professional life background, and who was interested in promoting a pain management practice here in Greenville. I was impressed with him, and happy to see another person who was not another plain vanilla white person in town. As we were getting ready to leave, he offered to pay the tab, and over my objections, pressed to do so. He offered a gold credit card to the waitress who said, "What is this?"

The waitress had never seen a gold credit card before because most folks paid in cash. I explained to Jeff that cash was a better option, and picked up the tab. I dropped him off at his B&B, and the owner there met us, inviting us to have evening coffee with her. While we were chatting with her, Jeff asked her very gently if there was a lot of anti-Semitism in town. To which she replied, "What is anti-Semitism?"

Let there be a long pause here as Jeff and I looked at her, looked at each other, and tried to process just how un-lettered this individual truly was. Or was it just pure naivety caged in a good Midwestern heart? Jeff explained and she understood, maybe. I went home and life around UMH began to whirl into a dark spiral.

The purpose of that vignette is to provide a clue for you to the naivety of the population that was now about to experience Jeff Askenazy, MD. They were truly nice people culturally unprepared to meet, in my opinion, a truly bad person.

One of the first things Jeff did was to "help" the hospital find a second OB/GYN. They already had a wonderful, skilled, kind, competent, hard-working, excellent bedside-mannered physician who was originally from Asia. His English was good, but he was obviously not American-born.

Jeff found a friend from somewhere back East, who came to interview. It was my understanding that the hospital decided that this person would be a good choice and a good idea because it would give the town a second OB/GYN.

I don't believe that the hospital ever asked the other OB/GYN if he wanted a partner or if he objected to competition. They offered the new doctor a practice, with staff and an office. It was my belief that he asked to have help purchasing a house, and the board said yes. Recall that the hospital had denied a similar loan to me when I moved back to Greenville.

Then it became my understanding that the hospital allowed him to live more than 20 minutes away from the hospital, despite the hospital's rule that medical staff live within a 15-minute response radius for emergency care and critical situations. I don't believe they offered this to the other OB/GYN. They made me pay rent when I joined the hospital, and I had to repay any advances they provided in my first year of practice, when a doctor needs financial support. They never offered to help me pay the mortgage on my house. I was up and running and profitable in less than one year without them.

From what I witnessed and heard from colleagues and patients, this new OB/GYN was horrible. He never sent a written report on any consult he ever did for any patient I ever sent him. I had the sense that patients didn't like him because he was arrogant and dismissive to women.

**Intersection of Racism and the Hospital Professional Medical Staff in Greenville**

One day, there was a holiday party in the summer for hospital medical staff, and all of us were gathered around, drinking, eating, and talking. Jeff and his friend, the new OB/GYN, began talking about being discriminated against because they were Jewish. The Asian-born OB/GYN and I looked at each other, then looked at them.

I remember our Asian American colleague spoke up first and said, "You can hide what you are for your religion, but we cannot hide what we are for our race, so you will never know true discrimination."

I recall being so surprised at the bluntness and the force with which he spoke, and I was so proud that he made that statement. If nothing else, it shut up Jeff and his buddy. I interpreted the first OB/GYN's statement as a way to get back at them for bringing in competition. In my opinion, the hospital insulted my colleague and invested in a doc who eventually left after a year. This was the start of bad times in Greenville health care.

Jeff Askenazy was a bold, visionary, greedy crook[7] because, as legal proceedings later revealed, he was willing to break the rules to earn money. I don't mind bold, and I love visionary, but linking it with greedy was a blueprint for disaster.[8]

He began practicing anesthesia for the hospital, as well as his spin-off weight-loss clinic and his pain management businesses. He began doing specialized procedures of a highly invasive nature, of which neither I nor the staff members with whom I spoke, had ever heard. He was inserting pain stimulator management devices into the spines of chronic pain patients. I understood that the devices were purchased by the hospital and inserted by Jeff. I witnessed that his procedures occupied two of the three OR suites in the hospital, took three of five days, and each procedure took more than an hour to accomplish.

I recall that he was getting pushback from all the other surgical specialists about the time and space he was occupying, but the hospital was billing out huge amounts of money and getting paid by Medicaid, Medicare, and private insurance companies[9] for his work.[10]

There was no stopping him. From my perspective, no one could approach this problem other than the CEO. I recall asking the CEO what value Jeff was to the hospital, and he told me that of the three million dollars in the bottom line, Jeff was generating a third of it.

It had to stop and, unfortunately, it did, the hard way.

One day, while inserting a device into a woman who was anesthetized, Jeff nicked a large nerve in her cervical spine, causing paralysis and respiratory failure. Resuscitation failed and she died in the OR.[11] Her family sued, of course, and the case was settled out of court.[12]

Meanwhile, the U.S. Attorney's office began a criminal investigation that led to felony charges against Jeff for fraudulently billing private insurance companies, Medicaid, and Medicare.[13] During the investigation,[14] his whole scheme came to light. It took a death and lawsuit to uproot him, but once he was gone, my conclusion was that the hospital knew what was happening and let it happen, because the bottom line was more important than good medical practice.

I firmly believe that hospital CEOs have lied to me. I hope things have changed now.

Eventually, a jury convicted Jeff on 34 of 37 counts of mail fraud related to his billings for unnecessary medical services.[15] He was convicted in December 1998, and was sentenced to 36 months in federal prison and was assessed fines and restitution.[16]

The hospital, which had been indicted, had to pay a criminal fine of more than a million dollars,[17] made an agreement to pay more than $750,000 in restitution as well as to reimburse the government for its expenses incurred during the prosecution.[18]

The hospital and the city of Greenville were tremendously embarrassed and shaken, and then got absorbed by the Spectrum Health system in Grand Rapids. That was a good thing because Spectrum made the right changes, brought in the right people, and fixed what was broken.

That CEO let the dollar cloud his judgment, and he let a criminal physician drive away good patients, demean good employees, create a cloud of hostility between other physicians and Jeff, defraud Medicare, Medicaid, and private insurance companies, and endanger the lives of countless patients, eventually killing one of them.

How many of my colleagues in medicine have similar stories to tell, I will never know, but I suspect the number is large. At least you have heard mine.

## DIGRESSION #22: GRANDMA, WHERE'S THE SEX?

Naturally there is sex in my life. My dear Grandchildren, your mother and aunt got born, so there had to be at least two times I found a way to get started on life's best adventure. Sex is so wonderful because it has the excitement of so many life experiences. Think of combining the feelings of a trip to Disney World with the excitement of a Las Vegas casino located in a war zone during a hurricane.

You can get such exhilaration, and then die if you do the wrong thing. The death can be actual, social, or emotional. I am not going to name my partners, just give them a number and move on. I hope there is a lesson in each of these instances for both of you, dear Grandchildren.

Number one was on campus at Wayne State University. The music was playing on the record player (yes, the thing DJs use in clubs) and it was Mose Allison, soft, smoky, sultry songs that encouraged people to turn off the lights, take off clothes, and shake off inhibitions. We had just come back from dinner and I went to his place because he asked me to. I was not smart, just curious. He convinced me that it would be OK and fun. This was my first time, and it was not horrible. I was lucky to have a skilled partner who was considerate of what I needed to experience. I must confess to complete enjoyment of every moment and every touch. After the first time, I realized this felt good. I was lonely, and now I discovered I was horny, too. After we finished, I went to my place—which was just across the street—hours later, very happy.

The next time I saw him, he said he had something for me. I went to his apartment expecting more of the same as before, only to find it was a pack of birth control pills. How he got them, I will never know, but I think it was a sign of either true love, social awareness, or self-protection. The last thing either of us needed or wanted was a pregnancy. I read the instructions and started the pills as directed, and stayed on them until after I was married. The pill revolutionized life for American women in the '60s, allowing us the sexual freedom men had possessed for centuries.

The development of the pill was an example of how western medicine experimented with people in underdeveloped nations, and how big pharma toyed with medication dosing for women.

The companies who made the pill had to get data from trial usage, but did not want to use American women. Most drug trials at that time were done on healthy white males between ages 18 and 30, so they were completely unacceptable to test drive a birth control pill. The proof that it worked would be the lack of pregnancy, so there had to be a population where there were lots of pregnancies occurring. Voilà, the island of Puerto Rico was deemed ideal. Women there were paid to take the pill, very little care was provided. Invasive testing was applied to determine if the pill was changing the nature of the endometrium (the inside lining of the uterus). No one cared about educating these women on side effects. The companies got the results they were hoping for, and the pill was subsequently also tested on women in Haiti (they're Black, so it must be OK) and Mexico (they don't speak English, so it must be OK). Once it was safe for American white women, the pill came on the market.

The first pills to market each contained a tremendously high dose of estrogen. The main one, Enovid, was a 2 mg tablet. The dose of estrogenic substance in birth control pills today is 20 to 35 mcg. This is an order of magnitude in metric units. Recall that one gram contains 1,000 milligrams, and one milligram contains 1,000 micrograms of substance. I think that Enovid was 100 times what is needed.

But who knew how much estrogen was needed to stop a pregnancy, and who knew what kind of side effects would occur at high levels of estrogen? No real records were kept of adverse events in the population of Black and brown women in the Caribbean; the companies only cared that the pill did what it was supposed to do—prevent pregnancies.

After many years and lots of side effects, they got it right with the development of low dose birth control pills. You will notice that the move to develop a similar medication for men has lagged behind over the last 60 years without a significant call for development. Men do not get pregnant, they cause it, and somehow that is deemed reason enough to exempt them from having any kind of pharmacologic restraint option.

How about an MOC—Male Oral Contraceptive for men?

Every once in a while, I read an article about how some company has finally developed one, but it has to be tested and then approved by the FDA. I can see how it will be a truly difficult development.

The goal is to get a person to take a medication regularly for a long time for a condition that will never happen to them—pregnancy. What is the motivation for a single man to do that? There are no penalties now for a man whose girlfriend gets pregnant. He can skip town and avoid child support payments. He does not need to get married. He can deny the child is his. For the married man, he can just defer to his wife and let her be in charge of family planning. His voice is taken away if she is the one in charge.

Families should be planned by the primary family members—him and her in traditional marriages. In those relationships that are same-sex, I am betting that they have already worked out who, what, when, and how to plan their procreative efforts. For same-sex couples, that must be a big consideration in their life plan. For the traditional male/female couple, it is just an event in the future to be determined at a later date in a lot of the cases.

How would a woman even know a man is on a contraceptive? Let's face the fact that men will sometimes lie about themselves in an effort to appear more attractive to a woman and convince her to have sex with them. So, how do you motivate a man to take the contraceptive medication?

Combine it with Viagra. Oh, yes, I laughed too when I wrote that, but on second thought, why not? The users of the contraception medication would be most likely single and young, so their incidence of cardiac and metabolic health problems is much lower. The population of men with Erectile Dysfunction currently is the group with cardiovascular and metabolic disorders like coronary disease and diabetes, and they are generally older and generally already married or have had a family.

The male contraceptive pill should therefore be aimed at the younger set. The next question is how will a woman know that her partner is actually taking a male birth control pill? There might be a subset of men who would say they are taking a pill, just to convince some trusting woman to have sex with them. The pill should cause some identifiable physical manifestation in the user. Maybe the man will glow in the dark if he is a true user of the MOC. I don't know; I'm just making stuff up.

Someone much smarter than me will figure out how this will work, and then the whole ball game will change dramatically. Family planning will truly involve the whole family—him and her on some much more equal footing. It is not just about sex. There are women who cannot take an FOC—Female Oral Contraceptive—because of problems it causes with blood pressure, blood clots, weight, or breast pain. There is a need to offer men the option of being in charge of how to plan a family, from prevention to spacing of children; it could be a truly joint decision.

In 1988, when pharmaceutical companies had real power and lots of money, and no one looking at how they spent it, I got invited to an all-expense paid trip to a medical conference in Scottsdale, Arizona. Flight was first class, the hotel was first class, the food was great, and the attendees were all physicians and their wives. We were required to spend the morning in lecture. We listened to a paid medical shill tell us how wonderful and safe the pharmaceutical company's drug was, and why we would be doing our patients a world of good to prescribe it.

But in the afternoon, we had the option of doing several things for relaxation. We could take a guided tour, shop, or sign up for extra sessions such as travel, sightseeing, pottery making, or fire walking. I signed up for the fire walking seminar. I was always willing to try anything dangerous once (but never do anything dangerous twice because that now makes it an addiction).

The two-day session began in the afternoon and lasted till just before dinner. The leader of the seminar was a former RAND Corporation think tank engineer-type person, very personable and very dynamic as a speaker. The day before the seminar, he demonstrated his fire walking, and I was glad I had signed up to learn how to do what I saw him do.

I took notes and paid close attention to what he said. I also noticed that some of the participants did not come back after the first break on day one, and more failed to show up at the start of day two. I persevered. What did I care, what did I have to lose? This is the kind of WHY NOT thinking that has gotten me to where I am today, good, bad, or indifferent, it is how I am.

On the start of day two, we had to gather wood and build a 12-foot-long fire pit before we settled in for our half day of cumulative seminar work. We had a break partway through and went back for the final portion. It was here that Michael (not his real name), the leader of the seminar, prepared us for our actual fire walk. He gently explained that no one is obligated to do a fire walk, and no one will be made to feel ashamed if they drop out at this point. About two more people stepped away and we all shared a moment to give them permission and our love before the remaining eight of us did our personal fire walk. I was not the first one, but I knew I would not be the last one to cross the blazing 12-foot-long bed of red hot smoking wood coals in front of us. Michael did his walk, and then from the other side, motioned to us and said, "Hold the thought of cool moss in your mind and come across."

One by one, we did. It was my turn, and I tossed off my sandals and stepped onto the coals.

I felt nothing on my feet. No heat nor touch, no pain, nothing. I walked; I did not run. I looked ahead, not down, and my mind was focused on cool moss. I crossed to the other side and was so elated at what I had done, I screamed and shouted with release and excitement. The remainder of us crossed over, and at the conclusion, we all gathered into a large bundle/scrum of men and women and hugged, cried, shouted, laughed, and surged with emotion at what we had done as individuals and as a group.

My mind was definitely on fire with the enormity of what I had accomplished. I felt peaceful, powerful, beautiful, expansive, filled with love and positive emotion, overflowing. I went to the main picnic area where dinner was being served and just had to tell someone what I/we had done.

The first person I told was a physician friend, and when I said that I had just walked on fire, he looked at me as if I had said I was Jesus Christ come back from the dead and had seen heaven. In short, he thought I was nuts or drunk, or both.

He smiled and said, "That must have been nice."

I had no reply, but I realized that no matter what I said, he did not see it, so he chose not to believe it because he still believed that fire will burn you, and you have no power to prevent that. Michael, in the seminar, taught that your mind has power to change what you believe, and you can control larger portions of your reality that you ever thought possible.

I turned away and shrugged, and "Caribbean Queen" by Billy Ocean was playing, so I danced to it by myself. I found my way to the bar at the hotel resort and Michael was there with a table of others who had also fire-walked. Music was playing, and he asked me to dance, so I said yes.

I was wearing a purple spaghetti-strapped dress with double side slits that showed off my legs, waist (I had a nice waistline back then), and my bust to the best advantage. He was a good dancer, and so was I. At some point in some song, later that night, he leaned into my neck and asked, in a sotto voce, "Do you want a lover tonight?"

I said yes.

We went to his hotel room and really got into each other, hotter than the fire pit ever was. After that wonderful night, I was really flying high on positive hormone emotion all the way back to chilly Michigan. I may have been in love, but I was still married.

I stayed in touch with Michael. We shared the same year of birth, and would call and wish each other happy birthday. One year, when I was chair of the committee that organized the statewide spring scientific seminar for all the DOs in Michigan, I invited Michael to be a speaker. He said yes, and we met again. He was an engaging speaker, and was also a most wonderful lover, with skills undiminished by time or distance.

Again, I thought I was in love, and this time I was divorced from Arney, so I thought there was a window of opportunity to be with someone else. Michael and I stayed in touch, and again I invited him to Michigan in the next year, hoping for a reunion and a chance to cement our relationship. One week before he was due to arrive, he called to tell me he could not attend because he had found "the love of his life" and needed to stay with her.

Needless to say, I was disappointed. Mostly crushed, but always the realist, I knew it was probably a doomed relationship from the start. So much would have to change on his part, as well as on my part, that it would never be long lasting or meet my expectations, not that I even knew what I expected to have happen.

Still, we maintained contact, mostly by email, but one day he called and we talked, and I must confess, I still felt a spark. Turns out, he had divorced "the love of his life," or she had left him after they had children. He was now living in a distant state, on some land owned by his mother.

Michael was always interested in planned conscious community building; what would have been called a hippie commune back in the day was the impetus of his work. To perform this goal of community building, he formed something called "The M Group" (I have hidden the real name to provide anonymity), and conducted an online program encouraging people to join in conscious community building, in which there would be love, trust, security, cooperation, etc.

He told me he had a partner, a lady who followed him from where he met her to the place in a distant state. She was still working, and he was building his "M" community, hoping to entice people to come and build homes on the land he lived on.

Time passed and we continued to speak on the phone, and I followed him online with his "M" emails. He really had great ideas and great thoughts about community building. But I think he never had any takers on his offer to come down and build on the land. Mainly, because he was not the owner; I think it would be difficult for a stranger to invest any sizeable amount of money in a place where there was no possibility of ownership. When Michael's mother dies, the land will be divided between him and his siblings. No sensible person/outsider would commit to such an investment where the guru-leader has no definite chance at unobstructed ownership.

I do not know if he sees it that way, but we do still call and talk. His most recent partner has moved on, and he is not with anyone as of this writing in 2020. He has no partner, no steady job, no takers on his planned community of loving, free-living people. He never fails to ask if he can come and visit (have sex with) me. I never let him know if I am alone or with someone, male, female, or not.

Michael was a sensational bed partner, but a failure as a life partner. I see him as a person who must latch on to someone and convince someone to take care of him while he keeps his head in the clouds with his community building plans. Very few women I know are going to be on board with that plan. I certainly was not, and will not, be one of them, no matter how much I loved him in the past.

Great sex is not the end-all, be-all of my life.

More than likely, my attitude about sex was formed by some very good, and also very bad, experiences along the way, from my very first kiss with a really yucky, sweaty-palmed white preteen to the present.

Let me count the men:

1. Sweaty-palmed white pre-teen.
2. Golden gloves Black boxer teen.
3. Wayne State University hot kisser Black guy.
4. Detroit hippie drug-smoker dirty white trash boy.
5. Italian Stallion Pontiac-driving hot guy.
6. My first (see above).
7. The campus Black stud who loved me.
8. My European rapist when I traveled there.
9. The Swede in the youth hostel I should have married.
10. Arney, before we married.
11. The Others after Arney and I broke up on campus.

12. Arney, after we got back together and married.
13. The intern I cheated with while married.
14. The classmate I cheated with while married.
15. Divorce.
16. The Black chef who was always late after I got divorced.
17. The Black insurance agent who was the tallest man I ever dated.
18. The last one, Michael (see above).

I do hope this list does not embarrass any of those who are mentioned. I would never give out their names, and if they are reading this, they will know who they are. I hope this does not bother you, dear Grandchildren, to know how I have been in my younger, sexually-active life. I learned a lot, and I suffered much because of sex, but I always found a way to enjoy sex, and so should you.

Rules for sex:

- Don't have it unless you have a condom and a reliable birth control method.
- You need both, because a condom is not birth control, it is STD control.
- Don't have it with someone who is cruel or unknown to your parents, because if you cannot tell your parents who the person is, you should not be in bed with that person.
- Don't have it with anyone who says, "Don't tell your parents we're doing this."
- Be loving and honest with your partner.
- Forgive your partner.
- Understand this is how babies get made, so be prepared to have a baby if you are going to have sex.

WE'RE BACK . . .

**Wage Slaves at Ingham Regional Medical Center**

I was so burned out by the Jeff Askenazy, MD, experience, the hospital, and the stress of divorcing Arney, that I made another geographic escape.

I eventually found my way to Lansing, Michigan after my divorce from Arney in 1991. Carol Monson, DO, my classmate, was practicing at Ingham Regional Medical Center (IRMC) in Lansing, and she was looking for a partner in her practice. We were actually all employees of the hospital system, and in fact, another classmate, Dave Neff, was in the next office across the hall from her. The building was a five-pod, multi-specialty clinic with three family physicians, three OB/GYNs, two pediatricians, and an X-ray facility on site for plain films only. Located next to the I-96 highway in Lansing, it had a great clientele, filled with a good mix of payors, and close to MSU's campus.

Carol and I trained residents, interns, and externs, and had a great time working together. I left Greenville, moved to the Lansing area, and bought a house on Hagadorn Road. The house was great, a 1970s ranch with three bedrooms, a sunken living room, two wood-burning fireplaces, a finished basement, and a huge backyard with a brick patio for my hot tub.

But IRMC was not as financially strong as Sparrow, the MD hospital in town. So IRMC was taken over by McLaren Health System, and its name and culture were changed. It became another health behemoth looking to gobble up practices and clinics and grow larger.

The leadership would brook no opposition from the interchangeable minions known as physicians. I advocated for a larger voice for physicians in the governance of whatever we were destined to become. I was a thorn in their sides, and they decided I must go. My friend warned me that my release was imminent, and he was correct because in early January 2000, I was told that the office was going to be downsized and I would be let go. I had a work contract, and they promised to pay me till the end of that contract, which was June 30th.

I packed my office desk in a cardboard box and was marched out to my car. I went home and cried. I was a doctor and I had gotten fired. How could that happen?

I moaned and mourned for about two weeks, searching for an idea of what I could do. I decided that I could work somewhere else, and I also decided that I had six months of paid vacation to find another spot somewhere. I called a friend who was working for the MEPS (Military Entrance Processing Station) in Lansing, and she said they were always happy to have contracted physicians who would do the examinations on the people who were being recruited for the five branches of uniform military services—Coast Guard, Airforce, Navy, Army, and Marines. The work was easy, the pay was good, and the hours were simple.

I enjoyed every minute of it.

The entrants were all healthy, and the exam was straight forward. They needed to be healthy enough to march, willing to kill, and smart enough to know how to be trained for both activities. I also saw how the recruiter had the power to override a medical disqualification, and that override was frequently applied if the applicant was anybody with a medical degree. A woman candidate for the Marine Corps was a dentist, and she had failed the visual test. Her recruiter was with me every step of the way for her exam, and when I informed him that she had failed, he merely smiled and said, "No worries, Doc, let me handle it."

He stamped the exemption sticker on her papers and she was on her way to Quantico, because as I understood it, the Corps needed dentists and that is what mattered.

I also gave a lot of time to searching for another full-time practice, and I opened the search to other states. I found recruiters were interested in placing doctors in practices all over the nation, so I did not have to do any of the hard work of searching; they did it for me. They hooked me up with a place in Wisconsin, the Gundersen-Lutheran Clinic, and it was the best place to be for a family physician, ever.

I got a call from Dr. Jorgensen, the director of the office in Prairie du Chien, Wisconsin, and we spoke on the phone and agreed to an in-person interview.

Suddenly, I realized if I went to another state, I would be alone. There would be no one from my family, no friends or relatives of any kind anywhere near me. That was a daunting thought, and I had never faced that kind of aloneness before. After sleeping on it, a strange thought came to me, and I acted on it the next morning. The thought was, *Why not ask Arney if he would like to move with me to Wisconsin?* He was no longer on the bench as judge, but was back in private practice and drinking as much as he could afford, coasting along and going slowly into the sunset of Who Really Knows.

I called him and we spoke:

"Hi, you wake?"

"Yeah, why are you calling?"

"I wanted to let you know that I got a job interview, and probably a lock on a really good job in a big clinic in Wisconsin."

"Wisconsin?"

"Yeah, a place called Prairie du Chien. It's on the Mississippi River."

"You gonna go there?"

"Yes. I want to know if you would come with me."

Long silence right about here. I could hear his thoughts moving from "no way" to "yes" in this fashion:

"Come with you? Go to Wisconsin? No way. But, what's there? Anyway, what would people think? What would I do there? I'm retired here, I could be retired there. Although, I suppose it would be OK if they thought we were still married. Hey, we're not getting re-married, are we? But even if we do or don't, on the other hand, I guess it would be a good move for me, and for you, and for both of us. So, YES, I will."

"That is great," I said. "We should plan to go together for the job interview. They will want to meet you."

We were getting the band back together.

Arney and I drove up and got a place in a local motel to stay, had the tour of the city and the clinic, and visited the main hospital in La Crosse. The hospital recruiter was so attentive. He and everybody else up there just assumed we were still married, and Arney and I never said anything to make them believe otherwise.

They made the work offer and told me they were only able to offer the median salary for a family medicine certified physician without OB, and that was $132,000 a year (that is $227,518 in today's dollars). I managed to keep my face still as I heard the offer. This was in 2000, and I had been making, take home, about $70,000 a year on my own in the clinic in Greenville, and maybe $90,000 at IRMC. Even better, that was just the cash pay; there was a generous package of benefits included with the deal. I put my head down, then slowly turned it back up as if I had been contemplating any other answer other than "Yes, fuck, YES," and said instead, "That is very generous and I accept."

**Becoming a Wisconsin Badger**

Time to move to another state.

I took the state board exams for Iowa and Wisconsin, and passed both. Both exams were required in order to work at Gundersen-Lutheran because the clinic complex spanned three states—Wisconsin, Iowa, and Minnesota—and included not only physician offices, but also ophthalmology and optical offices, plus the main hospital in La Crosse, Wisconsin.

My time there was wonderful. I had after-hours call one day a week, as well as every sixth weekend. I had to brush up on ventilator management and get recertified for advanced cardiac life support (ACLS), but I was ready when the time came. Not only did I get those skills upgraded, but I also found out that there was a wealth of information, valuable and solidly correct, from the then-burgeoning medical Internet sites.

No longer did I have to press everything into my brain and struggle to pull it back out on demand. If I had access to a computer, I could get it. Gundersen was fully computerized. In fact, one of the things they required of all physicians was the ownership and use of a Palm Pilot. Back in 2000, Palm Pilot was a top-of-the-line piece of hardware for management of all kinds of functions. I had a Nokia cell phone, a small Texas Instruments calculator, and a small digital flash camera to go with the Palm Pilot, as well as a Franklin Planner, so I felt really on top of the medical technical world. In fact, I quickly adapted to the computer and became known as the person to go to if there was a problem for any of the clinical users. My theory was that I was willing to mess around with anyone else's computer freely and frequently and do things to the office PC computer that would make me fall out of my socks if I dared do it with my precious Mac. I was fearless with the PC EMR, and quickly figured out how to navigate around and through the churning garbage that was laughingly called an Electronic Medical Record.

Gundersen-Lutheran did, however, have one feature that was a Godsend, which allowed clinicians to dictate their notes and did not force us to use pre-written macros or click through a hundred and one million damn drop boxes to input chart information. We spoke into a voice recorder that sent the information to a home-based transcriptionist, who then sent it back on the computer for our review. If we liked what we said, we accepted it, if not, we could edit the document from our own desktop. Plus, we had voice connection to the transcriptionist if we ever needed to speak directly to them, or them to us. Wonderful. No long day of typing after a long day of seeing patients.

The local hospital was a typical small-town place: one older man in charge, still calling himself the Administrator, a few top notch, hard-working RNs who actually ran the place, one crusty but wonderful RN who controlled the long-term care unit attached to the main hospital, and a bunch of nice people trying to do their best for the patients who came there. It was one big family. Except for the guys in ER.

The ER docs were hired guns.

They worked long, hard shifts a week at a time. Each one was as different from the other two as could possibly be. One was a DO who smiled and laughed his way through work and only called you if he was going to admit a patient. The other was a younger MD, originally from Canada, who was an outdoorsy-type, easy going fellow, who was not ashamed to ask for my opinion on any patient. And the third was a middle-aged MD, hard-edged, no bedside manner at all, who was a massive control freak. But they were all good at doing ER work. I admired their iron-pants attitude about their schedule: 24 hours for three days, then off for two days, then 24 hours for two days, then off for three days, all through the year.

With my arrival, there were now two DO doctors in PDC, the one in the ER and myself. But I was the only one that practiced any hands-on therapies. Once my MD colleagues figured out what I did, they quickly abdicated from the treatment of people who had any kind of chronic head, neck, or back pain, and rapidly made sure those folks found their way onto my schedule, forever and ever, amen, thank you, God.

"We want to make sure you have a full book of patients so you can get your clinic billing and numbers up to a good level," they all said. What they meant was, "These freaking patients have made my life miserable because I have no clue anymore about what to do with them, and they won't let me give them any more opioids than what I am currently doing, so you can have them."

I accepted all of them gladly. I had my OMT table for manipulation, the same one that I had ordered personally constructed for me when I started my clinic in Stanton, and which I still have with me today. I put patients on that table and I sat down at their feet on my exam stool and asked them to "tell me about why you are here and what is bothering you."

I learned that technique of where to sit from my ENT friend, Bob Quillan, DO, in Grand Rapids.

You would be amazed at how close to never that question gets asked of a patient in today's health care system, and if it does get asked, there is never enough time given to hear the full and complete answer. I managed to create enough space in my schedule to make time stretch so I could hear them. One of my trainers said, "If you let the patient talk long enough, he/she will tell you the diagnosis." It was true then, and I still believe it is true now.

These folks had never had any hands-on treatment by a DO. Some of them had been to chiropractors but did not get better from those treatments. As I progressed in the clinic, I decided to improve my OMM skills, so I signed up for CME classes at the Upledger Institute in Palm Beach, Florida. That area also happened to be where my good friends, Gerry and Mary Jean Teachman, lived, and it was the place where Arney and I purchased a small condo. So, my trips there were a combination of vacation, as well as CME activity. Besides that, Dr. John Upledger was the MSU professor who did my admissions personal interview, and later became my medical school advisor. He was weird, wise, wonderful, visionary, gently and spiritually guided with his hands-on work, and a powerful teacher. I learned so much, and I brought it all back with me to PDC, and all those patients who had head, neck, and back pain that had been unresponsive to my MD colleague's opioid management program.

They would sit on my table and talk to me about their problem. Next, I would ask them to lie on the table while I scanned their body energy. Then I would ask if I could place my hands on them. I would connect with them and scan down through the layers of tissue and layers of energy until I found the area, or areas, of discord and dysfunction. I would then begin corrections. The silence in the room was profound, and sometimes felt actually sacred. I do believe they joined with me in the healing of their bodies, because I had great results with 90 percent of them. My reputation grew, and I was a great resource to the clinic.

I was so glad that I was a DO, and so glad that I learned cranial manipulation from Dr. Upledger and from MSUCOM.

## DIGRESSION #23: DOs AND DCs MERGE

At some point in the future, the Osteopathic profession will make a fruitless and futile attempt to bolster itself by offering members of the chiropractic profession the opportunity to become DOs.

This is not unprecedented. In the late '60s, the MD profession in California offered all the state's DO physicians the opportunity to become MDs, with the provision that they could not capitalize the "M" or the "D," and must drop the DO from their names. The DOs accepted the offer, and went away for a long time from the California medical field, giving the MDs an unopposed control over health care in that state.

When the first DO college in California was established, that all changed, of course. But at the time of that merger, the DOs did not know how to counter the power of the MD lobby. So, they caved.

In some future yet to come, the DO community may decide to bolster itself by absorbing DC professionals, requiring them to become family physicians if they do a one-year hospital rotation, much like an internship year. The profession could more than double in size, and the increase in membership income and lobbying power would be a huge counterweight to the AMA.

Currently, whatever the AMA wants, the AOA goes along with it. If the AOA wanted to prevent being absorbed again, but on a national level, then seeking to add all the chiropractors would be a possible option.

Please don't laugh. Remember that John Palmer, the founder of chiropractic medicine, was a student in Kirksville studying for a year with Andrew Taylor Still. Palmer took what he had learned, absconded to Iowa, and opened his school of chiropractic. Much of what those two early professions did was therefore very similar.

But the AOA gradually learned that it must grow in the direction of pharmaceutical inclusivity, and not just remain a hands-on healing-only profession. The AOA has been in the shadow of the AMA for all of its existence and struggles with identity.

Absorbing the chiropractors back into the House of Osteopathy might be an option.

WE'RE BACK . . .

**Good Times at Gundersen-Lutheran Clinic**

Gundersen Clinic life was great. The town was small-town America on the banks of the mighty Mississippi. No one thought twice about being my patient, and in a very short while, I was immensely popular.

**Racism Reappears Once More Again as a Microaggression Racist Moment**

I was not only the sole DO, but also the only BIPOC (Black, Indigenous, and people of color) in the Gundersen Clinic, and probably in all of PDC. I thought I was OK, doing a good job, being professional, being friendly with my coworkers, and respecting them. Unfortunately, that was not the opinion held by one nurse who was, to put it mildly, a sheepish incompetent woman more interested in her nails and hair than in doing actual work. She was assigned to be my RN when it was my day to handle walk-ins and urgent care in the clinic. Each doc had this rotation, and generally was assigned one RN with whom to work. I was given her (like John McCain got Sarah Palin, she was the choice they gave me).

The front desk told us about a patient who was coming in and who was "having seizures." My RN became panicked. She paced back and forth, wringing her hands, and wondering out loud what would we do and why would that person dare to come here with seizures and not go to the ER instead. It was unsettling to see how jumpy and distressed she was. I must have spoken to her in a fashion she did not appreciate.

The patient came in, not actively seizing, and was seen, treated, taken care of, and sent home. I got through the day and finished my day on call. About a week later, the doctor told me that the RN manager wanted to speak with me and that I should just go to her office now. I did, and the RN manager closed the door and told me to sit down.

That is always a bad sign when they think they need to close the door and think they need to tell you to sit down.

She said that the RN working with me on my last on call day was very upset at my harsh words and unprofessional treatment of her, and that she was no longer comfortable working with me. Then, she went on to read more of the drivel written by that nurse before she put down the letter and proceeded to say that she could understand how and why this would happen because, the RN manager said, " . . . look at you, you are so large . . . "

What I believe she stopped herself from saying was, "And you are so Black."

We finished the discussion with the agreement that she would find another RN for me to work with because the other one was so fragile and could not possibly work with me again.

Later that month, I read an article in some entertainment magazine wherein a Black actor who is famous for his police/buddy/action movie series once said, "At the end of the day, I am just one more N*&&$ in Hollywood."

I know how he felt.

## The House in Okemos

My oldest daughter, Ophelia, came to live with us in 2003. A year later, we moved my mother in with us because her frail health did not allow her to live alone in her home in Virginia.

Then my classmate, Carol Monson, alerted me to the fact that there was a faculty opening in the department that she now headed at MSUCOM, and was I interested in coming back to Michigan and being part of her "crew?"

After discussion with Arney, I said yes, and we moved back to Michigan. I bought a house in Okemos, using cash from the sale of my house in Prairie du Chien in December 2005, and we took possession in January 2006. The housing market crashed in 2007-08, but I was so lucky because I did not have a mortgage. I just had an alcoholic husband with COPD, a disabled woman, a house that was a money pit of needed repairs and flaws, and a spring flood swamp hole disaster in the backyard.

The house in Okemos was just what I wanted. It was a ranch with a walk-out lower level and a huge backyard, perfect for pets and gardening. It was three bedrooms, with space for a mother-in-law suite in the lower level. We each had a bedroom and space for our two dogs. Arney used the smallest bedroom as his office, and I used the room off the furnace room as my personal office. We moved June, my mother, into an assisted living facility, and Ophelia had the mother-in-law suite on the lower level.

Then we found out about the problems. The first warning sign was the fact that the bank would not allow the mortgage or sale to proceed unless the sellers put on a new roof. Which they did, and they used the cheapest, sloppiest company they could find, because we discovered roofing nails in the lawn for all the time that we lived there.

The first spring in May, 2006, I came home to find my lawn had turned completely white. There were four trees, mock cottonwoods, that put out copious white fuzzy seed pods every spring, and those pods were responsible for the white covering that made my lawn look like high winter. I hired a tree cutter, Mr. Holman, at a cost of $1,000 per tree to get them cut down. He was slow and bad, and wanted to be paid before he cut the trees, but I knew better and refused to pay out front. I also insisted on paying with a check so I had a record. He and I argued, but I had dealt with wood cutters in Crystal, so I was ready.

I had to replace two doors at the side and front entry, and found a person who thought it was OK to send me a bill at the completion of the work, get paid, and then send another bill, because the first one was added up wrong. Thank goodness for Arney, the in-house consigliere, who told me that I should tell that person to get stuffed because the law said I only had to pay what they asked for.

Doors, trees, roof, the failed gas furnace, and the telephone wiring replacement, were actually minor compared to the lake in the backyard.

At the end of the first summer, I noticed a small, continually-wet marshy spot in the middle of the backyard, about one-third of the way to the back edge of the property. By January 2007, it was a large frozen spot of water, and in the spring of the second year, there it was, a small pool that never quite dried up. By the summer, it was obviously larger, and by fall it, had not gone away.

I had a lake in the backyard every time it rained. I was fearful that the water would fill up and flow back into the walk-out of the lower level and flood my home. I built a large raised garden bed around that door as a bulwark against flooding. But the problem persisted, and most days when it rained, I had standing water that was a foot deep covering the backyard from one side of the property line to the other. I had to purchase an outdoor sump pump and 200 feet of plastic drainage hose to handle the problem. Thank goodness for Ophelia and her efforts to help me drain the water. I cried when it rained, and I cursed when we had to spend a day pumping water out of our yard.

I explored other options, and found the real estate disclosure statement, part of which asked the sellers if there was ever a problem with water, to which they had marked NO.

Because the world has liars, the world also has lawyers.

They lied on the disclosure, and I knew they needed to make some correction.

For a couple of years, the case dragged on. I got a lawyer and sent a letter, which they ignored. I filed a suit and the legal paperwork kept piling up. I had the county inspect the sewer lines around my property trying to determine where the drain actually started and where it connected. I had to purchase hoses and sump pumps to remove the ever-enlarging lake of water that accumulated after any rain. Thank goodness Ophelia was living with us because she was the one who did most of that heavy work. I asked neighbors to sign affidavits stating they had seen the lake of water, and they had heard the previous owners stating the water was there.

As it turned out, the developer who built the subdivision excavated a small pond, and when my house was constructed, he placed the drain in to remove the small leak of water from the pond site. He ran the drain across the backyard, and made it take a 90-degree left turn out to the street where it connected with the city storm water system. But he also planted an oak tree at that turn. Over 30 years, that tree grew huge and the roots ran into the drain and plugged it up.

I decided to remove the tree because we were adding a deck, even before I knew the yard flooded. When the case was settled out of court (I won), I had the plumbing people come over and do a video evaluation, and they saw the root system. Well, the tree was gone now, but the roots remained. The company, Michigan Plumbing, hauled over a 900-gallon tank and used a high-pressure hose to blast the roots into perdition, and the drain was opened up and has run free and clear ever since.

If those previous owners had been willing to listen to my letter where I asked them to come and talk with the attorney and me, we might have decided on this kind of evaluation and solution, and saved them $14,000 in penalties, fees, and costs.

It was a glorious day in July when that happened, and I am so glad, because later, I was able to sell the house knowing that there was no water accumulation to haunt any other buyer.

**Working for MSUCOM**

The College of Osteopathic Medicine had a clinic in the Clinic Center. The payment structure was hugely unfair to the doctor who chose to work a lot of days in the clinic, because that doctor's share of overhead was higher than any other doctor who chose to work fewer days. Added to that was the fact that none of the staff was responsive to the doctor's needs, requests, or demands because they knew you were not the person who paid them, and they were all union members. Immovable, uncaring, and disconnected from anything but their paychecks.

The COM paid us a huge wage in our first year, then cut it in half in the second year, and expected us to gradually build our clinic hours up, billing up to the point that we would be earning what we used to get in the first year. No way was that going to happen. It would have required every physician seeing eight people per hour, and there are no logistics that can let that happen and still provide any speck of quality care, especially when you add the clunky EMR on top of the union workers in the nursing staff.

Overhead was unfairly distributed; in my opinion. For example, we were assessed for malpractice insurance based on the number of days in clinic. One lady was there five days a week, but one guy was there one day a week. The fact is they both needed insurance 24/7, and should have been assessed equally, but that was not the case. That is just one example of how assessments were not fair. The harder you worked, the more you got screwed.

## DIGRESSION #24: DPC GROUPS WILL PROVIDE 24/7/365 HEALTH CARE

Everywhere I have been, the patients are packed into exam rooms waiting to be seen by the doctor. I do not do group visits. I do individual visits. So why do patients just keep getting shuffled into another waiting zone? Habit patterns that are old are hard to replace.

That is why I am glad to see the arrival of Direct Patient Care. DPC can rescue doctors from the slave toil of working for a large health care institution or hospital, can reduce patient dissatisfaction with piecemeal care, and can drastically reduce costs. The administrative overhead in the C-suite is killing medicine. The doctor in the office, who is employed by the institution, is supporting a ton of people who are not putting an oar in the water to make the boat go forward, but who are sitting on the deck, asking and demanding to go faster.

There is the CEO, CFO, CIO, CMO, HR, PR, CNO, CDO, CCO, COO, few to none of whom are typically physicians, and all of whom make more than the highest paid/highest producing physician in the system.

I think you could provide top quality, primary care with 10 family physicians and one PA. And if you really amped up the video and technological aspects of care, patients could have on-demand care and real access 24/7, 365 days a year, and the doctors would not be worked to death, but would still make a good living.

Ten family physicians can create a schedule that allows the office to be open from 8 AM to 6 PM, Monday to Friday. Each day in the office, there are two physicians seeing patients, two physicians making house calls, two physicians making video/virtual calls, and two more physicians on call for night coverage. Two are off work.

On weekends, all patient contact is by virtual video care. A schedule I drew up gives each doctor two days a week off. The PA is the swing-in substitute when one of the doctors is gone on vacation or for CME events. The doctors' schedule, for face-to-face visits, is structured so that one doctor comes in early and works from 7:30 AM to 3:30 PM, and the second doctor works from 10:30 AM to 6:30 PM. The night call team of doctors splits the night with one working from 6 PM to 1 AM, and the second working from 1 AM to 8 AM.

The doctor team working house calls makes visits from 9 AM till 5 PM, starting and finishing in the office each day to log in their visits.

The doctors doing virtual care split the day so that one works from 8 AM till 4 PM, and the other works from 10 AM to 6 PM, Monday to Friday. This pair also handles all the lab reviews, refill requests, and other things that can be done electronically. On Saturdays and Sundays, the video virtual team works from 8 AM till 6 PM, and the night call team splits the night into two parts. Part one is from 6 PM till 1 AM, and part two is from 1 AM till 8 AM.

No patient is ignored or left waiting in a room. The office has two exam rooms, but each room is large and able to function for urgent care activity, as well. The Real Family Practice Office has reality in the Direct Patient Care (DPC) universe.

The rest of the building is comprised of modules that serve as medical, business, and supply storage in one module, lab/utility in a second module, X-ray and other diagnostics in a third module, and private office cubicles for 11 people in the fourth module. The clinical exam rooms would be the fifth module. The central zone would be the waiting/reception area.

The doctors would have to run their business, and each one would be assigned to one aspect of the business. Medical/pharmaceutical supplies and samples is one. Non-medical supplies is the second. Internet and tech is the third area. Tax, finance, payroll, benefits, and accounting is the fourth. Medical malpractice, licensing, and CME is the fifth. Operations, maintenance, building, and grounds is the sixth. CLIA, radiology, diagnostics, and compliance is the seventh. PR/outreach and med student training is the eight, and business contracting is the ninth.

When I was in charge of my own business, I had to be conversant with each of these features, and know what was going on in addition to keeping up with each patient.

The DPC model could require patients to pay on a basis much like the old country clubs used to run back in the day.

There is a yearly membership fee based on actuarial demographics of each person, and then there is a monthly drawn down visit fee. Assume a person pays $1,000 a year for membership, and $100 a month for visits. He/she draws down five dollars from the monthly fee that covers any encounter with any physician—face to face, text, video, phone, email, letter, etc. When that fee is exhausted, the charge for each service goes up to whatever is being charged out in the world of insurance medicine. This gives a person 20 visits/encounters a month with a doctor before he/she has to pay the exorbitant rates that are going on now. Some people will use all 20, while some people will use just one, but it seems more affordable than how people are being gouged by insurance carriers now. There are a lot of possible fee arrangements, and in DPC, the doctor decides which one to use.

I think it is possible to have a group that becomes skilled at not only taking care of patients, but also taking care of their business, and does not need the burden of all the drones in the C-suites.

When I was an employee of SHHS, I asked to see how they calculated my productivity. "Productivity" is a term tossed around by administrators to employed physicians. It is not the number of people you see, plus the number of dollars you bring in, minus the cost of paying you and your overhead. Here is what SHHS gave me.

Definitions for Productivity Report:

1. Total Productive Hours (TPH) = Actual worked hours
2. Total Productive Wages = Wages paid for worked hours
3. UOS Volume = Units of Service per pay period
4. Hours per UOS = Total Productive hours/UOS Volume
5. Earned Hours (*) = Actual UOS Volume x Budget Hours per UOS
6. Utilization Index (!) = Earned Hours/Total Productive Hours
7. FTE Variance (#) = (Earned Hours – Total Productive Hours)/80 hours per pay period
8. Wage per Hour = Total Productive Wage/Total Productive Hours
9. Wage Variance = Budgeted Wage per hours – Actual Wage per Hour
10. Cost Per UOS = Total Productive Wages/UOS Volume
11. Earned Wages = Budged Hourly Wage x Actual Earned Hours
12. Variance $ = Total Productive Wages – Earned Wages
13. OT Hours = Actual Overtime (OT is not budgeted)
14. % of TPH = OT hours/Total Productive Hours
15. Non-worked Hours = Worked hours – Paid Hours (given)
16. % of TPH = Non-worked Hours/Total Productive Hours
17. Total Non-worked Wages = All wages associated with hours in #15

None of this made any sense after number two, and no one was able to explain it to me, nor did they keep an accurate count of daily office visits. Even though I saved a copy of every face sheet for every patient for a month, we differed. They never counted the work I did from 2009 to 2010, when they calculated my "productivity bonus" for year 2011 and I got nothing.

I felt like I was screwed from behind without even a reach around for my efforts. DPC is the way for all physicians to go, and physicians should get the courage to walk away from the bovine manure handed out by health care institutions and their administrators.

One of my friends on staff, a pediatrician, told me that the CEO never paid any doctor a bonus in all the years he had worked there. She always found a way to cheat the doctor out of that money.

My advice is to never trust a hospital CEO; I believe they all lie.

See the index for a sample of the schedule that could be used by five family practice doctors and four employees to provide 24/7/365 care for a smaller group option.

WE'RE BACK . . .

**Working for MSUCOM Part Two: Family Medicine Clinic**

Life in the MSUCOM Family Med Clinic was fun sometimes, and tough most times. We were all colleagues, but not all of us worked equally hard. Those doctors who had managed to obtain outside consulting work had fewer days in clinic, but earned more money because the income from their consulting work was added to their side of the earnings balance.

The first month I was there, one of the staff MAs decided to file a grievance against my classmate, who was the department chair and clinic director. That took up a lot of time, and created a really tense situation in the clinic any day the MA was there. It witnessed the MA wearing headphones all the time, and being distracted from whatever you wanted her to do. I recall she was slow and she was angry. She eventually lost her grievance complaint and moved to another office.

The building was a fortress, built in the '70s when white people were fearful of the possibility of race-crazed Blacks, dope-smoking, anti-war white hippies, and their bra-burning feminazi girlfriends storming the campus to cause destruction. There was literally just one large window in the entire four-story building. The place was built with an abundance of odd angles so that, not only were the rooms closed in, but they were oddly shaped, and made the positioning of people and furniture very difficult.

But the international crowd was fun. The campus was very multicultural, and I enjoyed the variety of people who came in. But, nonetheless, there was the usual undercurrent of incipient racism in the patient population.

One day, a white woman patient came in, and when I knocked to enter and introduced myself, to begin the new patient process, she stood up and said, "I am so glad to see you." She went on to say, "My last couple of doctors were all people from India, and while those people are very smart, their English was just terrible. I never knew what they were saying, and I am sure they never knew what I was saying. So, when you showed up, I was so happy to see one of US was going to be my new doctor."

I did not know what the fuck to say. I am a large Black woman. What does she mean, "one of us?" In retrospect, it was just more funny than racist, but still it was racist.

There was continual conflict between the various deans and their schools. The MD school, the nursing school, and the DO school shared the facility and the costs. But they did not cooperate or share ideas, or share much else. So, it was always a power struggle at the top, and we peons at the bottom just dealt with the administrative fall-out and the turgid progress, if you could call it that, when there was need for improvement or change.

**VPA Life on the Road**

I decided to move on. Peripatetic is my middle name. I found work with a company called Visiting Physicians Association in 2006. It was started by two brothers who hired a physician who made house calls to care for their mother, and from that they developed a business which filled a great need for many homebound seniors unable to get to a doctor's office.

Every doctor had a car and a medical assistant. The assistant drew labs and did EKGs on a portable machine. Plus, the doctor could order home-based diagnostic tests via a mobile unit, and those tests were ultrasounds, sleep studies, pulmonary function tests, and dozens more that could be done in a hospital.

We were a small office located in Okemos, a small suburb near East Lansing. VPA was actually a large multi-state organization, and Okemos was just one of its local offices. I was one of four doctors; we were the bedrock of the physician crew. One day, we experienced an office harassment situation involving a physician and another employee, that required us staff members to stay away from the office for an hour after our official opening time.

On a regular day, my assistant and I would drive to eight to 10 locations, do an encounter, get back to the office, do charting, and go home. The day was nice. I rode in the back, reading charts and preparing for the visit, and usually got home at 5:30 or 6 PM every day. Not a bad life.

### Another Intersection of Racism in Medical Practice

Maybe this was just ADD meets racism, but who will really know? Once I worked with a medical assistant who seemed frequently distracted. She was with me at a patient's home, and I asked her for a pair of scissors so I could cut off a bandage from the patient's leg. My assistant, who was on the other couch facing me and the patient, tossed the scissors at me. I dodged to avoid getting stabbed in the eye or cut. I had no idea why she did that. Was it racism? How the hell would I know? Back at the office, I immediately requested a different MA , and our nurse manager quickly complied with my request.

Mostly, we were a good and happy bunch. We four physicians did our work, were socially connected, and happy with what we were doing with patients. The patients were so glad to see us and so happy to not have to travel to see the doctor. If I had it to do over again, I think I would do cash-only house calls for senior citizens. There is not a grandfather or grandmother in America who does not have a pair of $20 bills in their possession on any given Sunday, and who would hand that over for a house call visit.

Meanwhile, my life at home was going to hell. June, my mom, was growing more and more disruptive due to her personality disorder, while Arney was drinking more and more, and becoming more ill with his emphysema, heart disease, and diabetes.

**South Haven Health, Michigan—Blueberry Country**

Once again, I moved on. This time I think I just ran away from home and I took my mom with me to South Haven, Michigan. I am sure that was it.

I left Arney in the care of Ophelia and told them they only had to pay for their food and personal needs because I would handle the utilities from my location in South Haven.

Of course, they grumbled, but I did not care. I put Mom in a group home, which she hated and began to sabotage the owner with bad behavior and lies while skillfully engineering conflict between other residents and so forth.

There is not much about my working at South Haven Community Hospital, later called South Haven Health System, that I can speak of in a favorable fashion here.

The place was sinking into a quagmire of ineptitude and was being eyeballed for takeover by the local health care giant in Kalamazoo. The administration maintained that things were fine and told the board that the hospital was on good ground. Eventually the takeover happened, so that to me was an example of why I never believe CEOs of hospitals.

I spent time exploring the community and getting around the hospital, meeting people who would become my neighbors, coworkers, and colleagues. I found them to be open, friendly, hard-working, and dedicated to providing the best health care possible.

I also discovered that employees were unhappy and several told me why they decided to leave. Some cited lack of options for advancement or increase in pay. Some of my neighbors cited the ER's bad reputation and told me they were concerned that lawsuits would occur.

When I was there, at its height, the medical staff had two pediatricians, four family doctors, two general surgeons, two hospitalists, a psychiatrist, two orthopedists, three internists, and three obstetricians. Eventually over time, they all left. I was close to all of them and we talked a lot about how things were progressing.

Here I witnessed favoritism that bred resentment that I felt and heard from my colleagues. I also recall the departure of several physicians for a variety of reasons that included, from what I understood about their situations: impossible standards to meet requirements for bonus pay; refusal to write prescriptions for narcotics-seekers whom I believe were thronging around the hospital and that doctor's office; retirement; better job offers elsewhere; lack of board certification; failure to comply with basic job requirements that I remember caused a problem for me; and inadequate pay and coverage for vacation time.

I remember one very skilled physician who was from Africa and did all the hospital and office work and took call two weeks in a row every month. Then he went back to his other home in another city for two weeks. He was very friendly with me and one day over dinner laughingly told me that the administration never paid anyone a bonus.

One day he went on vacation to Africa, and while there, fell ill, returned home only partially well and never made it back to full practice. He died and the whole hospital community was devastated.

My office in Covert was a converted bank and my private area was actually in the old vault. It was a cute building with a great diverse population. One third were Black, one third were Latinx and one third were white. Many of them were significantly addicted to opioids due to the prescribing habits of the previous physician in that location.

That physician had become ill with some significant rheumatological problem and was out of practice for more than six months, necessitating my recruitment to his office. No one knew when he would return or if he could resume regular practice.

I met him after he recuperated and he insisted that he and I should practice together. He told me that he had been treating people for their chronic pain. He also told me not to trust anything told to me by the administration about him. But I had seen enough of how he "treated" that clinic's population to know such a union would be disastrous. His previous charts showed that he routinely handed out opioids and then added on some kind of amphetamine and then would back it up with a benzodiazepine. I decided not to abandon those people back to his open-handed, free-wheeling opioid prescribing habits. Eventually, he moved on to another city.

There was another specialist, who claimed to be a cardiologist, who would find any patient of mine who had any kind of heart condition and then convince them to let him perform a heart catheterization on them for "routine" check up every year. He never did any stenting because he was not trained in that procedure. The heart cath was just very lucrative and easy. I discouraged all my patients from this kind of activity. This person also dabbled in liposuction[19] and diet treatments. Eventually he got caught doing liposuction in a farm outbuilding[20] on a patient who coded and died.[21] He was sued and state officials suspended his medical license.[22]

One of the nicest family doctors was a person who, along with one of the OBs, had first met me and encouraged me to come work at South Haven. This young doctor had a great misfortune. It began when he agreed to begin issuing medical marijuana certificates and also converting his family medicine practice into a pain management practice. His office nurse told me this was at the insistence of high-ups in the administration. His real practice dried up and went away and he became the "drug" doctor. Eventually he was caught in a DEA sting for his opioid prescribing work and was suspended during the investigation that followed.[23]

I think I tried my best to support the hospital. I had ideas to make my clinic profitable. I proposed efforts to begin weight loss counseling and health education sessions, pain management education. I also offered to open the office for community meetings like AA or NA and to improve transportation between my office and the hospital. Everything I proposed or wanted to do, the administration told me NO, stating it would not be feasible or profitable. But somehow or other, the ideas I had were morphed into the structure of another clinic in South Haven where the internist was located.

I moved on because the administration saddled me with a mid-level provider who decided to sign my name to scripts for opioids without my permission or knowledge. The administration hired this person to work with me in a satellite clinic, so I was in two places each week—four days in Covert and one day in Bangor.

This mid-level medical provider never provided any real documentation in the charts. I know because I reviewed them each week when I was there. This abuse was really brought home when the pharmacist called me from the local discount megastore's pharmacy and wanted to confirm if I wanted to give Patient X a high dose, high volume opioid and said the name on the Rx was signed by the mid-level provider.

I was ready to explode! I left my clinic in Covert, drove to the administration office, and barged in on a meeting demanding to know WTF was going on with this mid-level provider and who gave permission for her to use my DEA number?

All I got was a mealy-mouthed, slick explanation of crap about how that was shocking and it was never the case and they were going to look into it and *blah, blah, blah*. I told them, sitting at the table:

"You can never fire me, because I'm quitting!"

At that point in 2012, I was sick to shit of South Haven and ready to retire. Arney had died in August of that year. My mom had passed away a year earlier. Veronica was in Ohio. Ophelia was living in the house in Okemos. My house in South Haven was nice, but I decided I needed to leave that city. I guess I was still trying to escape from myself, along with my internal fears and demons and weaknesses, with a geographic cure.

Plus, I was tired of the sorry state of things with the hospital. I think the Board of Trustees never really knew any of the reasons why medical staff were leaving, why employees were quitting, and why patients were going elsewhere. Maybe they were caught by surprise when the hospital was bought out by the big facility in Kalamazoo. I know I was not.

Some say small hospitals in America are closing because of pressure from declining populations, aging populations, economic downturns in rural communities and pressure from the need to meet government and insurance compliance rules and regulations.

I say you can add greed and lack of ethics on the part of administrations that force physicians to act against their own best interests or to behave unethically or illegally to the list of reasons why small hospitals are closing. And I think my time in South Haven cemented my mantra of Never Trust a Hospital CEO–I believe they all lie.

## DIGRESSION #25: HOW TO FIX THE CME PROBLEM

As of writing this in 2020-21, physicians are required to obtain a certain number of CME—Continuing Medical Education—credit hours each year to satisfy state licensing requirements. Each state is different. Michigan wants 150 hours in each three-year cycle. Indiana wants none. Wisconsin is happy with 50 hours in two years. There is no pattern or reason to it, much like the spotty response that has persisted throughout the COVID-19 pandemic.

If a doctor works for a large corporate health care organization, he/she is given a yearly stipend to cover CME. That stipend must cover the cost of signing up for the credits, attending the conference, travel to and lodging at the locale, and paying for the state license. The travel expenditures will take up 80 percent of the yearly stipend, and the states did not accept virtual digital CME credits. Also, the state and national professional organizations made money from hosting these CME events, and so they wanted doctors to travel and pay and stay.

The pharmaceutical companies were major sponsors and supporters of all these events because they knew they had a captive crowd of doctors in one place for three to seven days. Lots of money changing hands in the hotels and airlines made sure that stipend evaporated pretty quick. But if you did not have your CME, you could not keep your license, and then the hospital would not hire you. The hospital will never give you enough to cover what you need, so you end up paying out of pocket for the rest.

COVID-19 has caused a lot of changes, including how physicians obtain CME. All conventions have gone virtual. CME online is now acceptable in all states and by all professional medical organizations. CME from DO sponsored conventions is as good as CME from MD sponsored conventions, and equally accepted. We are not going back to the old way.

We should take the next steps and completely revamp how CME is done.

1. It should be virtual as well as face-to-face.
2. A set number of hours should be a minimum and acceptable by every state. Forty is enough.
3. Doctors could get four hours per month online for 48 per year.
4. They could also get another eight hours for any full day conference held face-to-face.
5. The virtual CME should be case studies, such as the ones done now on Medscape, because those actually teach something that is useful to people in practice.
6. The DPC clinics can write off the travel expense as a business deduction, just like the hospitals do now for their employee doctors.

This would remove a lot of pressure and eliminate a lot of bullshit in the CME game. At least it should serve as a starting point of discussion on how to change the broken system.

## WE'RE BACK . . .

### The South Haven Health System—Shenanigans Happening—Health Care Sinking

Let me offer another example of the intersection of racism, poverty, and health care disparities in this small clinic.

My office was just a staff of three: me and my two assistants. One day, a lady came in complaining of chest pain. I knew she was on metformin, which could have been given to her for her DM or her PCOS. As I listened and examined her, I decided that she needed to be triaged to the ER via ambulance because of her symptoms and her history. I was really sweating it because I did not have an Automated External Defibrillator (AED) on site.

Later that month at a general staff meeting, I asked to have an AED placed in my office. I recounted that story. I thought it would be a no-brainer to get an AED. The CEO, a white woman, and her medical staff advisor, a white man, said that I did not need one in my clinic. Their rationale was that the fire station and EMS supplies were just down the block from my office. It was a distance of 100 yards.

My administrative assistant was old, slow, and fat, and could not handle the alphabet effectively, much less make it down to the fire station in less than one minute. My medical assistant was a volunteer firefighter and trained EMS provider, but even with two of us, not having an AED would severely hamper our efforts if we ever needed to provide real CPR to a person.

I cogitated about how much time it would take for my administrative assistant to get up and get going to the fire station, and how much time it would take for her to explain in her usual flustered fashion what exactly we needed, and how much time it would take for them to decide to either run down or drive down with an AED to my office.

What would I be doing while those precious seconds and minutes were ticking by, and while that patient's life was slipping away while I had no AED?

I looked at the table of people, and I thought about the people who came to me—poor, white, Latinx, and Black—and I realized that here was another intersection of racism and capitalistic oppression with the practice of medicine. They did not want to spend the money for a piece of equipment that might save the life of a Medicaid patient who was poor. Jerks.

I had been around long enough to know that when a big bear is sharing something with a small rabbit, the small rabbit will eventually become the lunch or something much worse.

Remember the joke:

Mr. Bear and Mr. Rabbit are sitting on a log.

Both are taking a shit.

Mr. Bear asked Mr. Rabbit, "Does shit stick to your fur?"

Mr. Rabbit said, "No, it does not."

Mr. Bear said, "Thanks for sharing that."

And then, Mr. Bear picked up Mr. Rabbit, wiped his butt with Mr. Rabbit, and left.

Anyway, I quit.

**Moving to Indiana and Novia Care Clinic**

I looked around and found an ad for Novia Care Clinic. They were a provider of health care for employers who wanted a worksite-primary care clinic. The idea was great, and it was popular.

It was the last place that I worked in a stand-alone clinic, and it was with a group called Novia Care Clinic. They later sold to a paper mill company that had a medical care subsidiary called Quad Med. The owner of Novia Care got a golden parachute while everybody else got screwed, but that is another story, and is probably the rule in the business world of grow or die.

The headhunter who contacted me said the position was for the medical director position, so I applied.

I researched the work site clinic idea, prepared a clever PowerPoint, bought a good suit and nice shoes, and interviewed with them. They loved me, they praised me, they showered me with affection. They hired the local white guy MD.

They wanted everything I was not, but they knew they needed me, so they kept me as the lead physician in the main office in Fort Wayne. Their client was the Fort Wayne school system, huge and burdened with patients who needed health care. I was the doctor in the main clinic, and I had two NPs working with me. The secondary site was staffed by an MD who was by himself with just an office nurse.

I worked four 10-hour days, had three days off, and got good money. Patients had either 20- or 40-minute visits, so the schedule was open, and the EMR was workable. There was a dispensary for generic medications given free to patients, a CLIA-waived lab, and a draw station. No X-ray, but we did not need that because there were two large hospital systems in town, plus a free-standing radiology unit that was a privately-owned, stand-alone operation owned by the radiology group that was providing service to one of the hospitals. Talk about raking in the cash, coming and going; those radiology guys had it figured.

I loved my day. Early start, early end, and no call at night. All weekends off. I lived in a senior living community called The Townehouse, and I met people there who loved to play bridge. I think I was the token Black person, but that did not seem to be a noticeable problem at all. The Townehouse was filled with intelligent seniors who knew what was important in life, had overcome all kinds of mad, bad, dangerous obstacles to get there, and were totally unafraid to open a bridge hand bidding in fourth seat with 10 points, vulnerable with three passes prior.

The people were my joy. The house I rented was huge, 2,500 square feet, with a bonus space over the garage, and a concrete patio out back that overlooked an open grassy field.

My NP was a great, hard-working guy. The health and wellness coach was a darling young woman who made people do things for themselves and their health that were next to miracles. The MA could get blood out of anyone, in any condition or any age with one stick. However, the RN was a prime bitch in my opinion. I know she did not like me, nor—according to my observations—did she care to work with Black people—so I believe that the MA and I were on her automatic shit list—and it appeared that she was not interested in actual work. When she revealed to us that she was having a major flare of some rheumatological condition and got put on high dose steroids, she turned into Super Prime Bitch. We had it out most every day: eye rolls, snide remarks, sulking and skulking all day in the office. In my opinion, she took the joy right out of office life.

Even that was tolerable until they got a new EMR—the same piece of shit that MSU was using years ago and then sold out to Quad Medical. Everything changed for the worse.

In order to log in to a patient chart, I had to write down a series of 18 different steps to carry out on the computer. Operations office and staff were located in Indianapolis, a two-hour drive from Fort Wayne on a good day. Things slowed up administratively, and it became drudgery working there.

I became more depressed about high health care costs. Hospitals are focused on making money and less on making you well. I was on staff at Lutheran Hospital, which called itself Lutheran Health Network. All I had were walk-ins and talk-to-a-patient privileges, basically a medical visitor. That was enough. That status earned me the right to be on the mailing list for the *Med Staff Memorandum.*

The December 2013 issue featured front-page headlines about the hospital:

- Using the region's first specialized stent;
- Opening an advanced heart failure transplant satellite clinic; and
- Closing a tobacco intervention program.

Gee whiz. If they ramped up the stop smoking program, maybe cardiovascular and pulmonary disorder rates would plummet (maybe, hopefully), and the need for heart transplants and stents would also plunge. I am too simple. Maybe that is not correct, but I still think I am not wrong.

LHN had a competitor in town, an even bigger place called Parkview. They put out a brochure called *Focus on Health* in April 2013. The front page of the brochure loudly heralded, "Free Health Checks."

When I opened to the inner pages, I saw that blood chemistry tests were $32, A1C tests were $22, Hemogram blood tests were $8, Thyroid Stimulating Hormone tests were $20, Prostatic Specific Antigen tests were $20, and Vitamin D was $30.

Way down at the bottom was the free stuff—your height and weight, blood pressure, vision, plus a summary and referral.

This is just scamming people. Blood tests are not proof of health, and what they offered was not free. Just a way to get mo' money, mo' money, mo' money, mo' money.

**The Door to Retirement**

Veronica convinced me that if I were going to retire, then I needed to do it in Ohio and live near her. My dear Grandchildren, she had you two. Ezekiel, you were seven, and Magdalana, you were four. Veronica was working from home while her husband was working 16-hour days at a fulfillment warehouse for a large industrial manufacturing supply chain distribution company. He made good money, but the hours were killer.

I thought about what I was doing, why I was doing it, and what my future path was at my advancing age. The lure of being with grandchildren is just the strongest thing in the parental/grandparental universe. It is the ultimate bait and I fell for it, and I am so glad I did.

I went looking for a new place to live in July 2014. Veronica hooked me up with the real estate agent who found both her houses, and I was so fortunate to get Kathy Nerponi. She took me everywhere I wanted to go. I had spent a week developing a house evaluation checklist, and then I spent another week looking at houses for sale on the Internet, and got a list narrowed down, which I gave to Kathy Nerponi. She had even more places, and we weeded them down to the point where we could look at 10 each day for the three days that I was in town. For the life of me, I do not know how real estate agents have a life. Their schedule is as bad as a doctor on call. Any day, any hour, anywhere, they have to get up, get out, and get showing a place for people to see.

I settled for my home in a place that some people described as the place where the wife goes when couples get divorced later in life. I found three places. One was smaller, but had no deck, no finished basement, no finished kitchen, and no finished master bath. The other was larger, with a small dinky deck and no pleasant view, no finished basement, nicely finished kitchen, and master bath. The third one was smaller, but had a deck, a finished kitchen, finished master bath, and a killer view off the deck, plus the unfinished basement was an opportunity to make it in my own design. That is what I bought after I sold both my properties in Michigan.

In October of 2014, I moved into my new home. I used Two Men and a Truck moving company, stuffed my cat, Jane, into a carrying case, and drove her from Indiana to Ohio. We left at 5 PM, got in at 11 PM, and the truck followed, arriving just shy of midnight.

Those guys called in three other guys to do the unloading, and thank goodness, I had placed color-coded duct tape on the boxes so they knew where to place them in the house. For example, the boxes with tape imprinted with a mac and cheese pattern were headed for the kitchen, the boxes with solid purple were in the master bedroom, and so forth. One of the last items was my specially-made, personally-designed OMT table that had been with me since I opened my office in Stanton, Michigan in 1980. They were having trouble getting it down the stairs into the lower level.

I said, "You will find a way, because it is not going to be upstairs." And then I left. They found a way and that table is still with me.

I gave each man a $20 tip for the work they did, released the cat from the guest bathroom, and went to bed.

The day after moving in was total chaos, but it was good chaos. The weather was good and Dave Hawkins—the handyman, contractor, builder par excellence—had already been working on the lower level of the house, doing framing-in work. Dave was a self-taught, self-made construction genius who could eyeball an area and calculate the square footage, then calculate how much flooring and so on and so forth. He was meticulous and inexpensive, and he was fun to be around because he was absolutely down-to-earth honest. Plus, he liked football, baseball, and politics.

He and I had wonderful conversations about everything: politics, baseball, race relations, football, raising children, golfing, and so forth. He had done work on both homes that Veronica and her husband had purchased in Ohio, and was affectionately called by Veronica, her "day husband," because he was around the house all day working, before her "night husband," came home from work. He and all of us enjoyed the moniker.

Dave actually started working on the lower level three weeks before I was able to move, and he was there from September till January. People like him are the epitome of the adage "salt of the earth."

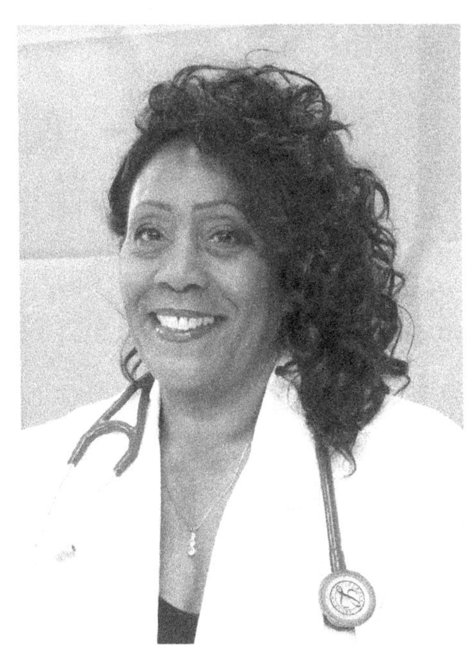

# SECTION FOUR
# AFTER THE END OF ACTIVE PRACTICE

## Daily Steps for Success

How do you know if you are successful?

Some people count stuff like their money, or their trophies and possessions, while some count the accomplishments that have been recognized by others. Some have nothing to count.

Maybe success needs a different definition. Maybe stating that you are successful is wrong, and maybe you should state that you are always moving into success as long as you are alive. Maybe looking back is not how to define success.

Over the years, I've cultivated a list of things I do every day to look back on my legacy, focus on the now, and look forward into the future with positivity.

I now share these Daily Steps for Success, especially for my grandchildren, to apply and use to reach your highest potential.

## Daily Steps for Success

- Know yourself by becoming aware of who you and what you want.
- Set specific goals and break them down into attainable parts.
- Plan solid strategies to achieve your goals.
- Get an accountability buddy or team to help you meet goals.
- Know that slow and steady wins the race.
- When you fail, learn from it, and try again.
- Identify whatever's blocking your success and remove those blocks.
- Keep It Super Simple (KISS).
- Invest your time wisely.
- Don't procrastinate.
- Understand the "why" that motivates everything you do.
- Choose friends who add and multiply value in your life.
- Create a daily routine and follow it.
- Schedule daily exercise and quiet time.
- Balance work and play.
- Get up earlier and make your bed.
- Go to bed earlier.

- Follow a schedule for eating.
- Have a beginner's mind, always open to learning and change.
- View challenges as a way to show how strong you are.
- Ditch the fear. Ask, *What is the worst that can happen, and can I live with that?*
- Be gentle with yourself.
- Don't try to be perfect; no one is.
- Write your thoughts and ideas in a journal every day.
- Watch less TV.
- Spend less time on your phone and devices.
- Monitor your progress.
- Reward your successes and share with others.
- Enjoy music by creating weekly playlists of songs you love.
- Switch it up; have variation.
- Get organized.
- Use lists for daily tasks and overall goals.
- Recite mantras to shift your mind into a positive place.
- Be productive during your commute time by reading, writing, and learning.
- Don't multitask!
- Always line your cooking pans.

You will notice that nowhere does it say to accumulate things, have more than anyone else, or wait for everyone else to say you are successful. It is very internally directed.

Thanks to these Daily Steps for Success, I count myself as a successful person. As long as I am alive, I can and will continue to work through each of these steps, and success will naturally be a daily accomplishment.

**Recuperation**

I left active full-time practice in October of 2014, walked away from the on-site worksite clinic in Fort Wayne, Indiana, and moved to a condo in Geauga County, Ohio. The place was excellent, and the location was even more so, because it was close to my grandchildren, Veronica and her husband.

I decided not to practice medicine. That was a big step. Once upon a time, I toyed with obtaining a license in Ohio, but I did not. The paperwork was too onerous, and I already had five other states that collected a fee every two years, plus a DEA license to maintain. I would have to keep up my CME activities and find a low-level kind of medical activity to justify having the damn things.

I found out about an opening in the Osteopathic College in Athens and applied to be on the family medicine staff. Long story short, I was not considered because I was not residency-trained. There is that old deficiency coming back to bite me in the butt. What is really funny about my rejection is that one of their deans, whom I recall was the relative of a very famous person, was not residency-trained either. But that was not a problem, and they accepted that person. Times changed, and they did not accept me. I never want to complain about what fate gives me, because fate knows what I need better than I know. I have no crystal ball and cannot see that getting my way now might be hurtful to me later. As Jimmy Hoffa is rumored to have said, "Never complain and you will never have to explain." I moved on.

Time to settle down and be more grandmotherly. That allowed me to focus on nest-building for my new condo. I was the second owner. The first owner lived completely on the first floor, never developing the lower level. The upper was a really compact, 1,600-square-foot space, just perfect for a single lady and her cat.

I hired Dave Hawkins, the same contractor who remodeled both of Veronica's Ohio homes, to build my lower level into a multi-purpose flex space for overnight guests, library books, and parties. I gave parties in my first two years, inviting everyone I met, and had a ball. I also became babysitter to my grandchildren, after their sitter went back to college full-time. What a joy it was to be with my grandchildren on a regular basis.

Except for my time with Ezekiel and Magdalana, I was bored to tears. I was never a housekeeper or homemaker, and even though cooking and cleaning were easy tasks, they were not at all fulfilling.

So, I went back to work, but this time as a Locums Physician, which meant doing temporary assignments for other physicians' offices. Maybe I thought I had something to prove. Locums seemed like a good option for work-life balance. I got to work when and where I wanted. I got good money for easy work, with no administrative stress. I wondered why the Direct Patient Care model was not available when I was starting out, because it is truly the best of the best kind of health care. Being a Locums doc was as close to that DPC model as possible.

I worked for McLaren Health System in 2017 and realized quickly why I hated traditional standard clinical family medicine practice. I got a job working for MSUCOM at a clinic, and realized why I hated clinical practice run by layers of administration. Next, I worked for another company, and realized clinical practice as it exists today, in my opinion, is just plain hateful. People need time with their doctor, as much as is necessary to find the answer and reach some kind of motivation. That is not possible in any system I have seen, except maybe in Fort Wayne.

Facing my own decline and eventual demise made me focus on recuperation, again.

In March of 2018, my classmate and good friend died. She and I had last seen each other in Detroit in late October 2017. I was filling in at the Popoff clinic, and she was working at Detroit Medical Center, teaching OMM. We had dinner at my hotel, the Westin downtown, and talked about our plans for next year. She was going to attend the American Academy of Osteopathy Convention with a former student, and I was going to attend Michigan Osteopathic Association Convention in Detroit in May that year. We planned to meet there and share a glass of wine, along with our other classmate. We shared dinner and a wonderful talk, then went our ways.

In late February of 2018, my friend sent an email asking for help deciding on what kind of surgery to have for her stomach problem. This was shocking and totally out of the blue. I had no inkling that she had any problems. Actually, she had survived a case of low-level lung cancer several years ago and was happy to be back on the path of good health. How she got lung cancer is a mystery, considering her non-smoking, healthy lifestyle.

She sent an email to me and our friend for advice. The three of us had been meeting at the state convention in Michigan for 20 years, so we were close. I told her what I could, and so did our friend. Her reply was that she was too weak to really do much research, and so she had to depend on us for the best advice. Eventually I learned that she had a complete eventration of her stomach, and had been unable to swallow food to the point where only water would pass through.

Eventration is where the stomach slips up between the muscle layers of the diaphragm and gets lodged in the space under the lungs. She had her surgery, went to rehab, and recovered just fine. I managed to speak with her during her second week of rehab. She was happy and upbeat, and told me she was glad she made the decision to be in rehab, and was working hard to get back home.

Weeks passed without hearing from her. I finally called her cellular number. Her relative answered, informing me that my friend was in hospice. Her lung cancer, which she had beaten six years ago, had returned with metastasis to her brain. She died in March of 2018.

I was devastated. She was one of my best friends. She was sweet and good and strong and smart. She was not supposed to die; in my opinion, that was the fate of some evil person, not her. My friend and I grieved in our own ways, alone, and I did not go to MOA that year or ever again. I preferred to remember the last time the three of us were at that convention.

The last time the three of us were together at MOA was in May 2017. We met in the lounge lobby bar and hoisted glasses of red wine, toasting life and us. Somehow, we got to talking with one of the waitresses who poured out her story of a sick grandchild. Each one of us shared a piece of advice with that lady on what to do, what to say, and how to connect with better care for that baby. She was so appreciative of our efforts. We felt like we were doing good work even when we were not working, because that is what we were trained to do. That moment of us together was precious, and it was one of the best times in my life of comradery with very beloved classmates. Going to another MOA convention would be ruinous to that memory.

**I Meet the EMS Crew in My Town, Nice Folks**

In June of 2018, I had a small gathering at my home for some people who had volunteered to be street reps for my condo association. After they left, I began having severe back pain on my left shoulder area. It was late, so I showered and went to bed. As soon as I laid down, the pain subsided. It returned when I got up to use the bathroom, but again subsided when I laid back down in bed. The morning of June 9th, I got up and went through my usual routine, but noticed that the pain was still present and worse with every step and activity.

Now I was afraid, and the pain was really intensifying. I called Veronica and then called 911. I was taken to Ahuja Hospital, placed in their observation bed, and kept there while a variety of cardiac tests were done. This included serial troponins, chest X-ray, EKG, and lab work, and then I was placed on a telemetry monitor.

Sunday morning, the 10th, feeling well, pain-free, and expecting to go home, I decided to just try walking around for a bit. I went back and forth from my bed to the bathroom, and the pain returned. Not only did the pain return, but I could see my read-out on the telemetry unit going up from 80 to 90 to 110 to 137 heartbeats per minute, when the nurse came for me and put me back to my bed. I was placed on metoprolol to slow down my heart rate, then had a lung CT scan and a cardiac vascular CT scan, both of which were normal.

The cardiologist and internist decided that I needed metoprolol to control my elevated blood pressure and subsequent tachycardia. I went home on the evening of Monday the 11th. I checked my blood pressure at home and thought it was way too high, but when I saw my internist on Wednesday the 13th, the numbers were great. Turns out my cuff was too small. One new large adult cuff later, I was able to check my pressures at home, and indeed they were now normal, thanks to the medication. I checked it twice a day, avoided excess sugar and salt, and continued my daily one-mile walk.

But God gets a good laugh when you make plans. On Wednesday, June 20th, I ended up in the ER at Hillcrest with severe gastroenteritis. I puked so hard that I called Veronica to take me to the ER. She came over and stayed with me till I was released, with some Zofran and Gatorade.

Things seemed OK for a while, but life had one more hiccup for me. On the first weekend of July, Friday the 6th, I was packed, dressed, and ready to travel to MSU for the opening ceremony as speaker for OsteoCHAMPS, when I felt strange and lightheaded, having pain in my back on the left side again. I waited for it to go away, but it did not. I decided to drive to Hillcrest Hospital, because I did not want to go back to Ahuja, but on the way, I decided that I should go to my doctor's office, so I walked up and asked if someone could check my blood pressure. The office did not open until 8 AM, and I was there at quarter of 8. The receptionist, however, found an RN who had come in early and asked her to bring me back. She did, and my pressure was up, I was having chest pain, and I was on my way to another 911 call and trip.

The fire department showed up, took me on the stretcher to Hillcrest, and I had another episode of 24 hours in observation. This time, the doctors decided to add lisinopril to my Toprol XL, and so I was home with more pills and another expensive test on the horizon. On the 12th of July, I got a cardiac nuclear stress test, which I passed with no evidence of blockage. The problem was that I knew the test was great at detecting late-stage disease, but not so good at detecting the 50 percent blockage, which is where most infarctions happen. I had to take the bitter with the better, and make a change in my life.

It is so hard to change. I cut down from two to one cup of strong caffeinated coffee each day, gave up adding salt to my food five days a week, took my Lipitor, Toprol XL, and Lisinopril as scheduled, and looked at things from the perspective of what was I doing with my life right then.

I knew I was not immune to illness, but I never thought those two episodes would come along some quickly, or one on the heels of another. My pressures had probably been probably bouncing up and down for the past six months, but had hit the danger zone in June. I am so glad it happened while I was home and not while I was on the road in Indiana working for Censeo.

The whole episode made me decide that it was time to scale back, and that I no longer had anything to prove as a working physician. I decided to let my Iowa and Wisconsin licenses go dormant and expire when they came due for renewal. I planned to keep my Michigan and Indiana licenses for a time longer, as they are my first and my last, but realized that that they, too, will eventually expire. It's a kind of sentimental thing.

Certainly, my perspective is different now. Life is sweeter. I am more willing to put up with bullshit from people now, because in the grand scheme of things, it is not really important to get angry with the dull or ignorant in the world.

So, I play bridge online, attend Al-Anon meetings via Zoom, work hard as a member of the board of managers for my condo association, and enjoy my cats. I read a lot every day, books and magazines, try to look at more sports on TV, have music in the house for relaxation, and navigate around Netflix and Amazon Prime.

There is no space for a real garden, but I carve out what I can for potted plants and outdoor container gardening. The neighbors are nice and seem to like me, but then they do not really know me. I am just their Tame Negro Lady Doctor in their community. I hope that opinion of me makes them feel good.

## DIGRESSION #26: THE KKK VERSUS DAIRY QUEEN

During late October of 2020, I drove with Veronica, her husband, Ezekiel, and Magdalana to the Rainforest Car Wash because they had a Halloween event going on where you could get your car washed while watching people in scary costumes ranging 'round outside and inside the car wash.

Because of COVID-19 restrictions, there was very little to do in terms of family Halloween activities. No one was going to do house-to-house trick or treating, and few neighborhoods were holding any kind of outdoor activities at night because there was still a curfew.

The car wash was therefore hugely popular, so we decided to go. It was a long way, but we had nice time chatting in the car. We got to the car wash and saw a line of cars stretching way down the street with police cruisers and officers directing traffic. This was not only a local community event; it was also a regional activity.

We had to wait in line for 50 minutes to get inside because we were in a long line of cars. The cars inched along at a slow, steady pace. But it was well worth it, with lots of laughter from us. We enjoyed looking at all the yard signs for the upcoming election. Some of the better ones read "Save the GOP – Vote Biden," or "Vote for Any Functioning Adult." We even saw one that said, "Unborn Black Lives Matter."

While we were in line and in the car, Ezekiel asked if we could go to the Dairy Queen when we got done because he had never been to one. Wow, 16 and still not ever been to the DQ? Of course, I said yes, Veronica said no and looked online to find a small, hometown, local, privately-owned, non-franchise ice cream shop nearby. She has a habit of changing any plan that anyone else wants to make. I, however, was ready for her this time. I told her that the place she found was located in a town where the KKK had a post.

"We should not go there," I said, adding an elaborate and fictitious trajectory about how the town's KKK leader had a brother who opened the chapter there and married the woman whose father started the White Citizens Council, and everybody knew this was true. I even quoted some phony magazine article about how the KKK would meet at this ice cream shop and hold rallies before going off to burn crosses somewhere. I sounded really knowledgeable and on topic.

My daughter, son-in-law, and grandchildren sat silently in the car, taking all this in as the mood grew sober. It took a while, but eventually, they realized that I was spouting fake news and we all had a nice laugh.

We went to the Dairy Queen, had a nice, sweet treat, and got back in the car for a ride home, enjoying the evening.

WE'RE BACK . . .

**Facing My Own Mortality**

Remember in Wuhan, China in November 2019, an outbreak began of a new, novel, viral, respiratory infection, which was highly contagious, remarkably lethal, and had no treatment? It attacked the upper and lower lung system and caused a cytokine storm that resulted in rapid death for the most vulnerable—those who were older, with underlying medical conditions, such as diabetes, those who take an ace inhibitor, women, and immunocompromised persons.

I had four of those five markers of mortality. It spread rapidly around the world, reaching the U.S. in January, and our 45th President dithered and lied. It spread quickly, and only the state governors responded adequately, not all of them, but at least the one here in Ohio. Everything was shut down—schools, shopping, eateries, and any place where more than 10 people would congregate, such as sporting events. Churches were exempt, but the smart leaders posted their services online or via a streaming function. The foolish ones gathered, prayed, became infected, and died.

My condo community began a program of self-quarantine. I stayed home, only going out for groceries, and wearing a mask and gloves when I did.

The loneliness was crushing. It was a slow process.

With nothing but time alone, I cleaned everything: bedrooms, closets, file cabinets, and dishes. I washed walls, painted floor quarter rounds, washed doors, pulled cat hair out of carpet edges, washed ceiling fan blades, cleaned all appliances, cleaned the entire basement, bagged up giveaway items, polished the silver, rearranged furniture, organized the bookcases, detailed the car interior, and washed the exterior. Kitchen drawers and cabinets were cleaned and organized. I washed everything in those drawers and cabinets. Fireplace tiles and floors were polished. I cleaned the computer and TV screens and walls. I dusted, washed, swept, scrubbed. The carpets were vacuumed and scrubbed. I cleared out dresser drawers, squeegeed hard wood floors, bagged up trash, cleaned my office and sunroom. I painted, disinfected, repaired the entire fucking house and car and garage, the small garden yard and patio, all from March 12th till March 30th.

Then I started calling people, and connecting via email with folks I had not seen or heard from over the years. I reread my old science fiction books and began to binge watch TV series I had enjoyed previously—*The Sopranos* and *Game of Thrones*—or not seen—*Orange is the New Black* and *The Crown.*

I was not good to myself in these times. I tried to use the treadmill daily, and was mostly successful, but my diet, which had been on a good trajectory, crashed on Easter Sunday, April 12th, when I enjoyed a brined Cornish game hen stuffed with an apple, mashed potatoes with sour cream, and a lettuce salad. I topped the whole thing off with a third of a bag of Lay's potato chips while I watched *Westworld.* The next day, my blood pressure was way up and I felt dizzy and weak. I took an extra Lisinopril, drank water, and rested all day, checking my pressure till I was sure it was coming down.

I do recall that when I used to work ER, every family holiday—Thanksgiving, Christmas, Easter—I would see the CHF (congestive heart failure) patients come in around 9 PM, after they had consumed a shitload of salt in their diets, with Virginia smoked ham, brined turkey with sausage dressing, etc. And now that I am an old fart, I did the same thing to myself. Actually, my pressure took a spike on the 1st of April, but I am not sure if it was as directly related to diet as it was on the 13th.

My own mortality comes in and out of my field of vision more cunningly and often each year, does it not?

But what does the coronavirus really care? It is the new apex predator for humans. Because we are led by politicians who want to keep power, they deny science, defy the medical experts, and have let people suffer and die. The Patriarchy does not think it will suffer as a result of this pandemic, but the world, at least the U.S., will not easily go back into its old rut of behavior.

While writing this in August 2020, the stock market has tanked, airlines are flying empty, unemployment is reaching 15 percent today and projected to reach 30 percent later this year, physicians and nurses are running out of protective equipment, there are not enough ventilators for the critically ill COVID-19 patients, small businesses are going out of business, telehealth services are expanding and being paid for by Medicare, and schools are struggling but functioning by using 100 percent online classroom learning. Anything that can work by digital process—Zoom, Duo, FaceTime, etc.—is doing so. These will not stop when the virus has had its final say over us.

Joe Biden is the only runner in the Democratic Party; Bernie Sanders dropped out in the second week of April. President Trump is on TV daily, but now no one wants to watch him as he lies and falters with the tatters of truth. He wants to fire Anthony Fauci, MD, the doctor who has guided him to do the right things to prevent the spread of this pandemic. I hope people remember that Mr. Trump let Americans die.

## DIGRESSION #27: COVID-19 SPEAKS

Here is an interview with the COVID-19 virus:

Welcome to *Meet the Pressure*, Mr. COVID-19. Thank you for taking time out of your busy schedule of increasing incidence and prevalence in our communities to come and speak to our audience. Getting to the point, let me ask, what do you hope to accomplish?

*Thank you, Human. By the way, just call me Sars, I like to keep things casual. It is so rare that one of my species gets to have real communication with one of your species. In short, my goal is self-replication, reproduction, spread, and life. Like any other living organism on this planet, I want to be around for as long as possible. This is, I am sure, a goal that you humans share, and that other species share, as well.*

Why do you kill us if you want to live?

*Your death is an unfortunate byproduct of my replication. I hurt myself when you die, and so I must share myself with many other humans in order to guarantee my species* in toto *will survive. I do not mean to kill you. Your immune response is so overwhelming to my simple cellular-busting actions, that you are actually killing yourselves.*

*You see, it's not me—it's you who are the killers of yourselves. Ideally, you would serve as my host, allow me to replicate, and then extend to another group of humans to continue my spread. I would settle down inside your system and become a part of you. Perhaps you would mount an antibody defense so that I do not flare up again, perhaps not, but my goal as a viral predator is peaceful coexistence in a compliant host that serves me as a vehicle for species spread. In that regard, I am much kinder than you are with other species that you have eliminated or threatened and brought to the brink of extinction.*

*Perhaps I am the revenge of Gaea? How many species have died as a direct result of human action, activity or greed? Carrier pigeons and Chestnut trees in North America, whole human civilizations in South America, the dodo bird in Australia, the aurochs in Europe, white rhinos in Africa, pygmy elephants in Asia, the list goes on and continues to lengthen. Why do you do this? You should ask yourselves why you are still killing off those who share this planet with you.*

Please, Sars, I am asking the questions here. Do you have political motivations?

*That is an interesting question. I have no political affiliation. I kill with equal opportunity; Red States, poor folks, blue states, rich folks, proud boys, Muslim, antifa, gay, evangelical, straight, Catholic, immigrant, trans, Jews, young or old, white or Black. What you see is the death of those who have been failed by your political policies and practices. The ones who are victims of failed education do not know that I am vulnerable to a simple hand washing. Those who believe your orange leader deny the science that says I spread by droplets, and a simple face covering will prevent my spread. I kill those who have been denied health care by your ineffective, inefficient, and unjust health care systems and policies. You make yourselves my victims, and I make all of you my hosts. It's your fault if you die.*

How will you react if there is a vaccine produced?

*I have no fear of a vaccine. Many of you will get a vaccine. Eventually, the companies will produce one that is truly effective, long lasting, free of serious side effects, and affordable and available to the majority of you. But there will be a nucleus, or greater number of those who say vaccines cause other conditions and problems, and will refuse to get vaccinated. Plus, your distribution will be spotty, uneven, inequal, and slow. So, I will always have a home in the bodies of the anti-vaxxers. And I will mutate.*

How will you react when there is a treatment for you?

*I do not fear your treatments. As I said, I will mutate. If you give me Vit C, I will mutate. If you give me Vit D with bleach, I will mutate. If you give me immunoglobulin, I will mutate. I will be with you in some form, the same as my distant cousin, H1N1, scion of the Spanish Flu, is with you. H1N1, or HeneryOne, is still here, still mutating each year. Maybe there will be a HeneryEight. It is the story of evolution, and you cannot live outside of that story any more than I can.*

Are you going to come back in the next year?

*I am never going away. After I have spread and mutated, I will be around forever. The Black Plague bacteria, for example, is still around. Herpes was written about by the ancient Romans; it is not gone. You still have HIV, and it is treatable, untraceable with certain drugs, but not curable, and certainly not gone. The flu is not gone. Why should I go quietly into the night? I'll be here as long as you will. Prepare for that.*

*This is only the first year of my appearance. You have no idea of what I can do, how fast I will change and spread, or how vicious and dangerous I can be. Thanks to your greedy politicians and reliance on "faith"—or drinking bleach, denying I am even here, to save you—I will be here always.*

Our time is up, and so we will close the interview on that unsettling thought.

WE'RE BACK . . .

**Think Like a Pharaoh**

Being older and alone now in the time of COVID-19 lets me have a lot of time to think. So, I have begun to think like a pharaoh.

Those leaders of ancient Egypt spent a lot of time focusing on being dead. For them, life was a process of returning to the dead. Since they were gods themselves, they were very calm about going back to that form, not to be burdened with being a man on Earth, when they were truly just gods in a human body.

The kings who built the pyramids made plans for the afterlife. I may not be a king or pharaoh, but I can make plans for my afterlife. I am not going to build a pyramid, but I am going to set my affairs in state, and set my life on a path of fulfillment and kindness as much as I can.

I do not want my children to scurry around in tears, trying to take care of my mortal remains or personal stuff. They should sit around and enjoy my money, have a great party, tell jokes, and talk about me while they eat and drink with friends, neighbors, and other relatives.

I set up a trust and made certain that you, my family members, knew about it. I wrote my own obituary and included plans for how to conduct the party after I am gone. The funeral should be simple, but the party should be worthy of a shindig at Versailles.

I was raised in a fairly religious household. My grandmother took me to church every opportunity she got. Most of that religious chit chat washed over me and rolled off. I never thought that the Black church did much for the people who supported it. The ministers seemed to get rewarded with fancy cars, their wives covered in furs and bedecked in jewels, and sitting in a nice church, but the neighborhood's needs were abandoned, and the people had nothing from the church in any concrete fashion. The whole concept of "you die and go to hell" for not following some set of arbitrary rules set up by a bunch of guys trying to get more for themselves was just such a turnoff.

Every once in a while, I look at the religious programs on cable TV. The Jewish channels are filled with people who talk all the time about incomprehensible aspects of life as defined by their Torah and other ancient teachings, and how those teachings are supposed to apply to life here and now. Hard to follow, even harder to swallow.

The Catholic channels are filled with ritual. People chanting the same prayer to dead saints, hoping and asking for blessings, whatever that may be. Whenever there is a question that poses a stumbling block, the whole thing is explained away as one of the Great Mysteries of God.

The Black Protestant channels are filled with shouting, sweating Black men, and singing, over-dressed Black women, gyrating their bodies in front of hypnotized congregants for some unknown purpose, but always ending with a call for donations.

The white Protestant channels are filled with funereal-looking older white men, and scrawny, heavily made-up white women, muttering and gesticulating their prayers in front of swaying crowds of equally hypnotized congregants. It always ends with an attempt to sell something to the home audience. Healing oil, a prayer shawl, a piece of blessed paper that will make your wish come true because you sent in a prayer gift. All this is tax-free and avidly watched.

Maybe I should join the church of the FSM—Flying Spaghetti Monster. I think it has as much validity as any of the other assemblies on TV. Hail, Pastafarians.

I think that life is the purpose of life. I think that we all go back to our component pieces when we are done. All the trace elements and atoms of me will disassociate in the ground and flow back into the creation of someone or something else. I will not know it, and I will not care.

If Heaven exists, it must be so wonderful that no one ever remembers anything of life here, because no one ever comes back and makes a report on conditions in Heaven. If Hell exists, it is already here on Earth. Look at all the suffering, loss, and pain that is perpetuated on humans, animals, and plants every day. That is Hell.

If I had a way to remove Hell on Earth, it would be to remove war, organized religion, and hunger from the face of the planet. That triad has been responsible for more death, devastation, destruction, and disorder, and is, in my mind, just short of the death caused by the volcanoes and meteor that wiped out the dinosaurs 65 million years ago.

Maybe the universe counts the number of positive events/energy/emotions and balances that number against the number of negative events/energy/emotions, and if the balance is on the positive side, a star is made brighter and the universe warms up. But if the balance is on the negative side, then a black hole enlarges, the universe has more entropy, and we move closer to the heat death of it all. Maybe the universe does not need a god or gods to make any of that happen; it just takes the energy that we generate from our minds and actions and uses it for creation.

Who knows? Well, as we used to say in the ER, "GORK"—God Only Really Knows.

## DIGRESSION #28: THE SHIP OF MEDICINE IS SET TO SAIL

Health care reform done my way: The Ship of Medicine.

When I was accepted to the advisory board of Ravenwood in 2018, I had a session with the CEO as part of my board member intake education. She mentioned how difficult it was to get the psychiatrists to see more than two patients an hour, how they were paid for lunch, and how low their productivity was. I spoke with her briefly about the mental mindset that is imposed on physicians when they work with an EMR and for an organization that does not understand their needs. One of the things I wanted to do was draw a simple graph to show this using a boat on the water analogy.

It goes like this:

Imagine a person in a sailboat, floating on a stream, coming to a large rock ahead, and a waterfall drop-off behind them. There is a rudder and an anchor in the water. Now imagine:

- The PERSON as the physician, whose job is to sail the boat along the river. This person brings skills, maintains licensure and accreditation, is updated in knowledge, and meets CME requirements.
- The RIVER is the patients who must be moved from the rough waters of illness to the calm waters of health.
- The SAIL is the propulsion given to the physician for this job. It represents the clinic, the billing system, the documentation method and tools, the physical plant location, and maintenance activities.
- The BOAT represents the support and staff used by the physician. That would be the nurses, techs, billing and coding teams, hours of operation, supplies, and equipment, cleaning and repair, and public relations.
- The FALLS represent disaster, the loss of income, and the closing of the clinic.
- The RUDDER represents the leadership, administration, board, CEO, CFO, CIO, CMO, etc.
- The ANCHOR represents regulatory and compliance requirements, and burdens from state, federal, and other agencies.
- The ROCK in the water represents legal hurdles and liability issues.
- The WIND in the sails represents change in the local and national political environment, public health needs, and medical scientific knowledge.
- The SKY represents the personal life of the person in the boat and all the pitfalls that could occur, such as illness, divorce, and so forth.

What the organization can change is the person, the flow of patients, the sail, the boat, and the rudder. A clever organization will find a way to optimize those factors and be on guard for the others, which may change from time to time. The wind, sky, and rock cannot be changed, just anticipated and planned around. The boat will always need cleaning and repair.

I wanted to give that analogy to the Ravenwood CEO, but never did. I wanted to tell her the following suggestions, but never did. Because I know now that people seldom appreciate advice not asked for, so I never spoke of this to her.

In addition to the boat analogy, I also had some suggestions about how to save money, improve productivity, and engage the physicians in these actions. Here's how:

- Stop paying for lunch. This might cost $86,000 a year in lost income.
- Hold a lunch for them on National Doctors' Day.
- Give them a quarterly reward for reaching a productivity goal in the form of a lump sum bonus.
- Let them work in stable cooperative teams.
- Give them an office separate from their treatment room. They are being required to see the patient in the same room that is their office. That seems like a truly uncomfortable working situation.
- Have yearly recognition prizes at the winter/Christmas holiday season.
- Hold a summer picnic.
- Give them a birthday lunch and gift.
- Give them yearly service pins and certificates.
- Fix the schedule so that patient flow is constant but interspaced with time for paperwork.
- Reduce paperwork.

Doctors want to be appreciated and well-paid. Doctors also want some say in how their process moves with patients.

In my opinion, the Ravenwood CEO was good, and even though

I never said those things to her, she managed to find a way to make the work flow better for the doctors as well as for the patients.

More importantly, I appreciate my late arriving wisdom of not telling her any of the above, and instead watching how she arrived at pretty much the same work improvement. She is the one CEO who has not disappointed me and I do not believe she ever lied to me.

Too bad other hospital leaders I have encountered did not see the ship of medicine as a true analogy, or used it to make life better for the doctors and nurses who worked there. It would seem to me that Direct Patient/Primary Care is going to be the true savior of medicine.

## WE'RE BACK . . .

### Allergies Cause My Alien Abduction

In May of 2020, I had another trip to the hospital for an overnight stay, and an upgrade in one of my diagnoses.

I struggled with a chronic daily productive cough, copious clear nasal drainage, and reflux at night for two years. Starting in July 2018, when I was ill with bronchitis, I began having these symptoms. At first, I thought it was just more of my seasonal allergies following hard on the heels of a lung infection. I was sick the week before I took Magdalana to Blueberry Camp in South Haven, and never really improved.

The problem was that the symptoms did not stop when the seasons changed. Prior to this, I would normally have spring allergies when the grass and trees budded out, and again when the ragweed flowered, and both times of the year, I controlled these problems with some Allegra or Claritin, and maybe an occasional Astelin nasal spray. Not this time.

Every day I would cough; every night I would cough; and I would cough in between. I coughed when I ate, when I drank, when I played cards, when I went outside, when I was inside, around cats, around dogs, when it was hot or when it was cold. I coughed so hard at night that when I laid down, I would frequently puke. I had an upper and lower GI consult and endoscopy, which confirmed that I had mild reflux and diverticulosis, and got another pill to take each day.

But still, I coughed. I was ashamed and embarrassed. I bought purses that were large enough to carry around all my inhalers, cough drops, and a box of Kleenex. I would not want to leave the house unless I had inhalers, Kleenex, and a plastic bag to carry the used tissues. I sat in the back of the movie theater so I could get up and leave when the coughing became uncontrollable. I choked and coughed if I ate dry foods like popcorn. Regurgitation was a common occurrence. I was miserable, and people could not help but notice.

On Monday, May 4th, I got dressed so I could take my car to the dealership for some simple service on the alignment. While I was up and walking around, I noticed that my chest felt tight and I was a bit breathless. I checked my blood pressure and it was OK, but I also checked my oxygen. I had a pulse oximetry unit from when I used to make house calls, so I put it on. Sitting down, at rest, it was 98, but when I was up and walking, 89. Not good.

I called 911. From here on in, my adventure reads better as a story of alien abduction and it sounds like this:

*My Medical Alien Abduction*

At 8:30 AM, three uniformed male strangers entered my garage and walked into my home office. They made me walk out to their conveyance, bedecked with red flashing lights, and then they strapped me to a hard cot and drove away. They placed a tight band on my upper left arm and kept inflating and deflating it. They put stickers on my chest and conducted a test that showed red wavy lines on paper. One of them waved the red and white lined paper at me and said words I did not comprehend.

At 9:00 AM, they hauled the cart into a large building and took me to a small, enclosed room. Two men and one woman entered the room. These strangers made me remove my upper clothes. One of them stuck a needle with tubing into the middle of my left arm, but did not connect anything to it. Another one kept asking me questions, shining lights into my eyes, pressing a metal piece connected to a tube that went into his ears against various places on my chest and abdomen. He felt my legs, showed me a picture, and asked me to explain what I saw in the picture. It was a woman washing dishes with her two children arguing in the background.

Then another woman came in and punctured the artery in my left arm. Another woman came in with a machine that shot radiation into my chest. Another woman came in and took blood from my right arm. They continued using the arm inflator/deflator torture band throughout all of this. Another woman took me to another room and placed me on a hard platform, injected a substance into my body that made me feel like I had a fever all over, and then turned on a machine with a rotating circular torus on it. She told me to hold still, told me when to breathe, and when to hold my breath, and exerted that kind of control till the machine stopped rotating. They demanded that I give them a sample of my urine. They stuck a long, hard tube into my left nostril and pushed it all the way to the back of my nasal/brain bone separation.

Then they gave me a tube with misty fumes flowing out of it and told me to inhale the vapors until the water chamber was dry. Then they instilled a substance into it using the first tubing needle, which had been inserted into my left arm. I was then taken through corridors via left and right turns till I was totally confused, and placed in a semi-dark cold elevator, taken to another corridor, and dumped into a hard bed in a room shared by another woman captive. Poor thing, she had been pierced in the back of her lower right lung, and they were sucking fluid from her. She was moaning and crying.

I lie there all afternoon. I could not tell where I was. The corridor was filled with white-coated women. They fed me. And then night came. They gave me pills to take, but the pills were not sleeping pills, nor were they pills I recognized as my own.

They put a tube in my nostrils and turned on a flow of vapor from a secret connection at the head of the bed and made me breathe it all night. In the dark, the room glowed with lights—a large, bright, unblinking and eerie neon-blue light, a smaller, unblinking red one, and a larger red one, which was blinking in a pattern that made no sense. The darkness deepened, and then the cacophony of noises rose up. The white-coated attendants in the corridor marched up and down, and laughed and talked all night. Sometimes they came in and did something to the woman in the bed next to mine. Sometimes they came in and tightened the band on my arm. The mattress in my bed kept moving and rising up in various random places, so that parts of my body were pushed by the pressure of the lumps.

The night wore on, and then the sounds of mechanical mayhem became more intense. The corridor was filled with buzzers, horns, beeps, and disembodied voices calling out strange announcements. One announcement was, "Code Violet on 4 North," as if it were urging some kind of night gathering of the white-coated attendees. There were ringing noises, steady noises, klaxons, ticking, knocking, honking, plunking, and chirping in various timbres, pitches, and rhythms—all at a multitude of volumes. Then there was an hour of silence. An attendant came in and took blood from me, and the noises started again. And then, a few minutes of silence, until my roommate began to moan and snore.

I finally passed out after a few minutes of crying, feeling depressed, and sobbing.

At 5 AM, I woke up. A new set of white-coated attendants gathered at the bedside. They gave me food, made me take more pills, and applied the hard, inflating band on my arm and the probe under my tongue.

I saw another white-coated woman, evidently of high status. She spoke to me as if she were explaining something before she left. The other attendants then called one of their male servants who took me down the elevator into the lower-most areas of this Borg ship building, in a twisty, turning direction that was dark and confusing. I was given more breathing tests, made to use another inhalation device, and then walked for six minutes, back and forth, in a seemingly aimless fashion, while the attendant monitored my finger with a glowing machine. I was taken back to my room, but only for a moment, before another high authority, white-coated woman attendant arrived.

This white-coated attendant, whose status was evidently higher than the first one, asked incomprehensible questions and sent me back to the lower level. I was turned over to another male attendant who made me breathe in several machines, but clipped my nostrils shut and shouted at me to exhale all the air from my lungs after he had filled them with another gaseous substance. These tests were completed, and I was left alone for a moment. I passed out into a fitful sleep of just one hour before I was taken up to the room by another male servitor attendant. Someone else came and took more blood from me. After the bloodletting was completed, I was given food and allowed to rest.

At 4 PM, the white-coated attendant of lower status told me to dress and sign papers, and then sent me in a chair pushed by one of their male servants. I was taken down to a covered exit, and my daughter was there in her car to take me out of that place.

Whew, time to get back to reality.

Do you recognize the ride in the ambulance, the ER bay with blood pressure cuff, nebulizer treatment, bedside chest X-ray, the CT scanner, the pulmonary function test, the pressure sore prevention inflating mattress, the roommate with a chest tube, and the $O^2$ saturation ambulation testing? My bet is that, to most regular patients, the time in the hospital is much like an alien abduction.

I was sent home with a new medication, Albuterol MDI. Goody, goody, more drugs.

**I Find OsteoCHAMPS**

Part of my recuperation was to become participatory in OsteoCHAMPS. This stands for Osteopathic Careers in Health and Medicine Program Service. I think they came up with the acronym, and then had to figure out a name to fit. But I digress.

Long ago, in 2000, people at MSUCOM realized that they needed to actively reach out to find qualified minority candidates for medical school. The students are definitely out there, and they are definitely bright and motivated, but most young Black people will go into IT or business, or anything else, because the money comes more quickly, and the life is less stressful on oneself and on relationships.

The idea for OsteoCHAMPS actually came from me. The person who sold the idea to the woman who launched the program was Norma Baptista. Norma and I were friends at MSUCOM, when she and I were both involved in the admissions program there. I was the chair of that committee, and she and I connected and spoke often about the lack of minority candidates.

I recall standing in the doorway of the old admissions office in East Fee Hall, speaking to Norma and saying how we had to go plant the seeds that we were going to harvest if we hoped to have any minority candidates at our school.

"We need to grow them ourselves," I told her. "Standing in our front door and shouting that we are open for minority candidates is not going to work. We have to go where they are and bring them to us, and we need to do this in high schools before they make a college or career choice."

My words struck her; they fell onto fertile ground. She took my words, polished them up into a proposal, and gave it to Margaret Aguwa, DO, MPH, a woman who later became an Associate Dean at the school, and who had the pull and vision to shape the rough idea into a proposal that won favor with the Dean and all the rest of the MSU administration.

Moving any new program through a major university cannot be easy, and to navigate the deep water required to get this kind of program accepted, funded, and staffed was truly a monumental task. Dr. Aguwa did it. She made it happen, pushed it into life, and gave it breath. I knew she had long advocated for something like this because I recall hearing her saying, "Where are the young Black men who should be coming to our medical school?"

She asked the question; I provided an answer and she heard me. So, they developed OsteoCHAMPS, which is a program of intensive immersion for one week in a mini-medical school experience for high school students in 11th and 12th grades. In addition to OsteoCHAMPS, the college also started Future DOCs, which targets younger high school students in 9th and 10th grades.

From the launch pad of OsteoCHAMPS, they can apply to MSU OMS (Osteopathic Medical Scholars). That is an undergraduate pre-medical school preparation curriculum that will guarantee automatic admission into MSUCOM, and also bypasses the need to take the MCAT. Wow, what a bonus. But, of course, a person must excel in the OMS program, or at least not fail.

I enjoyed every moment of time spent on campus with OsteoCHAMPS. Certainly, being on campus in summer, and being around smart, motived young people gets all kinds of seriously happy juices flowing. But more importantly, I was giving back to the community.

The program kicks off with an opening day keynote speech, then students spend the next seven days doing medical research, dissection in the anatomy lab, and case studies. They also learn about DPR skills—the Doctor-Patient Relationship, what used to be called bedside manner.

I was asked to do the opening day presentation. I told them about my three dads, and the setbacks on my road to becoming a physician in the first year. The second year of the program, I told them about my first patient, Mrs. H, and my worst patient, Mr. B, and how I overcame racism in the backwoods country of mid-Michigan. I also directed the DPR sessions. Together, with the Dean of Admissions, Katie Ruger, I wrote the case studies and planned the program. Each year we did it, it got better.

But one year, I could not go because my blood pressure was out of control, and the next year was COVID-19, which forced the program to become virtual/Zoom style. Not the same as being together on campus, but at least it was kept functioning.

One thing I did notice as the years rolled along was that the program attracted far fewer Black students. Originally, it was over 50 percent, but by the last time I was there in person, it was down to 10 percent. I cannot complain. The students are multicultural, multi-national, with lots of women participating. I am sure it will be good; I just wish it were more focused on the original group—young Black people.

Those students were so much fun. It was a joy to watch them go through the act of trying to function in a controlled model clinical setting. They had all the earnest looks that you want, and all the sweaty apprehension of teen life as they practiced their roles. But mostly, we had fun and we bonded.

I even got an email in 2020 from one young woman, whom I had in session back in 2019. She wrote to tell me that she had decided to go to MSU, and go into Osteopathic medicine, and that I was a determining factor because of my being a role model in OsteoCHAMPS. I was so honored and humbled. I guess there is a reason why I am still around.

But the best thing that came out of my involvement in OsteoCHAMPS, was the opportunity to meet and mentor Gabrielle (not her real name). My dear Grandchildren, you may recall that she came to visit us at my house one summer in July of 2019, from the 19$^{th}$ to the 22$^{nd}$, and was absolutely blown away by the Awesomeness of the Our Family Experience. She told me that Ezekiel, Magdalana, Veronica and her husband were so welcoming to her, and so funny, fast-paced, conversational, and just plain overwhelming, that all she could do was sit back, watch, and enjoy. She told me that she loved every minute of the time we were together.

Her path through medical school had been filled with grief and setbacks. She lost both parents and grandparents all during her medical school journey. She had to retake numerous exams and classes. She was seriously struggling academically. Dr. Ruger, the Dean of Admissions, called me to speak about this young Black woman, and asked if I would connect with her and give her some support.

I emailed her and we connected in February, 2019. She told me about family members' illnesses and deaths, including the loss of four people in five years as she tried to navigate through school.

She also confided in me that she frequently felt the sting of racism and rejection at MSUCOM—which was shocking to me, but I believe that what she told me was true. She recognized that her physical appearance was not up to what I believe are the unholy, unobtainable standards of *Vogue* or *Essence,* and she did not berate herself for her appearance, nor did she yield to what I perceive as the media's body shamers.

She shared with me her medical issues and allowed me to give her advice and suggestions on next steps to take to resolve them, or at least get competent help for them. We talked about everything: her birthday; the Essence Festival in New Orleans; her student life during her hospital rotations, and needing a place to stay in Detroit while she rotated there; her introverted personality; the adjustment to getting slowed down by COVID's shutdown of all hospital-based activities; and the forced transition into digital learning.

We celebrated her: passing the COMLEX 1 exam; getting her electives that she wanted; writing an article for the ACOFP magazine; vacationing in Jamaica; passing OMM and OB/GYN exams; getting a scholarship to Western Michigan University; being accepted for a rotation in Merida, Mexico for an OMM elective in February 2022; and major milestones for her family members.

She informed me that she had been shunted from person to person within the confines of MSUCOM's academic support structure, and was failed and disappointed by the majority of them. No teacher, counselor, or other administrative person reached her. I think she would have been tossed to the side of the academic road and flunked out of school if I had not been there to pick up her hand and hold it. For that, she and I must both thank Dr. Ruger, who saw the need, found the support, and put us together.

Gabrielle and I spent an hour on the phone one Saturday each month, talking via FaceTime, and enjoying hair styling tips (she is killer with rollers and weave techniques), recipes, current events, discussions, and family news and views.

She is my medical daughter, and I love her so very much. She was also a sensitive listening ear for me when I was struggling with personal matters, and Gabrielle's psychiatry background did good for me. Gabrielle will be a wonderful psychiatrist, and I know this is true because if she can help a screwed-up person like me, she can help anyone. She gave me as much good advice as I have ever gotten from my wonderful therapist at BetterHelp.

My relationship with Gabrielle, and my internal adoption of her to my medical family, makes me realize the need for connectedness in this world. That no matter how much I may know or have learned or experienced, I can still know and learn something from anyone else if I am willing to open up, connect to that person, and let that person share with me. I think that our sharing of support is exemplary of the Afrocentric life philosophy that is expressed in the seven traditions of Kwanzaa, an annual holiday from December 26 to January 1 to celebrate African American culture.

It seems that the Eurocentric philosophy encourages competitive forces, while the Afrocentric philosophy encourages cooperative forces. I am not a deep thinker in that regard, and do not have the rigorous training of a philosopher or historian, but my feeling is that there is a difference. If I am correct, then it is because I adopted the celebration of Kwanzaa into my life, and I think that was a wonderful thing to do, and to give to my grandchildren.

The fellow who developed Kwanzaa in 1966 is Ron Karenga, and his Afrocentric name is Maulana Ndabezitha Karenga. He had that rigorous training, and you should read his writings, or at least visit his website, where he discusses the elements of Kwanzaa and the African philosophies that underlie it. You can find him at www.officialkwanzaawebsite.org/.

This celebration, which highlights one of the seven principles each day and culminates in a feast, first intrigued me in 2017.

Where I live in Ohio is a multicultural place, which means the white people have five to 10 of every other kind of people in their schools, so that they can say they are diverse. When they teach Black History, it is always about MLK Jr., and what he did, but in such a bland, truncated fashion that I was not sure that my two grandchildren even realized they were Black People. Adopting the Kwanzaa tradition was a way to bring that awareness to the forefront, momentarily. Happily, both Veronica and her husband were on board with the celebration, and so we tried it.

Each year, I set up the Kwanzaa table, starting with the Kinara, which is Swahili for "candle holder." In its seven holes, I place one black candle in the center, then three red candles on the left, and three green candles on the right. Around that I place corn, a cup, and all the other things that go with the holiday. Then I try to engage my grandkids into a discussion about the seven traditions on a daily basis, after the Christmas holiday. It seems to help them think about the traditions in the context of current events.

Having had the Afrocentric awakening, I decided to pursue it into the medical realm.

It occurred to me that I should write something that merges the traditions of Kwanzaa with being and becoming a physician, because I see a connection. My love of the Kwanzaa holiday also encouraged me to develop the game of "!XO The Kwanzaa Game," which I named using X for kisses and O for the hugs I shared with my grandchildren.

Here I apply the seven principles of Kwanzaa in the context of Osteopathic medicine.

### 1. Unity – Umoja

Unity, the first principle of Kwanzaa, can be thought of as an Osteopathic concept, because it teaches that the body is a unit. Any action on one part will have an effect on another part. Similarly, all people are equal in the provision of care, deserving of being treated equally and equitably. Additionally, any action on one person will have an effect on another person in the provision of health care. The wise physician will recognize that her words, if properly chosen, will cause a patient to gain hope, and the patient's family to share that hope. Hope is the most potent tool a healer possesses.

**2. Self-Determination – Kujichagulia**

Self-determination is the act of choosing to be the kind of physician who allows you to excel, prosper, and serve. Every choice and every life-affirming decision you make will direct you down one path or another each day. You will decide to be self-employed or hospital-employed. You will decide to be solo or in a partnership. These, and every other decision, add to or detract from your character, based on the positive or negative energy generated by your decision.

**3. Collective Work and Responsibility – Ujima**

Medicine is not adversarial. That is the province of our sister profession, the Law. Medicine is always a collective effort of work, and a collective responsibility for bringing bodily coherence out of bodily chaos in our patients. The province also includes the work we do with our patients, and then with our partners in health care—nurses, technicians, housekeepers, dieticians, etc. The second part of the province is being able to accept responsibility for all our actions and their positive or negative outcomes throughout all the days that we serve as physicians. The tradition requires a physician to see that humility will allow work to be performed in a collective fashion, and courage will allow the physician to accept responsibility for the outcome.

**4. Cooperative Economics – Ujamaa**

Economy is defined as the "careful management of available resources." This definition avoids the confusing inclusion of money, cash, or wealth into the conversation. In medicine, we deal with many kinds of resources that are not based on wealth or dollars.

Hope, our team of coworkers, the patient's wishes, the family considerations, insurance requirements, hospital size, available time, and personal skill sets are some examples of resources that a physician must accumulate and manage. Kwanzaa asks that the community manage those resources to its own benefit, and physicians should utilize the concept of cooperativeness as we use our medical resources to the benefit of the community of fellow humans.

**5. Purpose – Nia**

When you choose the path and life of a physician, you are given a purpose. Specifically, it is to heal those who come to you, willingly or unwillingly, for your care. You are given their minds and bodies, and your purpose is to return these fellow humans to the state we call health, or failing that, to stand with them as they move to their final transition on this Earth, so that no one passes on alone, unloved, or in pain. Medicine is one of the "calling" professions, and the call to this purpose of healing is powerful and must be constantly honored and remembered.

**6. Creativity – Kuumba**

What more powerful tool can a person or physician have than that of creativity? How many times will the creative physician be challenged to find another way to fight the infection, another way to perform the surgery, or another way to move a patient into willingness to change? These common scenarios in the medical life cannot be accomplished by following some prewritten algorithm, medical cookbook, or copying what someone else may have done to a different patient. Your outlook as a physician must always include creativity.

**7. Faith – Imani**

Ultimately, you must trust that the body will do what you cannot do in so many instances. This is medical faith. It is not required that you have a specific religious belief, because the body has its own kind of faith. You must trust and you must know in your heart that all you do is still dependent on the body's inherent ability to cure itself. The instant you think you created health or you cured a problem, is the instant you fail.

I am so happy that I became a physician, happier yet that I chose to become an Osteopathic physician, and ecstatic that I performed my best role as a family physician. I look back at my life in practice and now ask myself, how often did I adhere to those seven great traditions and not even realize what they were or that I was doing it?

## DIGRESSION #29: TELEMEDICINE BECOMES A REGULAR PART OF LIFE

If nothing else, the COVID-19 pandemic of 2020 made tremendous changes in how medicine is conducted. There were efforts and skirmishes prior to 2020 with wearable tech, smart watches that could print out a single lead EKG strip, and various fun applications of tech in medicine. But in 2020, patients and doctors alike realized that social distancing required by the pandemic made telemedicine an expansive and necessary method of providing health care.

Home health visits via virtual care became open and routine. In fact, Medicare allowed telehealth as a codable, billable procedure. There is no way that doctors will want to let that go away. There was even a major chip in the armor of HIPAA when it was decreed that physicians can use methods such as FaceTime, Google Duo, and Zoom for communications. This removed the requirement to have a proprietary digital platform that gave a huge bolus of money to electronic developers and allowed them to restrict how doctors and patients communicated. Patients got used to instantly having a physician respond to a question, and used to having enough time to speak with someone, who in turn had enough time to provide good answers.

One of the first examples of the expansion of telemedicine into this void was the creation of a company called Medically Home. I have no commercial interest or connection with this company, as a matter of honest declaration. They announced and launched in early 2020, and I am certain they will not be the only purveyor of this kind of care as time goes on.

What the company does is provide medical care in the home to patients who would ordinarily be cared for in a hospital. They have partnered with major, large hospitals and insurers, naturally. The model they propose is truly brilliant and has been coming for a long time. When I made house calls, I, too, realized that home care was more comprehensive, less costly, more humane, and less traumatizing. It was a way to avoid medication errors and nosocomial infections, and was psychologically more soothing for most patients.

Eligible patients are those who would be high- and medium-acuity level of care, with common diagnoses such as CHF (heart failure), Chronic Obstructive Pulmonary Disease, Pneumonia, and some selected post-surgical cases and oncology patients. This development got the green light as Hospice showed the pathway of home health care, provided by groups like VPA, and payment models encouraged out-patient surgeries for more and more procedures.

In the old days of my active practice on staff at Sheridan Hospital, I recall scheduling a lady for a D&C. That is the process where the inside lining of the uterus is surgically removed for a variety of reasons—sampling to rule out cancer, prolonged postpartum bleeding, and dysfunctional uterine bleeding in perimenopausal women, to name a few. I admitted the lady to the hospital the night before the procedure, conducted the procedure the next day, and discharged her to her home on the following day. By the time I had moved on in practice and down the road 20 years, the D&C had been replaced by an in-office procedure called endometrial aspiration sampling. I learned to do that procedure, and for those women who had a lot of bleeding, I learned to give Provera tablets, a kind of hormone that shut off uterine menstrual flow. Time and money were saved on both sides of the equation—hospital and patient.

Today, we have Medically Home's method. They create a virtual hospital unit in a patient's home by setting up physician and nurse teams who see patients and stay in continuous contact with the homebound person. Medications and supplies are home-delivered, set up by pharmacies and medical supply distributors. They link not only a hospital, but also ambulatory surgical centers to the patient's home.

What this company promises seems just so revolutionary in how health care will be delivered, and it is about time. The company offers to:

- set up 24/7 physician and nurse practitioner oversight;
- bring mobile imaging into the home;
- provide nebulizer treatments every four hours;
- provide oxygen and durable medical equipment such as hospital beds and other medical supplies;
- obtain consults from specialists who will also make home visits;
- deliver care-appropriate meals and nutrition;
- monitor patients with remote continuous technology;
- provide infusion therapy for fluids, IV antibiotics, and other medications;
- provide physical and occupational therapy;
- manage medications; and
- obtain laboratory samples and tests such as EKGs.

I did a lot of this as a visiting physician with VPA, so it looks like the owners of this company have taken VPA's model to the next level, and it is really rewarding to see how this will change the majority of what goes on in a hospital and bring it back to the home and personal living quarters of people.

Imagine this service combined with the AI Nurse-Bot! This method would serve not only the acute, post-operative and sub-acute patients, but also the chronic care patients who hover somewhere between ER visits with short-stay observation, hospitalization, and nursing home admission.

I think that if the cost of this kind of care is $1,000 a day, it is still cheaper and safer than a similar level of care in a hospital. This is not the future; it is the present, and it has not come too soon.

Newsflash, Amazon now offers in-person and online medical visits. Look out, TeleDocs, you are on the killing floor. Since September 2019, Amazon Care has provided virtual health services across America, with plans to offer in-person services through home visits in more than 20 new cities in 2022.[24]

WE'RE BACK . . .

**Grandma Doc, Not Quite Papa Doc**

In 2014, I became a grandmother who is able to assist her family and spend time with my beloved grandchildren. I am living in the ritzy Republican suburbs/exurbs in a mostly white condominium association. It is a nice life. I get to see my grandchildren daily because Veronica and her husband still need help with a regular sitter. Ezekiel is 10, and Magdalana is seven, and they are the reason I am here.

At my place in Fort Wayne, Indiana, The Townehouse was so posh and nice. It had an exercise room, catered dining, all levels of care from independent to hospice, plus a great staff. And I had a large, 2,500-square-foot single story living area. But Veronica said it was too far away, and so she really decided that I should come closer to her. She was so right.

I do miss those wonderful senior people at the Townehouse. They played bridge every day, chatted about life every day, took naps, took walks, and enjoyed being retired and taken care of. But they had grandchildren in town, and my grandchildren were a four-hour drive away, so I decided to move; Veronica was right, as usual, and I am not unhappy.

I would sit at the dining table with my grandchildren after school and share dinner. I cleaned the house before they got home from school, fed the dog, washed the dishes, took care of laundry, emptied trash containers, and watered the garden. It was the life of nanny-housekeeper and it was fun.

The family dog, Riker, was a rescue, black lab that had been trained by incarcerated people in the prison training program. He was such a good pooch. Veronica bought that fish tank, too. She said it was a Christmas gift for her husband, but I know she got it because she wanted it. Those fish were absolutely fascinating. They floated around, and we sat and watched them. Who is the higher evolved species, them or us? Not really sure.

I enjoyed being that nanny person, and mostly I enjoyed watching and listening to Ezekiel and Magdalana talk about current events, and life in general. I loved sharing things that I think all Black children should know. Mostly, they should know that they are Black. Veronica and her family live in a truly wealthy suburb, and can do so because she and her husband have high-power, high-paying jobs. They have a 4,000 square foot home on a large lot in a gated community. Their life is definitely not ghetto.

I thought my grandchildren needed reminding of the reality of their lives. Despite attending a truly diverse school, someone somewhere will call them the N word, and I worried about how they would handle that.

One thing I instituted was the celebration of Kwanzaa. Veronica and her husband really took to it, and we began holding our Kwanzaa celebration with the candles, the traditions, and the dinners. My thought was that someone needed to discuss not only Black history, but also Black life and the future as a Black person. Kwanzaa was a perfect opportunity.

From that experience, I also worked on developing a game based on Kwanzaa, designed much like the monopoly game board, but using memes, names, and occupations more closely connected to Black American life. It was a project that I started in 2018, and had it ready for play as a beta test by 2020. Then COVID hit and I could not get a way to launch the game into the direction I had planned. I felt it would be nice to promote the game among people who also celebrate Kwanzaa, and that would be in any African American history museum, of which there are many in all the major metropolitan areas. One day, it may come to pass, but for now, it is what we do when we are together in the winter season, celebrating our lives as

Black people.

The murder of George Floyd in May 2020, and the riots that erupted across this nation and the world, made me certain that my little effort was truly in the right direction at the right time.

I made sure my grandchildren learned more about the Rev. Dr. Martin Luther King, Jr. (his real full name) and all the others who predated him in Black American history. Gradually, I think I made an impact on both of them. Ezekiel and Magdalana both seem more comfortable being Black, more aware of being Black, and better able to articulate what that means to their futures.

I enjoyed a few years in retirement, but in 2016, I felt like I needed to go back to work. Fool that I was, I did go back to work.

I first resumed teaching in the spring of 2016 at MSUCOM, in the Sensitive Exams, which is the practical teaching experience where medical students learn how to perform pelvic, rectal, and hernia exams on live people.

One of the hardest things for medical students to learn is the examination of genital areas in men and women. I think it is difficult because they may not be sexually active yet, and therefore have no personal experience. It is also one of the most intrusive kinds of interactions that a physician can have with a patient. So many barriers are not only sexual, but cultural, too, involving sexual exams.

I recall proctoring one exam where I had two young men as students and a paid female patient. The patient, a generously proportioned young Black woman, had been a paid patient for several years, and was very experienced in the process. The students, I fear, were both inexperienced with this exam, and seemingly with intimate relations with women in general.

The students all got a 30 minute group lecture, and a chance to practice on plastic models of breasts, rectal, and pelvic areas. These, needless to say, are nowhere even remotely close to what a real person is or feels like. After they had their lecture, they broke up into pairs, went to the proctor area, and were matched up with one of the practicing physicians. Once we entered the room with the paid patient, I demonstrated how to do the breast exam while my students watched. Then I let one of them practice the exam. He put on his gloves, stood by the patient's side, and gently, respectfully, carefully, and briefly applied a few light and quick touches to the surface of each breast. He was sweating profusely, but looked relieved to have completed his practice breast exam.

He only thought he was done.

The patient looked up at him and said, "Honey, I know you don't think you just did no breast exam. Let me show you how you 'sposed to do this."

She grabbed his right hand in a vice grip, pressed it deeply into her left breast, moved it in a circular fashion from the base to the areola, and each time pressing down firmly to the rib cage, until she completed the entire circle of her 52DDD breast. She then made him pinch up her nipple, put his hand into her axillary region for the lymph node exam, and when it was completed, she dropped his hand and said, "Now you good."

To his credit, he smiled and said thanks repeatedly, as he stepped back into the safety of the rear of the room, pale and sweating, but much more knowledgeable about breasts, breast exams, and this instructive woman. She was a fabulous instructor.

I, too, learned a thing a two from my students. One young student, a male who was from India, asked me how he should conduct himself when being introduced to a female patient, because his religion did not allow him to touch a female who was not a close relative. I had never heard of this, so I carefully thought about what to say, and decided that honesty was best. I told him that he should let the woman know he has this restriction, but that it will in no way prevent him from providing the best care possible. I think he was happy with that approach, and I trust honesty will serve him well with all his patients, female as well as male.

Being part of the faculty for the Sensitive Exams allowed me to drive back to East Lansing and enjoy my alma mater campus in spring. It was so beautiful. I was there for four days, and learned how progressive my school had become in teaching. They began integrating diagnostic studies, such as ultrasonography, into the curriculum, and provided hands-on experience for students. We never had this, and I am so glad students are getting it. They will be so much better as physicians if they continue to expand their circle of knowledge.

From that experience, I went back to Locums work. When physicians are short-handed, they contact professional headhunters in the Locums recruiting world, so I put myself in that pool. It was rich and deep, and I was needed in so many places as a family physician. I still had four active state licenses—Michigan, Indiana, Iowa, and Wisconsin—and so I could go to all those states. I put my Florida license in retirement, and never bothered to apply for an Ohio license. I also kept my DEA license active.

My assignment was in Michigan, in the northern portion of Macomb County, in a clinic owned by McLaren Health System. I had to spend one week learning how to use their clunky EMR, and of course, the trainers were two most excellent Black women. I got very close to them, and we actually spent some social time together. Why not? There were not a lot of Black people at that level in McLaren, so we naturally fell in together.

Then I worked in the clinic with an all-white staff and a mixed bag of patients from countries that made up the former nation of Yugoslavia. From the patients, I heard the languages of Croatia, Serbia, and Bosnia in that place, and enjoyed the different national dress that they wore. Once again, I was uplifted to learn that patients are patients, no matter where they are, and if you treat them with respect and compassion, they will respond with trust in you. All I had was a bit of training and a lot of empathy, and it worked just fine.

A man came in for a blood pressure check. He was a bit taken aback to see me, not because of my color, but because the regular lady doctor was absent. I went through the introduction and the exam, and told him that his pressure was a bit high, and also that I wanted to check his heart more completely. I thought I had heard an irregularity in the heartbeat, so I obtained an EKG, an electronic tracing of heart rhythm, in the office. It showed an irregular rate, but not too fast or too slow.

I spent the rest of the time with him explaining what I had found, what it meant to his health, how his blood pressure was related to it, what type of treatment was needed, and the specialist who would be consulted for higher level of care. I made sure to ask him if he was sure he understood my meaning and my plan, and asked him if he had questions. I answered all of them. Then I left the room, set up the consult, and returned to let him know that I wanted him to return for follow up, because I, too, was concerned and needed to be sure he was not getting worse. If I had been in my own clinic, I would have medically cardioverted him, but I knew the safest course as a Locums was to refer him to cardiology.

He got to the cardiologist, was cardioverted, and when he returned for a follow-up with me, his heart rate had been corrected. I told him that it was now functioning properly, and his blood pressure was also much better. He looked at me and said how much he appreciated what I had done for him. I thanked him. He continued saying that no one had ever spent so much time explaining and answering questions, and he wanted me to know that he appreciated all I had done for him, and then asked if I would be remaining in the area. I had to let him know again that I was just the "fill in" until the regular lady doctor came back from maternity leave, but I did very much appreciate his comments.

One concept behind DPR—doctor-patient relationship—is empathy, and the best definition I've heard for empathy came from Chris Voss, a former FBI hostage negotiator, who said in his book, *Never Split The Difference,*[24] that empathy is demonstrating, understanding, and describing the needs, interests, and perspective of your counterpart without necessarily agreeing with them. I suspect that gentleman never really got a lot of empathy from the busy staff and physicians at the clinic because they were pushed and pressured to just rush people through the gates to make money, wellness be damned.

The staff knew not to push me because I could not be fired, so if I wanted to spend time with patients, I did. Fuck their schedule; I was there to get people the help they needed and THAT TAKES TIME. There is no way around that fact.

I stayed at a crappy motel about five miles away from the clinic; it was an extended stay facility. I hated that life. One moderate-sized room with a cook top, fridge, microwave, sink, bath, table, TV, bed, chair, and a heating system that did not ever work, no matter how I tinkered with it or how the hotel manager tried to fix it either. Oh, well, the pay was great.

I made $14,000 for a month of work. I was amazed at that. I also ended up increasing my income to the point where I had to make payments in anticipation of taxes going into the next year. But I could see where working Locums would have been ideal if I were young, single, and willing to move around.

No overhead, lots of money, and travel. Maybe if I am reincarnated, I would try that. But as a retired family doc, I was not going to pursue it.

My next Locums work was for a company that did Medicare exams. Medicare advantage plans have to prove to Medicare that their members are getting proper care. So, the plans hire companies, like Censeo, to send around physicians who assess Medicare recipients in their homes. Basically, I just checked their meds, blood pressure, and history, and advised them to keep their visits with their regular physicians. But it was wonderful to sit down for two hours with a person and go over every aspect of their health history. I only had to see five people a day, and got $100 per person. The company paid for my meals, hotel, and rental car. I would never get rich, but I would get fulfilled by doing what every family physician should be doing.

However, it was life on the road, and so I realized that I had nothing to prove, did not need to earn the money and no longer felt that patient care was important to do.

I quit Locums life in 2017, just about the time my high blood pressure raised up to strike me down with a reminder that I, too, can be a patient on the edge of mortality.

Meanwhile, I have always wondered what it would be like to create the ideal family practice office. I came close several times in real life. My first office in Stanton had a great location and staff, but I was inexperienced in medical office business management, and my time was spread too thin by trying to do 48 hours of work in a span of 24 hours.

My Fort Wayne clinic was closer because of the time I was allowed with patients, but the staff sucked, except for my medical assistant. The EMR went from bad to worse in the second year I was there.

No hospital-owned clinic was ever anywhere close to being good, much less a model of the ideal clinic. As far as I am concerned, no clinic owned by any hospital will ever be ideal, because the hospital is concerned with making money from illnesses, and the clinician is concerned with moving people into wellness.

## DIGRESSION #30: THE IDEAL FAMILY PRACTICE OFFICE

I have long thought that the arrangement of the family practice office was inefficient, and just wrong.

The typical arrangement is to have a certain number of exam rooms for each physician. The plan is to load the rooms up with people who were waiting in the waiting room, but who can now wait in an exam room. The patients are seen by a check-in clerk for payment purposes, a nursing aide to obtain some vitals (occasionally done incorrectly), then a nurse to review medication and provide a basic reason for the visit, to then finally be seen by the physician. By this time, the patient's scheduled appointment time has actually expired, and the 15-minute visit with the physician is down to five minutes. The patient leaves in frustration, while the physician leaves to finish computer charting. Repeat this awkwardness 30 times a day all throughout family medicine offices in America.

Every part of that farcical parade, prior to the face-to-face meeting with the physician, can be eliminated. First of all, the actual exam room should be huge. It should be large enough for the doctor to provide all the skills and set activities he/she possesses. Minor office surgeries, manual medicine techniques, casting, splinting, injections, counseling, detailed physical exams, video consultations, and biopsies should occur in that space. Do it all in one large 20 by 30-foot exam room.

Just outside of that is the intake space—a private chamber where the patient's vitals are obtained. One door opens in from the waiting area; another door opens into the exam room. The intake chamber has a scale in the floor, a laser level to measure height, a blood pressure/pulse $O^2$ saturation finger-tip reader, a head swipe thermometer for temperature, and a respiration dongle to count breaths. There is a toilet so the patient can provide a urine sample. There is a sink for hand washing. There is a baby scale, while another scale on the floor can accommodate a wheelchair-bound patient. Moms, as well as a nursing aide, can connect the monitoring devices to their infants, without risk of germs from unwashed hands on their child. When this automatic intake is complete, it is automatically entered into the computerized chart by flow over digital process, not keyboard entry.

Now let's look at the waiting room. Today, patients sit there staring at the receptionist or ignoring the commercially provided television with health information blaring at them. They wait and fume silently. A reception room can be educational, relaxing, informative, and functional.

Let them enter a comfortable, well-designed space, with chairs, couches, bean bags, benches, and tables of all arrangements for their enjoyment. They will go, first, to the private kiosk and begin their check-in. This large space should have headphones, charger cables for iOS and Android devices, VR (virtual reality) headsets designed for patient education series, recliner chairs, wide body chairs, a mobility-impaired zone, a special area for nursing mothers, a well child zone, and a sick child zone. Greenery, such as a terrarium, fish tank, or fountain enhance the atmosphere. If there is a TV screen, it must be connected to headphones.

Additional amenities would include table games, a fresh snack bar, a water station, a music channel through those headphones, and walls displaying artwork, preferably done by patients.

They pull up their chart and go through each of the sections to verify demographics, insurance, or method of payment, to review allergies, medications, surgeries, family history, social history, and a complete review of systems. Yes, they can answer all these questions just as they do now, on so many other platforms with the help of a voice-activated assistant to guide them.

They then provide their chief complaint, and are guided through the steps of the HPI—history of the present illness. Regarding their problem, answer questions regarding: when did it begin, how long does it last when it happens, how often in a day does it occur, what makes it worse, and what makes it better.

If pain is involved, not only does the screen develop a pain scale, but it also provides a gender-specific figure with an electronic pen that the patient uses to show the location of the pain. All of this is captured for the chart and is seen by the physician, in real time, as the patient is writing it. So that when the patient moves from the waiting room kiosk to the intake chamber, the physician has read all of the information and is prepared to dive directly to the heart of the problem. No one is between the doctor and the patient, and the two of them can work on the problem together. They have the room and the time to do so.

Once in the exam room, there are various arrangements. There is a pair of chairs for talking, a desk for writing, an OMM table, a GYN table, and a surgical table. Equipment is stored in cabinets to the side, or in a rolling cart for small hand instruments. There is also a large giant screen on one wall, which is the video communications link, so that the physician and patient can have a conference with any specialist anywhere in the world.

This is just like the concept behind Nighthawk radiology, which is that some radiologist is awake somewhere in the world and can read any digital film from anywhere else, applying it to other consultants. Dermatology, rheumatology, neurology, and cardiology are easy and readily accessible. The physician can perform the exam while the consultant watches, coaches, etc. The patient can ask questions directly to the consultant. The patient swipes his/her credit card to pay the consultant, and the visit is completed. It is recorded in the chart as a video clip. No scribe needed. No notes to decipher. No typing to do. The physician dictates his/her notes as the patient is in the exam room.

The patient exits the exam room, leaving via the exit to meet the doctor's nurse/assistant/receptionist person at the check-out desk. The patient can schedule a follow-up visit at the check-out desk, or go home and make a visit for himself/herself online by looking at the physician's open schedule. At check-out, the patient is given a thumb drive or DVD of the video visit.

Think of all the better care that can occur in a place where there is plenty of room to function.

American family physicians are highly trained, and then told to go sit in a room and just make referrals to specialists. Family physicians should be able to screen for colorectal cancer by administering a camera capsule, doing a digital exam and stool occult blood, and performing sigmoidoscopies or colonoscopies. They should be able to screen for glaucoma with a digital tonometer, the same as the ophthalmologists use.

Bladder cancer could be found with a urine examination and urine cytology. Skin cancer is found by having the completely undressed patient examined under a special magnifying glass with an excisional or incisional biopsy done on-site.

Cervical cancer is done with a pap and pelvic. Ovarian masses can be found with bedside ultrasonography and a pelvic exam. Oral cancers are screened with vinegar/five percent glacial acetic acid washes, which reveal leukoplakia and are being done in dental offices all over.

Lymphomas are often found with a palpatory diagnosis of groin and lymph node locations. Blood disorders and cancers are revealed by a CBC with differential. A Chem 24 will show liver and kidney electrolytes and trace element values, and if you add lipase and amylase, the pancreas is also evaluated.

Blood tests for HGBA1C and glucose levels, lipid and cholesterol screenings, HIV, and Hep B and Hep C are simple to obtain. And now, the advent of the IDx-DR device makes it possible to detect diabetic retinopathy in primary care. They're using it in CVS drugstores[25] now.

The device uploads photos of a patient's retina to a cloud computing AI, which can determine if retinopathy exists or not. There is an overread function performed by a board-certified ophthalmologist. Mammograms, chest X-rays, and CT scans are more complex and would not be part of the FP office of the future, but should be readily available on demand to any patient who requests such a test, and who can pay for it. This requires that the physicians who perform those radiology procedures be disconnected from servitude to any hospital, and be allowed to function as free-standing, independent operators.

Finally, look at scheduling. Even with Cleveland Clinic's MyChart function—a secure, online program that enables patients to access their electronic medical record—it is still hard to get an appointment at the time and day I want. That is because I cannot book myself into my doctor's schedule.

When I was new in practice, one of the older doctors in town (in Stanton, Michigan) had a scheduling system that was awesome. He made no appointments in advance; everyone was a walk-in. People would walk in, find an open time on his paper appointment book in the reception room, slot themselves in for that time, and leave, returning when it was time to be seen. Now that would be a major HIPAA violation today, but the premise seems to be sound. It could be done electronically. Just show the day's schedule and let people take the time they want. Extend the schedule for one week. Everyone gets 30 minutes.

I think the doctor who did it this way would be busy all day and doing fruitful work, happy to see his/her people, every day, all day. This is where Direct Patient/Primary Care is taking the profession. It is only a matter of time before the DPC doctors figure out all the details that will make them the go-to providers for all of us.

WE'RE BACK . . .

**Gratitude Sets In**

The year 2020 was a roller coaster for me and for this nation. We were all blindsided by the COVID-19 pandemic, and so woefully unprepared. Thank goodness I am where I am, here in Ohio, when this all began in March with the first lockdown.

I think that if I had been working as an employed physician or even a Locums physician, I would be dead from COVID-19, or dead from something else, stress-induced.

In November 2020, with a chance to look back to Patient Zero—who came in here in December 2019 through January 2020, bringing this virus—I have seen people behave like angels and others behave like devils.

I have decided to be more grateful for every day. I will also be gentler with everyone I interact with. You can never know what disaster awaits you. I am always hearing from people I know about sudden crises, such as the sudden onset of a terrible illness, a fall that causes broken bones, and even a shocking divorce initiated by a chauvinistic husband because he wants to have fun after a half-century of marriage.

I am so lucky. I am so blessed. Never forget what you have; and never forget that what you have can go away in a hot second. Cherish each day and each person who is in that day with you.

Part of being blessed is being able to forgive the wrongs that were done to you, and to make that act of forgiveness as a person and as a member of the Black community.

I think that we Black Americans will have to save those white Americans who are hellbent on destroying all of us.

Joe Biden was confirmed by the Electoral College as President on December 14th, 2020, and a small portion of the 49 percent of voters (70 million) who voted for Donald Trump went off on a tangent of hate and violence. Joe got 80 million votes, but the nation is still mostly 50/50 on everything else of importance. However, the loyal Trump base still believes that the election was stolen. They marched in Washington, D.C. on January 6th, 2021, and ended up causing a riot, with people getting stabbed, injured, and one killed. Some of the Electoral College electors in Nevada held their meeting via Zoom to avoid being physically targeted by Trump supporters, and the angry, hate-filled actions they take in these rallies.

**Understanding the Fearful White Racists**

I had a long conversation with a relative in California while all this was playing out, and we asked ourselves why some white people are behaving like this. Why are they voting for a sociopath who refuses to follow the law? And why are they so violent?

I had an answer, and it stems from watching a movie documentary called *Out of Darkness*[26], which explored the development and cultural pathway of Black people in the world, and our contributions to the world in terms of science, math, medicine, law, religion, music, food, sports, and pretty much everything.

It occurred to me that if some white Americans may be filled with fear that there will be a wave of angry, armed Black people, who will come for them after January 20th, 2020, and try to kill them and rape their women. This thought has been placed, I think, in their heads by the sociopath in the White People's House, and by his masters and cronies, to gain and keep power and money.

Some white people also may fear being eliminated, and there is strong evidence that this process is actually happening. The American Urological Society released a report that found sperm counts are decreasing in all westernized countries and locations. That is pretty much west Europe and all of North America. They, the fearful white racists, do not know why.

The U.S. Centers for Disease Control and Prevention released a report[27] that showed white Americans between the ages of 45 and 55 were dying of suicide and drugs at a higher rate than any other demographic group. They, these fearful white racists, do not know why.

Birth rates in white American teens have been falling. They, the fearful white racists, do not know why.

Intermarriages between white Americans and non-white Americans increased from 3% in 1967 to 19% in 2019.[28] The fearful white racists do not know why.

Gay white males and females are increasingly emboldened about coming out of the closet, forming not only civil unions, but also true marriages, and then adopting children who are non-white. The fearful white racists do not know why.

Cities and urban areas are increasingly becoming more diverse as Black Americans and immigrants proliferate, and young white rural Americans move to the cities and abandon the farm country. The fearful white racists do not know why.

Their fear has been continually stoked by those who make racist policy, who control the wealth of the nation, and who promote the lies that divide us. So if you are a white person who sees these trends, you may become even more fearful. That increase in fear allows you to create a backlash and become a fearful white racist.

Fearful White Racists, the FWRs, will support anti-abortion laws because that is how they will preserve white babies. But once any Black baby is saved from abortion, that baby is abandoned by the FWRs and left to suffer from economic, medical, educational, and institutional injustice. That Black baby will grow up and be hounded and left to the mercy of the criminal justice system, and then killed by the same FWRs, who now espouse the death penalty and laws that are tough on crime and promote the for-profit prisons, because that is how they get rid of Black babies that were not aborted. Truly, prison is just late-term abortion in the Black community.

Those FWRs will support their second amendment rights because they think they will need guns to shoot Black and brown invaders, whom they "know" are coming for revenge, retribution, and rape in white communities. They will support the militarization of the police for the same reasons. They will support the death penalty for increasingly trivial crimes as long as those being killed are not white.

FWRs will support policies and institutional powers that punish gays, male or female, and trans individuals, because those people, if they are white, are viewed as guilty of betrayal of the prime white directive, which is to produce white babies. Those who intermarry with non-whites are also lumped in as betrayers.

FWRs probably thought that Viagra would also increase sperm count numbers along with increasing erections, and thereby increase their ability to make white babies and increase the number of white people. Interestingly, FWRs supported the move to quickly approve cheaper, generic prescription programs for Viagra, but opposed prescription programs for birth control pills and Plan B morning after pills. Would that be evidence of any sexism mixed in with racism in the world of FWRs?

FWRs will resist any immigration policy that allows ingress of any non-white peoples. They will argue that jobs are being taken by these immigrants. They will argue that they are not racist, but are looking at the economics of the situation. Yet, I challenge you to find large numbers of FWRs who are actively seeking work in landscaping, grocery stores, delivery services, cooking, home construction, the picking of food crops, and other low paying, transient jobs that offer poor wages and no benefits to the same extent that I have seen Latinx, Muslim, and Indo-Asian people do this kind of work.

FWRs will oppose needle exchange programs, drug treatment centers, decriminalization of minor drug possession charges, and criminal justice reform that includes stopping the automatic plea bargain instead of a real trial. FWRs will support for-profit prisons and the death penalty. This is how FWRs get rid of Black and brown "troublemakers." If a few "white trash addicts" also happen to get sick or die from drug abuse, Hepatitis, or HIV, so be it, as long as it preserves the best white people for reproduction, and reduces the

Black and brown populations in America.

FWRs will support government that ignores the homeless, undereducated, the mentally ill, and those who are medically underserved, because they know that these are the reservoirs of Black and brown people at the lowest end of the line of survival. If a few white people die along with large numbers of Black and brown people, so be it, in the name of preserving the white race in America.

These FWRs are consumed with the horrific thought of extinction. They will barely whisper the word outside of their own special, secret gatherings, but the thought is there, throbbing in the undercurrent of white America, in places like Q-Anon, the dark web, the KKK, and ReTHUGlican super PAC donors. This extinction fear is a tool, a nail-studded club wielded by the masters and economic controllers in white America, because they know that as long as they keep poor people separated by their color, those poor people will never thrive and will always believe the lies they hear that make them hold on to hate.

Black America has a huge task in the reversal of this fear, and the requirement to lead our brothers and sisters in the world of FWR out of darkness and into the light.

## DIGRESSION #31: THE END OF TRANSPLANT SURGERY

You are valuable just for your parts nowadays.

Your heart, lungs, liver, kidneys, corneas, pancreas, bone marrow, and skin are all implantable. The work of transplantation is truly marvelous, but truly expensive, and not at all fair and balanced. The waitlist for a new kidney is complex, and the sickest one may not get the kidney.

The advent of 3D printing and in vitro organ growth is on the medical horizon. Once these techniques become truly possible, transplant medicine will be completely transformed and may go away entirely.

Stem cell therapy exists now. It is making scientific advances in Europe, it is facing hurdles in America, and it is being done commercially in South America, without regulation of any kind. Some of it is bogus; some of it is groundbreaking. The point is that it is going on, will continue—Pandora has opened the box—and once stem cell therapy joins commercially, in a financially viable setting with 3D printing, the transplant problem is solved.

Need a kidney? No worries. No longer do you have to buy one from a person who was executed for political crimes in a country where an underground market sells human organs. Instead, just provide a swab and your local lab will grow one for you. No need to sign up for organ donor status at the DMV. No more waiting on a list for a kidney or heart donor who is in California while the recipient is in New York.

If the neediest person is in New York, the second most needy person is in Chicago, and the third most needy person is in San Jose, and the donor died in San Francisco, that kidney goes to the San Francisco recipient, because time counts and every second outside of the body is tissue death for the donor organ.

That California kidney goes to the third most needy person, merely because that person is closer to the donor. The first most needy person loses out due to an accident of geography.

## WE'RE BACK . . .

### My Water Filter Installation Demonstrates Sexism and Racism

In April of 2019, I got rid of my expensive, salt-using water softener because I had installed a Scale Blaster to descale my water. Go look up Scale Blaster by searching for Scaleblaster SB 75 Hard Water Conditioner online at any of the big-box home improvement stores. But I wanted to be sure I had all the crud removed because I live in a community that has well water.

I purchased a Pentair Water system filter that cost $2,000, but required no filters and no attention from me, plus it had a five-year warranty and a 15-year lifespan. I thought that was a good idea, and asked a well-known plumbing company to go ahead with the installation.

The thing worked well until October 31st, 2020, when the drain hose worked its way back up and out of the floor drain, spewing water all over the floor that night. I was appalled to see the wet floor the next morning, and with visions of flooding reminiscent of my backyard in Okemos, I called the people who installed it.

The first guy came over and repositioned the drain hose, videotaped the floor drain down to the Y connector, and said things were good.

It failed again, and in three days I had more water on the floor. The second guy came over and repositioned the drainpipe, taping it to the other pipes that also flowed into the floor drain—hot water tank, gas furnace, and humidifier—to secure it.

It failed again in three days, and the third guy came over, repositioned all the pipes, and taped it down with dragon tape. I also added 17 pounds of rocks in a bag on top of the pipe and 10 pounds of rocks on the mid portion of the drainpipe. He tried to pin it down with a curved metal collar that required screws into the concrete. I could see that the screws were not long enough and he could not get the drill to bite into the concrete because the flooring just dissolved into powder. We agreed to just apply the rocks and go from there.

It lasted about eight days before it failed again, but not nearly as badly as before, because I could see that the drainpipe was just laying horizontally over the floor drain. The rocks and tape were working, just not perfectly.

I called, and they sent their manager. Nice guy, mid-30s to early-40s, licensed master plumber. I explained my theory of why this was happening, why it was happening now, and how to best achieve 100 percent success. My solution involved sticking the drainpipe into the floor very deeply, taping it at the entry of the floor drain, and laying one bag of rocks on the neck, another bag of rocks on the mid-point, and applying dragon tape across the pipe at six to eight locations.

My theory said that the pipe had been incrementally working its way up and out of the floor drain because the pipe was spurting water obliquely against the wall of the floor drain. The force of the water would then push the pipe up and out. The drainpipe was rigid and would not bend, but it could be positioned into the hole below the openings of all other pipes and weighed down. My theory said all three planes of motion had to be prevented. Rocks on top, rocks on the side, and tape across would do that, so I reasoned.

The master plumbing manager listened briefly and said, "No, it needs to have a metal collar installed over the neck."

I told him I did not want that because I had been told by the condo association that if there was damage to the floor, the association would not pay for it if I caused it. We were at an impasse. He agreed to reposition the rocks, and then he left.

I then taped the hose at the neck with Alien Tape as it entered the floor drain, as well as two other locations along the length of the pipe. I made sure the rocks were on top and along the side of the pipe. I also marked with a green sharpie the location of the pipe at the edge of the floor drain.

It did a cycle on November 5th, 2020, and the next morning, I checked it. The floor was dry and the green line had not moved back.

It seemed to be secure.

It also seemed to me that the master plumbing manager was severely challenged by a woman, who was also Black, telling him how to fix something that he was supposed to know how to fix. Maybe he was right and I was wrong, but he was shut down emotionally and intellectually, and did not want to hear or see any of what I had to say or show. His status as a white person and as a male was under duress, and he needed to leave the field of combat because I was, first of all, a customer, and he could not risk losing a customer.

## Intersection of Racism and Sexism at a Neighborhood Party

I believe that some white people need to be saved, and that Black people can serve as their saviors. But saving them will be difficult because they don't know they need to be saved, and if they did know, they would resist efforts to be saved by BIPOCs (people who are Black, Indigenous, and people of color). If they know and don't resist the efforts, they may still just decide to fail and die because the change required is too hard, complex, and painful.

The problem is that most white people do not know what they don't know. They live in a soft, cocooned world of ease and privilege, and never see or hear from folks who are not just like them.

The racist geography of home ownership has resulted in all the discrete islands of discrimination and separation. But I have lived in the middle of those islands and have had many opportunities to see how clueless my white neighbors really are.

A good case in point happened in one location where I lived, at a party that I attended at a beautiful home. I wore a long, brightly-printed, bohemian-patterned skirt, a white spaghetti-sleeve top, a white long-sleeved sweater, and white sandals, with a yellow cross-body bag to hold my car keys.

My hairstyle was a long, curly, modified Mohawk with sweeping curls down in front of each ear, a curly point of hair slipping over my eyebrows, and a long string of curls gathered on top of my head, running down to the nape of my neck. Add some long swing earrings and my best makeup, and I was all set for a stylish, fun evening.

When I arrived, I was met by a woman who insisted on showing me her Christian-themed artwork on her iPhone, telling me about the visions and voices that inspired her artistry. Then, when finally I maneuvered away from her, a man literally rushed me with both arms held out, shoulder high, as if he were ready to grapple and grab me. I put both arms up in front of me and held them in a crossed position so I could push his arms out and prevent him from completing the tackle. The Christian artist lady came up beside him, like an OLB (Outside Line Backer) assisting in the tackle, with her left arm held up and out, directed at my head and hair. I was stunned.

He said, "You know what's wrong with your hair style? It's not curly enough," before he moved forward to complete the tackle.

Then she said, "I love curls," as she continued to reach for me.

I stepped back—out of the pocket with no defenders, so it was a Fran Tarkington QB scramble for sure.

I said to her, "Don't touch my hair."

There was no "please" in that statement. She dropped her hand, and the man stopped trying to grapple me. I stepped back some more and looked at what I was facing. Three other guests were watching the interaction, but they lacked awareness of what they were seeing—a microaggression in which white people feel it's OK to touch and comment about Black people's hair and bodies without understanding that it's an offensive and dehumanizing violation of our personal space, boundaries, and dignity. As a result, none of them came to assist me.

I believe this involved another reason as well.

I am a Black woman, and I was unaccompanied by a man. The Black couple who arrived shortly after me did not undergo any of that group microaggression. The woman was with her husband, and so was protected by the unspoken cultural taboo against touching another man's female partner.

I believe that these white individuals accosted me because I was an unprotected, unaccompanied Black woman. Now, if you were to ask them, did they know this was a full-on racist, sexist assault, they would say no way, no how, not me. Then I would ask, if it wasn't a racist sexist assault, then what the fuck was it?

The rest of the party was fairly uneventful. I positioned myself next to the hostess and we spoke about this and that, and made nice cocktail conversation.

I had every right to be angry, but I was not, and every right to feel something negative about those two, but I did not. I recognized their deficiency, socially, culturally, and racially, and forgave them for their ignorant trespass. The man who charged at me had dementia. The Christian artist lady was hampered by lack of history and lack of cultural exposure to people who are not white. They are limited, not evil or mean. How can I hate them? They are the examples of what I mean when I say they are the ones Black people have to save.

## DIGRESSION #32: THE REFORM OF MEDICAID

Maybe this will happen before any of the other ideas come to fruition. I think it is time to make it happen, because in my humble opinion, the Family Independence Agency (FIA) is too costly. I believe that it does not keep families together, it makes women powerless victims, and it continues the practice of keeping Black families separate and dependent on outside agencies.

I give you the example of three women for whom I cared when I worked in one small town. All three were Black. One had six children by multiple fathers, one had a baby as a young teenager, and one had her third child in her late thirties, by yet another father. All three women were on Medicaid.

The one with six children by multiple fathers was so nice, so poorly educated, and so needy of emotional support that I understand how she would throw herself at a man, any man, as just the ticket from her emotional and financial despair. They all used her and left her. Her parents failed her; her public education was a joke, so what choice did she have but to convert her uterus into a method of support? If she had been male, she would have been in the school-to-prison pipeline. Because she was female, she was in the school-to-Medicaid pipeline. Dependent, uneducated, and fearful of her own security.

The young teen mom was failed by the example of life in a single parent household, a public school education that was a joke, and a man who took advantage of her beautiful innocence and virginal body. First, according to my understanding, he abandoned her, and then her girlfriends abandoned her when it was no longer fun to be around a crying infant. In my opinion, her mother took advantage of her by becoming her paid assistant, getting funds from Medicaid to watch the grandchild, while the daughter went to school to finish her ed-JOKE-cation. Learning nothing, becoming nothing, perpetuating the sadness.

The woman who had a baby in her late thirties already had a 19-year-old and a 10-year-old child, so a baby at nearly 40 years old keeps her on track for continuous Medicaid payment. As one child drops out of eligibility, another comes along every 10 years. With "luck" and help, she could have another child at age 49, staying on Medicaid until age 67, when she will then be eligible for Medicare. If she learned how to work the system, she may have been able to get her last child declared "handicapped," and then she would have the child's income to manage as its lifetime legal guardian. No job, no husband, no education, no life, no better hope.

Shame on us as a people, as a nation.

All of this blame should fall on what I believe is the device created by institutionalized racism and known in Michigan as the Family Independence Agency and whatever institutional governmental clone it has in other states. I believe it has not promoted the family in the Black cultural experience, it never wants independence for women, especially women of color, and it is not just an agency of the government, but also an agent of cultural destruction.

Black family life, when I grew up, was rich, vibrant, and strong. In your family and in your neighborhood, you were respected for your character. Guess what—it is still that way. The problem is that Black cultural neighborhoods have been systematically impoverished, politically disempowered, and cut asunder by the development of the prison-for-profit system that takes men and women away from each other and their children. And don't even get me started on how gerrymandering takes away political voice for Black people.

The FIA would not let a woman and man live together if they were not married. The woman would lose all health and support benefits if she were married. Being married takes more than a suit, a ring, and a minister; it takes effort, time, and the ability to support and sustain each other.

Men, who feel as if they are hunted by the System, may be fearful of exposing women to the same fears. Who knows? I cannot say, but I certainly did see good Black men and good Black women, who loved each other, stay away because, by getting married, they would be denied the scant support of money and health care given to the women by the FIA, provided she remain single. Then she is forced/rewarded to have children to gain an extra amount of money. Her reproductive ability becomes her resource. But then she is criticized and castigated for her reproductive action. She is then forced to have sterilizations (yes, that went on early in my medical life) or forced to get a second opinion because she wanted to have a sterilization procedure (but no white woman with money/health care had to undergo such a hurdle).

See, if you are Black, you cannot win for losing, because no matter which choice you make—to be sterilized or not to be sterilized—you are going to be punished for it. The men were not required to get a second opinion before a vasectomy because racism takes a back seat to sexism in this instance.

But many of the Black men I have seen in my professional life avoid anything to do with doctors for a variety of reasons, and most of them would shy away from something as misunderstood as a procedure on their genitals. I totally understand that reasoning, given the history of how Black men have been treated by the white medical establishment.

Racism, sexism, fear, and ignorance intersect in such a destructive quadrangle. I cry to see it.

## DIGRESSION #33: THE NEW REPUBLIC OF COVERT

I practiced in South Haven, Michigan from 2009 to 2012, and found it to be a fascinating ethnic mix. Approximately one third of residents were African American, one third were Hispanic, and one third were white Appalachian descendants. All were poor and all, except for a very few, were on Medicaid. I would joke with my medical assistant, that what we really needed to do was have Covert secede from the Union, become an independent nation, but remain a "client state" of the USA, and set up an entirely new set of rules and laws to correct all the BS that was going on in the times.

Here are some of those rules and laws that I developed for the NRC—New Republic of Covert:

*Health care*

Citizens are encouraged to follow good health practices.

The NRC will provide a yearly stipend to each citizen for health care—dental, pharmaceutical, podiatry, optometry, audiology, mental health, hospitals, physicians, and all therapists are included in the definition of health care. This grouping is reviewed yearly for inclusion or exclusion. To earn the stipend, each citizen must spend a certain amount to obtain catastrophic coverage from a private insurance company.

Each citizen has a Medical Health Spending Account (MHSA) in a qualified banking institution. The NRC will determine and provide a list of qualified banking and insurance companies. This list is reviewed for inclusion and exclusion yearly. Each citizen may add personal funds at any time in any amount during the year to his/her MHSA. The amount will bear interest. The MHSA's unused amount will rollover into the next year. Children have an account in their own name, but linked to their parent/designated guardian's account.

Citizens who are unable to manage their own account due to mental or physical infirmity will be assigned a dedicated social worker who is charged with maintenance and administration of the account. The NRC will hire these social workers, who are called advocates, pro bono.

Each citizen is also required to maintain an updated medical record on a secure web hosting site. These sites will be evaluated by the NRC for inclusion and exclusion yearly. Each citizen is required to update this record once a year, to provide proof of updates before the NRC will disburse funds into the citizen's MHSA.

Each citizen is required to have a yearly physical exam and provide proof of this before the calendar year ends, or submit a reason for exemption. The NRC will provide additional funds into the accounts for citizens who meet certain thresholds for a healthy lifestyle. The NRC will provide a list of the acceptable markers and the monetary bonus for each one on a yearly basis. An example of the list of markers would include: HGBA1C, BP, negative HIV test, VDRL, TB, skin test, flu shot, shingles shot, other vaccinations, mammograms, and PSA tests.

For children, the list would include vaccinations at age-appropriate intervals. Adults will be rewarded for each recommended adult immunization received.

Citizens may seek care with any licensed provider in the NRC. Citizens pay providers directly from their personal MHSA or their private funds. The NRC does support and encourage no fault auto insurance laws, and supports and encourages workers compensation insurance laws.

Providers may design a variety of payment models, but they are required by law to post their charge schedule in clear terms and plain language. Providers who give charity care receive a tax credit equal to the amount of care that would be charged. This must be clearly documented each year in the medical record. Citizens who have retired from the active workforce or are working less than full-time receive an additional retirees' subsidy into their MHSA if they meet income requirements (no more than X amount earned in a year). This amount is adjusted by the NRC yearly. People who have no MHSA (prisoners, visitors from abroad, homeless, etc.) will have charity care provided to them.

In the event of a medical mishap that results in an adverse outcome for any patient, the event will go to an arbitration board. All citizens will also contribute half of one percent of their annual gross income to the National Arbitration Board and its patient compensation fund. All pharmaceutical companies pay half of one percent of their gross corporate income to support this board and fund, as do medical device manufacturers. (For me today that would be $225.) The arbitration board is composed of lay citizens and members of the involved medical specialty, surgery, family medicine, dentist, NP, etc. This panel is arbitrated by an attorney, who may cast a vote only in the event of a tie decision.

If the medical professional is deemed to have made a preventable error, the practitioner will undergo education and mentoring, and will be removed from active practice until after the education/mentoring is completed. The patient will receive health care services from the compensation fund until the problem is corrected, if correctable. If the problem is not correctable, the care will be provided via the patient's comprehensive catastrophic insurance fund. This system is designed to remove blame, remove legal efforts to obtain high cash rewards for frivolous suits, and remove incentive to sue. The system will instead educate and correct medical providers to prevent errors.

*Citizenship*

The requirements are threefold. A person who requires citizenship via immigration in the NRC must be free of any felony conviction, must have a high school education or its equivalent or higher, and must have a job and/or a marketable skill that is needed within the NRC.

All citizens, native-born and naturalized, are entitled to all privileges and rights. All citizens are required to perform their responsibilities, which include jury duty, voting, and military service.

*Immigration*

All immigrants must meet citizenship requirements. Marriage to a citizen by an immigrant does not automatically confer citizenship on the non-citizen immigrant. We do accept refuges if they are vetted by our national security agencies, and also meet requirements for citizenship. All other resident non-citizens must apply for residency status determination. Categories of residency are: A) seeking citizenship; B) non-citizen temporary for less than six months while not seeking citizenship; and C) temporary for more than six months while not seeking citizenship.

Those who enter the NRC illegally will be returned to their country of origin. If they apply for refugee status, they must wait in their native country while the process continues. Employers who knowingly solicit illegal workers will be fined and penalized.

*Military*

The NRC maintains a national military/security force. The military armed service provides security for our borders, and is also the local policing agency inside our nation. All qualified citizens must serve one year of military service. They may opt for additional years of volunteer service after that. Their first year of service must occur between ages 18 and 25. There is an alternative option, the Civilian Service, which consists of a civilian-based community service in the fields of environment, infrastructure, agriculture, education, and social work.

The armed service provides protection from national down to local units of government. Service in either section may be deferred for legitimate reasons—health, family hardship, etc.—as approved by the Military/Civilian Services governing board.

The NRC military arm serves as the local policing force. Personnel are stationed in their neighborhood of origin. Troops who elect to serve beyond one year, and also want to earn a college education, may apply, and if approved, will earn six months of tuition for every year of service after the required first year. This is for college tuition above the Bachelor's level.

*Language*

The official language of the NRC is English. All citizens will be proficient in English, reading, listening, writing, and speaking. All commercial, educational, communications, government, legal, and health care activities are conducted in English. All citizens are also required to study a second language for 10 years as part of their primary education, and to develop speaking proficiency in that language.

*Death Penalty*

The NRC does not have or support the death penalty.

*Education*

All education in the NRC from pre-K to grade 12 is private pay. The teachers work for themselves, either alone, as self-employed/ self-organized groups, or as private tutors for private academies. College and skilled trades schools are free and run by the NRC.

Students entering secondary education—college or skilled trades—must pass examinations beforehand. There are five national examinations from K to 12, and one exam given by the college of the student's choice.

The state exam is given in third, fifth, seventh, and 12th grades. Students who fail must obtain remedial education and retake the exam. All primary schools, academies, and tutors must report their failure rate on a public website. Remedial education is offered by any school, other than the one attended by the student. The schools that failed to educate them does not deserve to have them back as students.

The exam given by the NRC may consist of true or false questions, multiple choice questions, or an essay. Additionally, it may consist of artistic endeavor, performance, dance, oral questioning, or any combination of these methods.

All K-12 students are required to speak one other language in all four phases of proficiency—writing, reading, listening, and speaking. Exceptions are made for non-living languages such as Latin, Aramaic, Sumerian, etc., where the student must be able to read and write only.

All K-12 students are required to participate in a sport or physical activity in all 12 grades.

Education is conducted in English. Non-English speakers must hire a tutor privately and pass a proficiency exam before entering K-12 levels.

Special education is offered by schools which are exclusively devoted to that student population, and may offer either K to 12 or K to Bachelor's level. Special education schools receive evaluation by the NRC, and are partially or completely funded by the NRC based on the student's family income.

Secondary education at the Bachelor's level is free and paid by the NRC. All matriculated students must maintain passing grades to remain in school. The passing level is set by the college being attended. All students must also pass an entrance exam determined by the school.

Tertiary education, Master's, Doctoral, etc., is privately paid, or by scholarship and loans. Loans can be obtained from the NRC or from private lenders. NRC government loans are available at a three percent interest rate. Private loans are held to a maximum of two percentage points above the government loan rate. Government loans are kept at a restricted number and are based on competitive scores.

Those parents who cannot afford a private pre-K to 12 school will send their children to a co-operative school. Each private academy donates teachers to the co-operative schools on a rotating basis. Parents pay a percentage of their gross income to the co-operative school. The percentage is determined by the income level of the parents.

Education in the NRC is not funded by property tax, where people with children do not pay into the system because they rent, and where people without children pay because they own. Also, schools set their own curricula, schedules, hours of operation, rules, and tests. These private schools may eliminate the need for bus drivers and winter sessions. Schools are free to use multiple methods of teaching—in classrooms and on field trips, as well as through distance learning, focus camps, digital learning, on demand courses, and webinar sessions. While they are allowed labor unions, they are not required because teachers own their schools or work as private tutors.

Schools compete for students. Schools strive to get students educated so they can go to a college and pass the national proficiency tests. Colleges still select students based on their own standards. Trade schools are considered equal to academic colleges for this purpose.

*Governance*

The President and Vice President must run for election separately.

The winner of each contest is limited to two terms of four years each. The person who receives the highest number of votes is the winner.

Campaigns begin four months prior to start of the term. The person who receives the second highest number of votes becomes Vice President. In the event of a tie, there will be a run-off election.

There is one house of Congress. Each state gets five members in this Congress. All members of the national congress are selected from the jury duty rosters. All members serve for two, four, or six years. All who are selected must pass an additional filter to demonstrate a lack of felony convictions and evidence of mental health competency.

All national representatives get one million dollars yearly for salary, have paid-up life insurance policies, and have guaranteed preservation of their pre-selection employment, plus all expenses are paid for their residence and official government travel. All national representatives must reside in their district for 300 of the 365 days each year, and must have open office hours, totaling a minimum of 60 hours per week, open to any resident in their district.

No lobbyist can meet with any national representative in secret in the district. When lobbyists meet with the national representatives in the capital or in the district, the meeting must be published, announced, and electronically broadcast, listing the attendees and sponsor of the meeting.

All national representatives will have communication via the most appropriate and most advanced method available, so that they can communicate with each other while they are present in their districts. National representatives meet in a committee as a whole in the capital, as required for votes that concern taxation, warfare, constitutional changes, or confirmation of judiciary or cabinet officials.

No national representative can be exempt from any law passed by the national legislature. Any benefit given, legislatively to a national representative, must also be given to all citizens of the New Republic of Covert. All meetings held in the capital will be broadcast and recorded to the general public. No national representative may ever serve as a lobbyist after serving as a national representative. All national representatives are subject to the same laws as apply to citizens.

No national representative can be reelected to the term she/he currently serves, but may be elected to one of the other terms, after being out of office for a number of years equal to the number of years in the term served. For example, a person is elected to a six-year term. That person must be out of office for six years before they are allowed to run for either a two- or four-year term.

The Supreme Court Judiciary is appointed by the President and confirmed by the national legislature. Appointments last for 25 years, then the judicial appointee becomes an ex officio member. Ex officio members of the Supreme Court may serve as advisors to the national legislature and/or to the President.

Voting in national elections is held and conducted over the course of three days. All citizens can vote if they are over 18, and are a citizen by birth or naturalization. Polling places are open for 24 hours during that three-day term.

*Homelessness*

It is the hope of the NRC that no citizen will be homeless. But in the event of that occurrence, the NRC has a program of government, non-government, and community resource cooperative management for those who are without a place to live.

The NRC believes that a safe living environment is a right for each citizen, and the responsibility of all citizens and of their government.

Commercial and residential properties that are unoccupied or abandoned are eligible for use as residential centers for those who are homeless. Each residential center will house one family, or three unrelated, same-sex individuals. The owner of the RC will be given a moratorium on taxes in exchange for providing payment for one of the following services: heating, electricity, water/sewage, or IT/ communications. The other three services are paid for by those who live in the residential center.

Each residential center will be refurbished so that it can comfortably house a family or a residential group, by providing at least three bedrooms and one and a half bathrooms in the structure. The people who wish to live in a specific residential center will provide sweat equity labor on their place, and will be joined in the project by skilled contractors who will provide labor, materials, and assistance to the people who will be living there. These contractors will be paid by the NRC, and the residents of the units will repay the NRC over time for this refurbishing.

The people who occupy the residential center must be free of substance abuse problems and must be employed. Any member of such a group who develops a substance abuse problem is first reprimanded, then on second offense, ejected from the unit and removed to a substance abuse treatment facility. Residents will agree to random, on-site saliva or urine tests for substance abuse.

Each residential center will also be assigned a social worker, a pro bono advocate, who will provide and arrange for counseling, education, job training, transportation, and medical care for the members in the group. Additionally, each residential center is partnered with any one community organization or commercial venture, which shall provide official mentoring and support to the members of the residential group.

*Religion*

The New Republic of Covert does not have any official state-sanctioned religion. Citizens may worship as they chose, as long as that form of worship does not harm themselves or others.

WE'RE BACK . . .

**Ohio Life**

My life in Ohio settled down into a few activities. I played bridge, took care of my grandchildren, decorated my house, and had parties. It was very strange being off the clock 24/7. A retired patient once said to me, about retirement, that "every day is Saturday, and then the last one is Sunday." I was afraid that I would be bored, but with two grandchildren, boredom was quickly washed away.

My dear Grandchildren, you two are the world's best grandchildren. Each day that I can spend with you is a jolt of life and a breath of fresh air, even if you are being difficult. I do think I am fortunate and privileged to be in your lives, no matter how large or small the effort; it is worth it.

I must tell you both that you better not do drugs, because I will come back from the grave and spank you. I also know that I would be willing to destroy anyone who hurt you. I wonder if I were so adamant about things like this when my own children were young? I think not; I think I was a depressed workaholic who ignored the joys and journey of parenthood because of my life with an alcoholic. I was so flawed, not that I am perfect now, but I can say I am on a pathway to improvement now, whereas back then I was heading for disaster.

I have discovered that I have some creative juices. As I said, one expression of creativity is the development of a game called "!XO The Kwanzaa Game," which is based on the traditions of Kwanzaa.

Another expression of creativity is my craft room in the furnace room. I have developed a passion for making doodads and decorations from pieces of anything. Now that I have a glue gun, I am really dangerous with crafting. Each year, I make a gift to give to my friends in Al-Anon and the condo association, and the gift, no matter what, is a smile-bringer. I have developed a nice reputation as a result of this tinkering.

**My Day as an Old Person**

Retired and old and into a total routine:

Get up.
Pee.
Drink water.

Start coffee.
Open curtains.
Light candles.
Take a shit.
Read my ODAT.
Have coffee.
Pee.
Make more coffee.
Pee.
Drink more coffee.
Take my medications and use inhaler.
Pee.
Have breakfast (the same every day, and includes prunes).
Pee.
Take a second shit.
Clean up the kitchen.
Pee.
Get dressed.
Put on makeup.
Groom and play with the cat.
Clean the cat box.
Check the basement for problems.
Pee.
Check phone for texts, emails, weather, calendar events.

That is the first hour and a half of my day. Or more succinctly put:

Urinate.
Hydrate.
Defecate.
Caffeinate.
Medicate.
Meditate.
Ingest.

Get dressed.
Do my hair.
Do cat care.
Plan the rest.

The rest of the day after cat care is varied. Lady Jane gets groomed with treats, and then I scoop her litter box and clean up around it. At night, she gets play time with the fishing pole toy, and we look at something to stream on TV.

Following morning cat care, I check the weather and email, and either go for a walk if the weather is good, or walk on the treadmill if the weather is bad or if it's winter.

Then what happens from 9 AM till 4 PM would be my "workday." After that, it is time to plan dinner, feed the cat, and settle in for the evening to watch something streaming on Netflix or Amazon.

Not exciting, but if I wanted excitement in my eighth decade of life, I would continue to work, including delivering babies, taking shifts in the ER, smoking Kool Milds cigarettes, and looking for unattached men in bars. Been there, done that.

**A New Definition for ADHD**

Part of the joy of retirement is the opportunity to read, reflect, and write about the messiness of medical life for my colleagues who are still in the struggle. I've read many articles about a Great Resignation by doctors, surgeons and administrators who are leaving hospitals to seek employment elsewhere.

One article described a mass exodus from one particular hospital, quoting unnamed sources who lay the blame on the ACA/ Obamacare (yeah, blame the Black guy), which is certainly fair, but the ACA is not the only culprit.

A common theme is that hospital administrations are disconnected from the medical staff and de-emphasize academics, even at teaching institutions, while placing a higher priority on making money. Let's see, that emphasis would be, "Ignore the docs, screw the residents, forget quality care, and make mo' money, mo' money, mo' money."

Sadly, some hospitals respond with an inflexible strategy of refusing to raise physicians' salaries while firing complainers. What a Powerful Methodology for correcting problems, don't ya think? Hospitals then respond to media interviews with statements written in pure "Administralian," which may be as hard to decipher and understand as Minoan Linear A and Linear B, or Mayan stone hieroglyphics.

Just for Shits and Giggles, suppose the hospital focused on things that made sense, not only in English or Spanish or any other real language, but also that made sense medically. Three popped into my mind, and I would implement them if I were the administrator. They are:

1. Reducing hospital-acquired infections.
2. Reducing medication errors.
3. Reducing wrong-site surgery.

There are more, but these would possibly impact patient satisfaction and patient outcomes.

But then, I am just a woman, a Boomer, and a physician, so I am prone to having silly, simple, logical thoughts like that. Call me an old-fashioned curmudgeon, but I sincerely doubt that Gen Xers and Millennials would go for this kind of bovine manure management style either.

I have also read about complete disrespect for physicians and their concerns, along with sexist attitudes toward female leadership in hospitals.

Let's consider this scenario as if it were your car dealership. The dealership would replace the owner with a person who has a degree in the philosophy of automotive engineering, but who has never sold a car, worked on a car, and who does not drive a car because he has a chauffeur. Then the sales staff would be cut in half to provide focus on the strategic direction. The repair crew would not be paid a salary, or even hourly rate, but would be paid on an RVU basis (Rapid Vehicle Up&Out) system, which would drive metrics forward. Finally, the front staff would be replaced with an AI robot voice machine, with recorded messages and responses to questions to provide accountability. WOW.

Non-physicians in charge of a hospital filled with physicians.

Employed physicians losing respect from the non-physician administration.

Physicians, who care about providing good care, leave rather than compromising.

The result is that patients suffer and are at risk for all kinds of harm, and good hospitals are destroyed by bad administration, again.

I have worked for places like this, and have seen hospitals get sued, get closed, lose money, and lose good people repeatedly because money became number one. That trend is going on every day in health care because health care is driven by profit first, and there is no second or third. So Sad.

Therefore, I am proposing a name change. Put this in the ICD-10. ADHD now means Administrators Destroying Hospitals Daily. It has more utility than the old name, and is certainly true.

## DIGRESSION #34: THE MALE HIERARCHICAL DOMINANCE

So much of the harm in the world seems to be due to our holding on to the idea of male hierarchical dominance (MHD). It seems to me that the supremacy of the MHD form of rule rests on three principals. One is pressure to reproduce. Two is achieving control. Three is glorification of the acquisition of material goods.

MHD was probably necessary when muscle power was the only form of energy available for humans. The strong survived; the weak did not. The strong mated and prospered. The strong banded together and supported each other. The strong made the rules. Over time, those who were not as strong developed the concept of religion and promoted it to the strong to prove their right to rule by the law of God. These purveyors of religion knew that their ascendency depended on being in the good graces of the politically and physically strongest ruler.

Look at the failed or long-gone nations of antiquity; their religion has gone the way of their political moiety. No Roman empire, no Roman gods. No Assyrian empire, no Assyrian gods. No Mayan empire, no Mayan gods. Do you not see that, if those gods were truly viable, they would have survived the downfall of the politicians who espoused their worship? Religion kept the Egyptian kings on the throne for five millennia. The fallacy of religion kept the subjected people from sharing in the advancement of their civilization's inventions, education, and development. The best of the material world went to the strongest, and their religious lackeys who fed the propaganda of God Knows Best to the not-so-strong. If you convince the leader that he is a god himself, and convince the subjects of that idea, the system is almost impossible to change.

The pressure to reproduce is not just what has been foisted onto women. It is also what men must do to insure their survival, via their lineage. Thus, we have the notion of kings and princes and royal lines of succession. The bride, wife, queen, and mother must be carefully selected, and only the king may produce a child from her. The king may produce children from other women, but none of their progeny will be royal. The queen may not produce any child except that of the king, or she will be cast out along with her non-royal offspring.

Furthermore, the poor must reproduce in large numbers to guarantee their survival at the end of their reproductive years. Their children must care for them as they cared for the children, in order to live, because there is no societal/political support for the old in most societies, even today. Women are victimized if they do not have children, do not have enough children, have children that are not perfect, or are defective in any fashion.

Women who refuse to have children (including some lesbians)

or who cannot have children (infertile) are ostracized. They are perceived as a threat and will be labeled as witches and killed. Or they are perceived as useless because they cannot conceive, are labeled as worthless, and are killed or cast out. I wonder how many of the women who died in the Salem witch trials were actually gay or infertile, or just too intelligent to give in to men who demanded sex from them?

Controlling others is a mainstay of corporate, cultural, and political life today all over the civilized world. It springs from desires to be supreme over your peers, and to have the ability to possess women who give the strong man reproductive control. Just as the gay woman is useless to the MHD structure, so is the gay man. He cannot be bribed with the offer of breeding with females from your family or threatened with loss of reproductive rights. Further, the MHD male fears he may subvert their sons and take them out of the line of reproduction. Being in control allows the controller to exempt himself from multiple onerous responsibilities and to insert himself first in line to receive benefits.

Hard on the heels of control is the glorification of acquisition of material goods. Here is the manifestation of MHD visible for all to see. The strong man who has the best or most of any- and everything, will feel superior to all other men. The need to feel superior must be what drives men locked into the MHD structure to want more and more of every material thing.

More material things, more women as sexual partners and more control over other men, makes for a potent cocktail of destruction in this world. Muscle power is not the prime power any longer. If anything, it is intellectual proficiency that rules, or so it would seem evidenced by the rise of Silicon Valley tech billionaires.

The desire for material goods has made us destroy our planet. Forests, animals, rivers, and oceans, and the land below our feet, are all harvested, wasted, polluted, slaughtered, or depleted so that some few of us, not everyone, can have a better THING. We seem to be determined to raise a nation of envious, workaholic, spendthrift consumers—people who know how to shop and buy, but not work and save, nor do they know how to rest, relax, enjoy each other, or pursue intellectual ideals.

We cannot seem to be at peace with ourselves, much less at peace with each other.

Shame on us. One day, when the alien space invaders come, they will not care about our petty religious, linguistic, or cultural differences. They will not care about the variety of skin shades we possess. They will not care about us because we will only be useful, harvestable commodities to them, the same as we have made commodities of all other species on this planet.

We are doomed by Male Hierarchical Dominance.

WE'RE BACK . . .

**Our Current Political Chaos in 2018**

In this nation, I think there are 10 topics that are important politically: (1) economy, (2) taxes, (3) immigration, (4) guns, (5) abortion, (6) employment, (7) cultural identity, (8) environment, (9) health care, and (10) foreign relations.

The 45$^{th}$ President, Donald Trump, managed to focus on taxes, immigration, guns, abortion, and foreign relations as his favorite push buttons. His comments and policies in these zones kept us inflamed, divided, fearful, and angry. He and his cronies benefitted. The rest of us suffered.

I think this list is actually compressible down to just three, which are sexism, racism, and greed. Sexism forces us to make abortion an issue. Racism encapsulates immigration, guns, cultural identity, and foreign relations. Greed is the focus for economic policy, tax law, employment figures, environmental decisions, health care, and, again, foreign policy.

A better way would be to look at the 10 items that should be of greater concern to us and our national political leaders, in my next list:

1. Health care should be available for all, but not free.
2. Infrastructure needs another effort, like the old WPA or CCC, to rebuild our system of connectedness.
3. Drugs—everything about drug rehabilitation, drug abuse prevention, stopping the influx of drugs into our nation, and more, should be on this list.
4. Revitalization of our cities as a federal initiative needs to happen, because demographically, more people are moving into the cities, but many parts of our cities are unlivable, cramped, and lacking services and jobs for them.
5. Agricultural methodology and food distribution need attention. We let agribusiness pollute the land, poison the animals we eat, spill fecal material into our waterways, put small farmers out of business, and deny the importance of organically grown alternatives. Meanwhile, large numbers of people are forced into hunger and food insecurity, while we throw away 40 percent of what we produce.
6. Education. Beyond STEM is the need to become more aware of history, not only the general history of this nation, but the history of all the ethnicities who came here, and who originated from here. Then weave that into the general history of our world. Furthermore, our population needs to be 100 percent literate in English, and at least 50 percent of us should also learn a second language, or possibly, a third language.
7. Homelessness is a national shame. Currently there are six empty residences for every one person who is homeless. Why? The main reason for homelessness is that people cannot afford their homes, even when two adults in a household are fully employed.
8. Employment is always important to any nation. We should count all people who are looking for work, as long as they are in the eligible pile of workers. Currently, we stop counting them after a certain space of time and call them chronically unemployable. I think that is BS.
9. Foreign relations: what has happened now must be repaired or we will shrivel and die under the onslaught of the Chinese hegemony, and a unified Europe.

10. Wealth equilibrium. The distribution of wealth should be a bell curve. It is not. One percent of the population holds 32.3% of America's wealth (as of 2021), while the lower 50% of income earners have just 2.6% of the country's wealth, according to Federal Reserve data on Wikipedia. In addition, the U.S. Census Bureau reported that in 2020, the median household income was $67,521, which was a 2.9% decrease from the 2019 median of $69,560.

Nearly 13% of Americans live below the poverty line, which is defined as $13,590 income per year for one person and $27,750 for a family of four, according to the U.S. Census Bureau. I do not ask the rich to give up their wealth; I just ask that those who have the wealth, to stop denying wealth—by making opportunities for income improvement to those who do not have the wealth. Tax law, credit card management, debt laws, and lending laws need to be corrected so we stop punishing those who have nothing.

Removing racism, sexism, and greed from the political fray allows us to see the true concerns of a democracy, and would let us focus on those things that make us stronger, not those things that divide us and lay us open to dismemberment by our enemies, or those who are just envious.

In the third week of December, 2019, another U.S. President was impeached by the House of Representatives. He, number 45, was charged with bribing/forcing a foreign nation to dig up dirt on the son of a potential political rival. He is guilty of that, and so much more. He became the first American president to be impeached twice, when it happened again on January 13th, 2021.[29] So much time was wasted with impeachment, that nothing was done regarding homelessness, hunger, drug abuse, health care inequity/unaffordability, climate change, racism, sexism, or antisemitism.

I think the New Republic of Covert would have another way to deal with such a disreputable dog.

In November of 2020, Donald Trump was defeated by now

President Joe Biden, whose Vice President Kamala Harris has a Jamaican father, a mother who was Tamil/Indian, and a husband who is Jewish. What a new life on the horizon for her, for women, for the men in this nation, for the children growing into maturity, and for all of us.

**Closure at Last**

Well, I have so many more stories that come into my mind every time I edit or revise this memoir. I must have seen thousands of patients over the 35 years I worked in five states. I had more than 100 classmates who shared all my dreams, traumas, and dramas. The teachers and friends at MSU, WSU, MCC, and CMU certainly made my life great. The neighbors in all the cities where I lived probably deserve their own chapter, maybe even a book. There are family members who are not mentioned, some because it would not be right, others because it would be wrong, and some because I just don't know where to put them. There is a lot that I cannot put into this book because it would be slanderous, or because I just forgot the details.

Ezekiel and Magdalana, what you have from me is the best I could do. As for those who did not make it into this memoir, rest assured, they are in my head and in my heart, and that may be the best place to leave them.

There are lots of jerks (and worse) who need to be exposed to the light, but that would take more time, paper, and effort than I have, or that they deserve. If someone tells you they read this and wonder why they are not here, I apologize, or you can apologize on my behalf.

If someone you know tells you they are here and wonder why they are, then I also apologize. I am not sorry for the cuss words or language.

This is written for my beloved grandchildren, who have heard me say these things in the past. Sorry—NOT GONNA DO ANOTHER APOLOGY.

If the things I write make some people call me a ravening, reverse racist, politically naïve, godless, ranting, neo-liberal, potty-mouthed harridan, then I gratefully accept all those labels, and will wear them with pride. You, the others who read this, remember that you have the right and freedom to write your own book.

Just remember how I earned all those accolades (I will not call them epithets because I deserve each one). My life was not easy or sweet, and I know I am shaped by my genes as much as I am by my experiences, so I will admit that many of those terms are true, and so what? I will no longer deny the validity of my own experience.

Naturally, I know that I am not perfect, and one nice thing to discover when writing about yourself is that you learn about yourself. I learned:

- I tended to run away from my problems, thereby showing cowardice.
- I trusted people who did not have my best interest at heart, showing naivety.
- Love is blind, showing emotional ignorance.
- I am a hard worker, showing ethics and skill.
- I am too defensive to seek another partner, showing an ingrained lack of trust.
- I failed to take advantage of precious opportunities, showing timidity.
- I was a frightened child, showing loneliness.
- I was an angry parent, showing my unloved life as a child.
- My imagination is boundless, showing me to be an avid reader.
- I was outspoken in private and quiet in public then, but not now.
- I was harsh with many people who did not deserve it, which was defensive posturing.
- I doubted myself, which allowed people to use me badly because of a poor self-image.
- I have a wicked sense of humor and I love puns, showing I am

funny and optimistic.

- I am more of a cat person than a dog person, showing just what it says.
- I am not a religionist, but rather an agnostic.
- I am an antiracist and must also be a realist.
- I am a fiscal conservative, showing my caution.
- I am a social progressive, showing my optimism.
- I am proud of my cultural heritage from both African and European sides of my family.

I was born as a female, developed into a woman who is Black, and got to be a doctor. But as I have matured, now I am happy to say I am a Black Woman Doctor.

My Blackness contains a pocket of rage, to which I am entitled, and from which I draw upon for a special kind of crazy courage.

As a Woman, I have a pool of tenderness that allows me to show compassion, which is that special tenderness all humans deserve.

As a Doctor, I have the right to an opinion and am free to give it. Be warned; I will say what I want because I don't work for you, I'm not married to you, and I don't owe you any money.

Ezekiel and Magdalana—you two can call me Grandma, all others must call me Doctor Mustonen. Because, at the end of the day, at the end of my life, that is who I am.

Next, please.

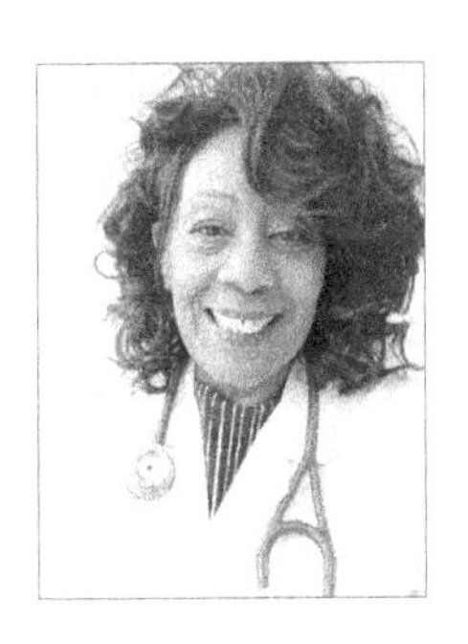

# ABOUT THE AUTHOR

Sylvia Mustonen, DO, has led a fascinating life with two illustrious careers: first, as a high-profile TV news reporter who earned exclusive coverage during the 1967 race riots in Detroit; and second as a physician helping patients in hospitals and in private practice in multiple states.

In addition, she was interracially married to a judge and has two grown daughters and two grandchildren.

Now Dr. Mustonen shares her remarkable life story and innovative vision for the future of medicine in her gripping memoir, *New Medicine for a New Millennium: A Memoir Looking Front to Back in Time at a Black Woman's Life in Medicine.*

In the book, she exposes the racism and sexism that she experienced as a Black female medical student and physician in usually all-white hospital and smalltown environments. She also shares heartwarming stories about the patients she has helped, the colleagues she worked with, the fraud she witnessed, the lessons learned, and the unique populations she has served.

Dr. Mustonen does not sugarcoat her story or the realities of her world; she bares all in sometimes graphic language that conveys the drama of each experience.

She describes growing up in Detroit, attending Wayne State University, and later medical school at Michigan State University College of Osteopathic Medicine.

While many parts of her life seemed idyllic and charming, like when she and her husband purchased a country home in rural Michigan and enjoyed the cozy-warm glow of a burning stove, her husband's alcoholism created an undercurrent of angst. She coped for decades by attending Al-Anon meetings for family members of alcoholics.

At times heart-wrenching, other times hilarious, Dr. Mustonen is a skilled storyteller sharing the rich moments that comprise her 70+ years.

Now retired, she offers unique observations about the medical field, and her vision for how technology, robots, and unique devices may transform the field of medicine in the very near future.

After learning journalism by observing her high-profile mother, June Brown, working as a popular columnist at *The Michigan Chronicle*, Dr. Mustonen became a television news reporter at Detroit's CBS News affiliate, WJBK, Channel 2. There she pioneered new ground as a Black female reporter, and excelled as one of few Black journalists in Detroit.

After the deadly 1967 riots in Detroit, she and her husband, Attorney Arney Mustonen, who had Finnish ancestry, left the racial tensions of the city to raise their biracial daughters at their country home.

Then she attended the Michigan State University College of Osteopathic Medicine in East Lansing, Michigan.

She became Board Certified in Family Medicine and a Fellow in the American College of Osteopathic Family Physicians.

Dr. Mustonen has a very distinguished career as a medical instructor, medical administrator, and Family Physician.

She has served patients in many Michigan cities, including: Lansing; South Haven; Covert; Bangor; Greenville, where she was also the Medical Director for United Memorial Hospital; and Metro Detroit. She has worked in Prairie du Chien, Wisconsin.

Dr. Mustonen has also been Associate Professor in the Department of Family and Community Medicine at the Michigan State University College of Osteopathic Medicine. She has provided instruction for Family Practice Residents at Detroit Osteopathic

Hospital and at Botsford Osteopathic Hospital in Farmington Hills, Michigan, and was an Associate Professor (Adjunct) for the College of Osteopathic Medicine and Surgery in Des Moines, Iowa.

In 2007, Michigan Governor Jennifer Granholm appointed Dr. Mustonen as a member of the State of Michigan Board of Osteopathic Medicine and Surgery.

Dr. Mustonen is also an Associate in Healthcare Risk Management and Quality Review (AHRMQR).

Dr. Mustonen created a board game called !XO The Kwanzaa Game to celebrate the Kwanzaa holiday.

Now retired from practicing medicine, she enjoys spending time with her grandchildren and gardening, as well as working in the toy store owned by her youngest daughter and son-in-law.

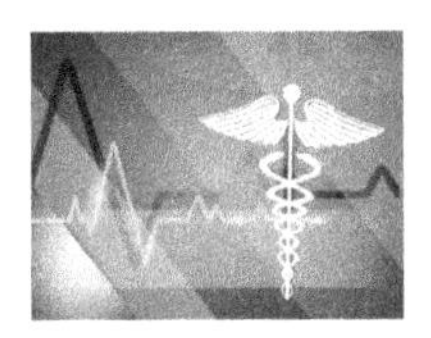

# CONTACT THE AUTHOR

You can contact Dr. Mustonen at her website: www.kwanzaagame.com as well as via email: sgmdomybook@gmail.com. Dr. Mustonen occasionally will post a VLOG on her You Tube channel. Find her at Sylvia Mustonen Speaks @ You Tube.com

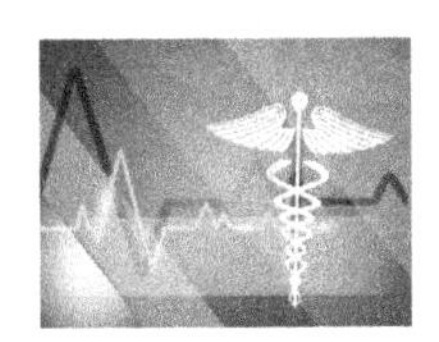

# APPENDIX 1

A Schedule for five family doctors and four staff members to provide 24/7 DPC Care:

| | | |
|---|---|---|
| A | slot | On call Monday to Sunday from office close to office open |
| B | slot | Works the weekend in the office |
| C | slot | Early shift in the office |
| D | slot | Late shift in the office |
| E | slot | House calls Monday to Friday |

| Monday | Tuesday | Wednesday | Thursday | Friday | Saturday | Sunday |
|---|---|---|---|---|---|---|
| A slot – phone call coverage | | | | | | |
| 7P –7A | 7P-7A | 7P-7A | 7P-7A | 7P-7A | 7P-10A | 6PM-7A |
| B slot weekends only | | | | | | |
| Off | Off | Off | Off | Off | 10A-6P | 10A-6P |
| C slot Early office | | | | | | |
| 7A-3P | 7A-3P | 7A-3P | 7A-3P | 7A-3P | Off | Off |
| D slot Late office | | | | | | |
| N-7P | N-7P | N-7P | N-7P | N-7P | Off | Off |
| E slot House calls week | | | | | | |
| 8A-5P | 8A-5P | 8A-5P | 8A-5P | 8A-5P | Off | Off |

Week by Week for August 2021

| | 1 – 7 | 8-14 | 15-21 | 22-28 | 29 – 9/4 |
|---|---|---|---|---|---|
| Doc | Slot | Slot | Slot | Slot | Slot |
| Jones | A | B | C | D | E |
| Smith | B | C | D | E | A |
| Brown | C | D | E | A | B |
| Miller | D | E | A | B | C |
| Green | E | A | B | C | D |

No doctors do hospital rounds. Minor urgent care is handled in the office. The EMR is custom designed. Office procedures are bunched on one day to simplify the doctor's day. House calls may include one nursing home, no more than one. While the weekend is brutal, it is just phone chat with computer access, via Zoom, and video treatment is possible. All diagnostics are outsourced (free standing radiology, LabCorp). Mobile diagnostics occur on the day after the house call was made. One staff member drives with the house call doctor, one staff member works with the weekend doctor, and two staff members work with the early and late doctor in the office. The phone is answered by everybody in the office, docs and staff. The building is a rental with the option to purchase. There are two large exam rooms and a small waiting room. A few CLIA-waived tests are done in the office. CME and vacation ideally occur on the five days off stretch. No one is overworked. All patients can see all doctors. Everybody gets paid well.

# REFERENCES AND RESOURCES

Citations for My List of Trends in the Future of Medicine


**ONE: MD and DO schools and professions will merge**

"AOA ACGME Update," Michigan Osteopathic Association, email from kmcfatridge@mi-Osteopathic.org, Saturday August 3, 2013.

"Work continues toward unified graduate medical education accreditation," William D. Strampel D.O., Dean, in *Communique* magazine, Michigan State University College of Osteopathic Medicine, Fall 2013, Volume 40, number 3, page 2, 2013.

"Comlex-USA and Acceptance for ACGME Fellowship Program Applications," National Board of Osteopathic Medical Examiners, email from communica-tions @nbome.org, Monday January 18, 2016.

**THREE: Physicians will become automated Cyborgs**

"Da Vinci Surgical System," Wikipedia the free Encyclopedia, March 21, 2013.

"The Coming Medical School Bust," www.hcplive.com; June 27, 2016.

"New MSUCOM research shows live videoconferencing can be an effective tool in higher education," Laura Probyn, *Communique* magazine, Fall 2013, page 3.

"For High-acuity patients in a home setting on demand acute medical care," Medically Home Group Inc., www.medicallyhome.com, April 28, 2020.

"Brave New Worlds in Diagnosing Diseases," Your Health, *AARP Bulletin*, page 8, May 2015.

"BIO 1158 What Do we DO when The Medicine Runs Out?" Moina Tahnee Snyder, OMS III, Lindsay Karlin, OMS III, Andrew Smythe, OMSIII, Taisei Suzuki, OMS II, Al Turner DO, A.T. Still University School of Osteopathic Medicine in Mesa Arizona, *The Journal of the American Osteopathic Association*, March 2013, Vol. 113, Number 3 pages 235, 236.

"Cultivating common sense – a band of Seattle computer scientists is on a mission to make artificial intelligence actually intelligent," Carl Engelking, *Discover Magazine*, April 2017, pages 33 to 39.

**FOUR: Medical School enrollment will be open to all who can afford it**

"Musings on Humanism, Medicine and Medical Education," Ronald V. Marino, DO, MPH, *Journal of the American Osteopathic Association*, March 2013, Vol. 113, Number 3, pages 196, 197.

**FIVE: Hospitals will deploy robots instead of nurses for the majority of care**

"Parkview's Tugs," *Fort Wayne (Indiana) Monthly* – Health, 2012, page 19.

**SIX: Nursing homes will become automated also**

"A Failing Business Model – COVID 19 has revealed and worsened weaknesses in nursing home finances," Harris Meyer, Special Edition Nursing Homes, *AARP Bulletin*, December 2020 pages 26-28.

**SEVEN Government will drop Medicaid and move to Medicare for All**

"Physician Quality Reporting System," CMS.Gov, www.cms.gov/Medicare/Quality-Initialves-Patient – Assessment – Instruments/, March 27, 2013.

"It's Showtime for health care reform," *Consumer Reports Magazine*, special section, November 2013, pages 30-40.

"Obamacare open enrollment: Here's everything you need to know," Jan Christensen, *CNN Health*, www.cnn.com, September 26, 2013.

"Medicare Discloses Hospitals' Bonuses, Penalties Based on Quality," Jordan Rau, KHN Staff writer, *Kaiser Health News*; www.kaiserhealthnews.org, March 27, 2013.

"Does Rigorous Quality Process Reporting Guarantee Superior – Quality Health Care?" Gary Seabrook MD, *Journal of the American Medical Association*, July 17, 2013, Volume 310 Number 3, pages 316-317.

**Eight: The EVE – Extra Uterine Viability Environment device will be invented**

"Commercial Surrogacy in India," Wikipedia.org, 9-2-2019.

**Nine: More Physicians will move to total Concierge Medicine**

**Ten: Physicians will form independent corporations**

**Also: Digression 4 Customer versus Patient**

**Also: Digression 24: DPC groups will provide 24/7/365 Health Care**

Colonoscopy beats "camera pill" at catching color cancer, but less invasive detection method still shows promise, scientists say, Alan Mozes, health day reporter, usnews.com,/health, July 15, 2009.

"Commentary – Doctor – Workers Unite!" Howard Waitzkin, MD PhD, WWW.Medescape.com, May 20, 2016.

PCP status, compensation poised to improve, Bert Berenson, MD, *Medical Economics*, October 25, 2012, pages 52-58.

"Should Medical Practices Charge Subscription Fees?" David Doyle, www.physicianspractice.com/blog, April 13, 2013.

"My Transition to a Direct-pay Practice," Robert Lamberts, MD, www.physicianspractice.com/pearls, April 3, 2013.

"Concierge Medicine as a Consumer-based Quality Measure," Wayne Lipton, www.physicianspractice.com/blog, March 14, 2013.

"How to Test the Waters of a Cash-Only Practice," Jeffrey J. Denning, *UnCommon Sense*, www.medscape.com, 2012.

"Physician Independence May Die by a Thousand Tiny Cuts," James Doulgeris and Nicholas Bonvicino MD, www.physicianspractice.com/blog, March 21, 2013.

ACO Insider: a prescription for rising health care spending; Julian D. "Bo" Bobbitt Jr. J.D., *Family Practice News*, p.50, March 1, 2013.

"Plato versus Hippocrates," Craig M. Wax, DO, Medical Economics, page 3, February 25, 2013.

"As hospital ranks swell, salary pressure could, too," Steven Podnos, MD, MBA, CFP, Medical Economics.modernmedicine.com, January 25, 2013.

"A physician's toughest choice: Accept an offer or remain independent?" Craig M. Wax DO, Medical Economics, page 3, December 2012.

"The Hospital: Your Best Frenemy?" Bob Keaveney, www.physicianspractice.com/blog, March 26, 2013.

"Disappointed Docs Say: MIPS Is Not Worth It!" Elizabeth Woodcock, MBA, FACMPE, CPC, www.medscape.com; August 20, 2019.

"Medicare Discloses Hospitals' Bonuses, Penalties Based on Quality." Jordan Rau, KHN Staff Writer, www.Kaiserhealthnews.org, December 20, 2012.

Concierge choice physicians, advertising flyer: "You want to grow your practice . . . not have someone take it over . . . ," 100 Merrick Road, Suite 410 W, Rockville Centre, NY 11570; www.coice.md.

**Eleven: NPs will become totally independent health providers**

**Digression 20 – The future of NPs and Pas**

"The Federal Government Wants to Replace You with a Nurse," Ralph J. Nobo Jr. MD, President/Chairman, Board of Governors, Florida Medical Association, 1430 Piedmont Drive East, Tallahassee, FL 32308, May 27, 2016 via email.

"Ready for Autonomy," N.C. Aizenman, *The Washington Post*, reprinted in the *Fort Wayne, Indiana Journal Gazette*, Sunday April 7, 2013, Section H, p. 1.

"Race Model 2: AANP President Weighs in on Full Practice Authority Laws," Robert Duprey MD, www.authenticmedicine.com, September 18, 2019.

**Twelve: Physician Assistants will become health providers in underserved areas**

"Physician Assistants Given Autonomy Under New IHS Policy," Madeline Morr, www.clinicaladvisor.com/, August 29, 2019.

**Thirteen: Patients will be able to order their own labs and X-rays without an order from a physician**

"LabCorp Bypasses Doctors, Reaches Out to Patients Directly," Doximity Family Medicine from Nasdaq, www.doximity.com, August 29, 2015, via email.

Flyer from The Community Open MRI Group, "Insurance: low out of pocket rates, no insurance: low cash rates," www.fortwayneopenmri.com, 2013.

**Fifteen: The Medical Record will be a video Document**

**Digression 9 – Why the EMR sucks**

"Patients Peer into the NICU," Bytes, *The Week News Magazine*, August 23, 2019.

"Telemedicine: Patient demand, cost containment drive growth," Beth Thomas Hertz, *Medical Economics*, February 10, 2013, pages 37-42.

"The Doctor is In (well, Logged in)," Joshua David Stein, www.nytimes.com, March 19, 2013.

"Scribes can help document care, boost efficiency," Maxine Lewis, CMM, CPP, CPC-I, CCs-P, President Medical Coding and Reimbursement, Cincinnati, OH, Medical Economics, October 10, 2013.

"EHRs: The real story," *Medical Economics* magazine, February 10, 2014, entire issue.

"Taiwan's Progress on Health Care," Uwe Reinhardt, www.economix.blogs.nytimes.com, July 27, 2012.

"Denmark: Electronic Patient Records," Economist Report Executive summary: future proofing Western Europe's health care, *The Economist Magazine*, October 10, 2013.

"Physicians make inroads in EHR use," Daniel R. Verdon, Group Editor, Primary Care, Medical Economics, March 25, 2013, pages 30-32.

Sylvia Mustonen's visit with Christina Muha, CNP Chagrin Falls Cleveland Clinic Family Health Center, progress notes of August 21, 2019. She never did any of the physical exam findings that were documented in the chart.

**Sixteen: The biophysical basis for OMT will be discovered.**

"Better Nature," Gregory Mone, *Discover Magazine*, "Tensegrity," April 2013, pages 35-36.

**Nineteen: A cure for HIV will be developed**

"A game changing HIV implant?" *The Week Magazine*, Health and Science section, August 9, 2019, p. 21.

**Twenty-one: The etiology of autism, irritable bowel disorders, attention deficit/hyperactivity disorder, celiac disease, Alzheimer's and other neurodegenerative disorders will be proven to be an environmental/toxic etiology**

"Hidden Invaders – infections can trigger immune attacks on kids' brains, provoking devastating psychiatric disorders," Pamela Weintraub, *Discover Magazine*, April 2017, pages 47-55.

"Protein Boost Halts Huntington's," Jill Neimark, *Discover Magazine*, January 2, 2013, p. 68

**Twenty-three – There will be vaccines for cancer of the lung, bowel, bladder, breast, prostate and bone**

"PsiOxus Therapeutics Comments on Phase III Results from Amgen's Oncolytic Vaccine," *Business Wire* and posted by www.marketwatch.com, March 20, 2013.

"Checkmate – how an iconoclastic cancer researcher gamed the immune system and unleased a potent new weapon against the disease," Kenneth Miller, *Discover Magazine*, November 2016, pages 47-51.

"Anti-cancer vaccine suppresses tumors", Melinda Wenner Moyer, *Discover Magazine*, January 2, 2013, page 57.

**Twenty-four – Tort Reform will encompass a national no fault initiative**

"Bitter Pill," Steven Brill, *Time* magazine, Vol 181, No. 8, March 4, 2013, pages 16-55.

"Law and Medicine: Tort Reform," S. Y. Tan, M.D. J.D, *Family Practice News*, March 1, 2013, p. 12.

"Serving as legal champion for the medical profession," Steven J. Stack MD, AMA Board of Trustees Chair, *American Medical News*, Vol. 56 No. 6, March 25, 2013, p. 25.

**Twenty-five – Mega retailers will install self-care automated medical diagnosis and treatment centers based on super AI computer interfaces.**

"Commentary: Supercomputer becomes physician assistant," Sherry Boschert, *Family Practice News*, March 1, 2013, p. 59.

**Additional Resources for the remainder of the writing follow here.**

1. "Western sperm counts 'halved' in last 40 years," www.nhs.uk/news, Wednesday July 26, 2017, originally published in the journal *Human Reproduction Update.*
2. "What it means to be an Osteopathic physician," Thomas Benzoni DO, *The Journal of the American Osteopathic Association*, December 2013, Vol. 113, Number 12, p. 880.
3. "Correlates and Changes in Empathy and Attitudes Toward Interprofessional Collaboration in Osteopathic Medical Students," L.H. Calabrese DO, J.A. Bianco Ph D, D. Mann PhD, D. Massello BA, M. Hojat PhD, *The Journal of the American Osteopathic Association*, December 2013, Vol. 113, Number 12, pages 898-901.
4. "A Degree of Difference – the Origins of Osteopathy and First Use of the DO Designation," Norman Gevitz PhD, *The Journal of the American Osteopathic Association*, January 2014, Vol 114, Number 1, pages 30-40.
5. "The Diplomate In Osteopathy from School of Bones to School of Medicine," Norman Gevitz PhD, *The Journal of the American Osteopathic Association*, February 2014, Vol 114, No. 2, pages 114-124.
6. Fort Wayne Community Schools 2014 Health Plan Options for Employees, general summary of benefits, <u>Medicare for all.</u>
7. "Direct Patient Care – more for you;" this is a letter sent by email to a 3rd year student at MSUCOM who was externing with me at Popoff clinic and who had asked me about <u>direct patient care</u>. I sent it to him on Monday December 4, 2017.
8. Digression 4 Patient – v- Customer. "10 Ways to make sure you don't have enough business," Paul and Sarah Edwards: lifestyles for the millennium, in The Costco Connection, March 2015, p. 13.
9. Digression 1 – Trends in the future of Medicine. "The Future is Here;" This is an email sent to me by Unknown, maybe my classmate Bob Snyder, September 6, 2016. It is scarily accurate and is tasty mental fodder.
10. Digression 29 – Telemedicine becomes a regular part of life; Novia Care Clinics Appointments 3-13-2013 my schedule. I marked the patients who could be seen by a virtual visit, or in a minute clinic or a regular office visit. Of the 14 people, 7 could have been virtual, 3 office visits, and 4 minute-clinic patients.
11. Digression 29 – Telemedicine becomes a regular part of life. "Florida medical home may offer a model for the future of senior health care," Jay Wolfson, DrPH, JD, interviewed in Medical Economics February

25, 2013, pages 76-77.

12. Digression 29 – telemedicine becomes a regular part of life. “Phoning in care a dangerous idea,” Matthew A. Shehan, MD, Omaha NB letter to the editor in *Medical Economics*, December 25, 2012, p. 16 letter to the editor.
13. Digression 30 – The Ideal Medical practice. “Patient engagement remains cornerstone of primary care's future,” Daniel Verdon, Group Editor, Primary Care, *Medical Economics,* February 25, 2013, pages 20-28.
14. Digression 13 – physicians will be automated cyborgs, Neil Blomkamp interviewed in *Discover Magazine*, “A Fanboy's Flight of Fancy” on Transhumanism in the movie Elysium, *Discover Magazine*, September 2013, p. 64.
15. Digression 31 – the end of transplant surgery. “FDA Oks AI Device to Detect Diabetic Retinopathy in Primary Care,” Megan Brooks, www.medscape.com, Friday, April 13, 2018.
16. Digression 31 – the end of transplant surgery. “Physician guide to Pharmacogenetics,” Kevin Hardy, Geneticpathways.com, 512 940 0018, 2500 N. Houston St. Dallas, TX 75219, email to me on Friday March 29, 2013.
17. Digression 33 – the Male Hierarchical System. My personal writings for my Google blog, “The best 100 years for White Male Privilege in America” and “The Male Hierarchical system and why it hates homosexuality,” both in December 16, 2015.
18. The End of Fee For Service as we know it? Beth Thomas Hertz, *Medical Economics*, August 25, 2013, Vol 90, no 16, pages 14-23.
19. US Primary Care System Under Strain Survey Shows., Alicia Ault, www.medscape.com, December 8, 2015.
20. When the Post Office was Cutting Edge, reprinted from Politico, in The Week Magazine, September 22, 2017, pages 40-41.
21. Medical Tourism and e-hospitals rising in the absence of regulations, Jeff Rowe, www.continuumof carenews.com, June 01, 2016.
22. Racial, health care disparities found in hospitalization for psoriasis, Jonathon I. Silverberg, www.healio.com, Hsu DY, et. al. J. Am Acad. Dermatol 2016; doi: 10.1016/j.jaad.2016.03.048, May 31, 2016.
23. Overcome Regulation Overload, Pamela Lewis Dolan, *American Medical News*, May 20, 2013, pages 23-24.
24. How the ACA is reshaping Medicine, Beth Thomas Hertz, *Medical Economics*, February 25, 2013, pages 30-39.

# ENDNOTES

[1] Kathleen Steele Gaivan, "Nursing home staff turnover up to 25 percent from last year: survey," *McKnights Senior Living,* last modified August 01, 2022, https://www.mcknightsseniorliving.com/home/news/business-daily-news/nursing-home-staff-turnover-up-25-percent-from-last-year-survey/#:~:text=Last%20year's%20overall%20turnover%20rate,experienced%20greater%20increases%20in%20turnover

[2] "Neuralink," *Wikipedia,* last modified November 14, 2022, https://en.wikipedia.org/wiki/Neuralink

[3] "Surrogacy in India," *Wikipedia,* last modified September 19, 2022, https://en.wikipedia.org/wiki/Surrogacy_in_India

[4] Kenneth P. Miller, "Malpractice: Nurse Practitioners and Claims reported to the National Practitioner Data Bank," *Science Direct,* last modified October 2, 2011, https://www.sciencedirect.com/science/article/abs/pii/S1555415511003448

[5] Paige Minemyer, "Nurse practitioner malpractice payouts are on the rise; opioid prescription liability an emerging hot spot," *Fierce Healthcare,* last modified November 15, 2017, https://www.fiercehealthcare.com/finance/malpractice-claims-nurse-practitioners-payouts-are-increasing-opioids IS THIS WRONG?

[6] Robert R. Stauffer "Criminal Plea Agreement by Michigan Hospital Highlights Needs to Respond to Internal Complaints," *Jenner & Block,* last modified March 2005, https://jenner.com/system/assets/publications/8467/original/Hospital_Plea.pdf?1327352545

[7] Shellie Karno, "The Criminal Prosecution of a Medical Malpractice Claim," *Lowis & Gellen LLP,* last modified March 11, 2005, http://low-is-gellen.blogspot.com/2005/03/criminal-prosecution-of-medical.html

[8] Robert R. Stauffer "Criminal Plea Agreement by Michigan Hospital Highlights Needs to Respond to Internal Complaints," *Jenner & Block,* last modified March 2005, https://jenner.com/system/assets/publications/8467/original/Hospital_Plea.pdf?1327352545

[9] "U.S. v. United Memorial Hospital," *casetext,* last modified July 22, 2002, https://casetext.com/case/us-v-united-memorial-hospital-wdmich-2002

[10] Shellie Karno, "The Criminal Prosecution of a Medical Malpractice Claim," *Lowis & Gellen LLP,* last modified March 11, 2005, http://low-is-gellen.blogspot.com/2005/03/criminal-prosecution-of-medical.html

[11] Shellie Karno, "The Criminal Prosecution of a Medical Malpractice Claim," *Lowis & Gellen LLP,* last modified March 11, 2005, http://lowis-gellen.blogspot.com/2005/03/criminal-prosecution-of-medical.html

[12] Shellie Karno, "The Criminal Prosecution of a Medical Malpractice Claim," *Lowis & Gellen LLP,* last modified March 11, 2005, http://lowis-gellen.blogspot.com/2005/03/criminal-prosecution-of-medical.html

[13] Shellie Karno, "The Criminal Prosecution of a Medical Malpractice Claim," *Lowis & Gellen LLP,* last modified March 11, 2005, http://lowis-gellen.blogspot.com/2005/03/criminal-prosecution-of-medical.html

[14] Robert R. Stauffer "Criminal Plea Agreement by Michigan Hospital Highlights Needs to Respond to Internal Complaints," *Jenner & Block,* last modified March 2005, https://jenner.com/system/assets/publications/8467/original/Hospital_Plea.pdf?1327352545

[15] "U.S. v. United Memorial Hospital," *casetext,* last modified July 22, 2002, https://casetext.com/case/us-v-united-memorial-hospital-wdmich-2002

[16] Robert R. Stauffer "Criminal Plea Agreement by Michigan Hospital Highlights Needs to Respond to Internal Complaints," *Jenner & Block,* last modified March 2005, https://jenner.com/system/assets/publications/8467/original/Hospital_Plea.pdf?1327352545

[17] Robert R. Stauffer "Criminal Plea Agreement by Michigan Hospital Highlights Needs to Respond to Internal Complaints," *Jenner & Block,* last modified March 2005, https://jenner.com/system/assets/publications/8467/original/Hospital_Plea.pdf?1327352545

[18] Robert R. Stauffer "Criminal Plea Agreement by Michigan Hospital Highlights Needs to Respond to Internal Complaints," *Jenner & Block,* last modified March 2005, https://jenner.com/system/assets/publications/8467/original/Hospital_Plea.pdf?1327352545

[19] *News,* last modified April 27, 2017, https://www.fox17online.com/2017/04/27/two-liposuction-patients-of-dr-bradley-bastow-recall-it-as-a-nightmare

[20] "Doctor facing federal lawsuit for pole barn liposuctions," *Fox17 News,* last modified December 20, 2019, https://www.fox17online.com/news/local-news/lakeshore/allegan/doctor-facing-federal-lawsuit-for-pole-barn-liposuctions

[21] Michael Oszust, "Lawsuit blames pole barn doctor for woman's death," *WoodTV News,* last modified May 19, 2017, https://www.woodtv.com/news/lawsuit-blames-pole-barn-doctor-for-womans-death/

[22] John Steckroth, "Michigan doctor's license suspended after allegedly

performing liposuction in unfinished pole barn," *ClickOnDetroit.com,* last modified May 16, 2017, https://www.clickondetroit.com/news/2017/05/16/michigan-doctors-license-suspended-after-allegedly-performing-liposuction-in-unfinished-pole-barn/

[23] Meagan Beck, "South Haven doctor suspended after office searched by drug team," *MLive News,* last modified February 2, 2018, https://www.mlive.com/news/kalamazoo/2018/02/south_haven_doctor_suspended_a.html

[24] "Amazon Care now available nationwide as demand continues to grow," *Amazon News,* last modified February 8, 2022, https://www.aboutamazon.com/news/retail/amazon-care-now-available-nationwide-as-demand-continues-to-grow#:~:text=Amazon%20Care%20combines%20the%20best,Care's%20unique%20hybrid%20care%20offering

[25] Chriss Voss, "Never Split the Difference: Negotiating As If Your Life Depended On It," *Amazon Shopping,* last modified May 17, 2016, https://www.amazon.com/Never-Split-Difference-Negotiating-Depended/dp/0062407805

[26] Christopher O'Donnell, "Diabetes can cause blindness. A trip to this pharmacy could help." *Tampa Bay Times,* last modified March 9, 2022, https://www.tampabay.com/news/health/2022/02/21/diabetes-can-cause-blindness-a-trip-to-this-pharmacy-could-help/

[27] "Out of Darkness," *Amazon Prime Video,* https://www.amazon.com/Out-Darkness-Dr-Umar-Johnson/dp/B083C6FDQ9#:~:text=Out%20of%20Darkness%20is%20a,Umar%20Johnson%2C%20Dr

[28] "Disparities in Suicide: Suicide rates differ by age," *CDC Suicide Prevention,* last modified November 2, 2022, https://www.cdc.gov/suicide/facts/disparities-in-suicide.html#age

[29] "Interracial marriage in the United States," *Wikipedia References, Note 3,* last modified November 3, 2022, https://en.wikipedia.org/wiki/Interracial_marriage_in_the_United_States#cite_note-3

[30] "Donald Trump becomes the first U.S. president to be impeached twice," *PBS Politics,* last modified January 3, 2021, https://www.pbs.org/newshour/politics/majority-of-house-members-vote-for-2nd-impeachment-of-trump

CPSIA information can be obtained
at www.ICGtesting.com
Printed in the USA
JSHW031024090323
38672JS00001B/2